Progress in Pain Research and Management
Volume 14

Opioid Sensitivity
of Chronic Noncancer Pain

Mission Statement of IASP Press®

The International Association for the Study of Pain (IASP) is a non-profit, interdisciplinary organization devoted to understanding the mechanisms of pain and improving the care of patients with pain through research, education, and communication. The organization includes scientists and health care professionals dedicated to these goals. The IASP sponsors scientific meetings and publishes newsletters, technical bulletins, the journal *Pain*, and books.

The goal of IASP Press is to provide the IASP membership with timely, high-quality, attractive, low-cost publications relevant to the problem of pain. These publications are also intended to appeal to a wider audience of scientists and clinicians interested in the problem of pain.

We will achieve high-quality publications through careful selection of subjects and authors, well-focused editorial work at several levels of production, and a smooth flow of materials. In addition, we believe that we can restrain costs and prices by employing the administrative resources of the IASP central office and by obtaining grant support for selected publications.

Because we will keep the price of our books low and their value high, they will reach a wider audience than do similar books published by for-profit companies. Furthermore, our access to leaders in the field of pain research and treatment guarantees an outstanding selection of material and excellent editorial oversight.

Progress in Pain Research and Management Series

Pharmacological Approaches to the Treatment of Chronic Pain: New Concepts and Critical Issues, edited by Howard L. Fields and John C. Liebeskind

Proceedings of the 7th World Congress on Pain, edited by Gerald F. Gebhart, Donna L. Hammond, and Troels S. Jensen

Touch, Temperature, and Pain in Health and Disease: Mechanisms and Assessments, edited by Jörgen Boivie, Per Hansson, and Ulf Lindblom

Temporomandibular Disorders and Related Pain Conditions, edited by Barry J. Sessle, Patricia S. Bryant, and Raymond A. Dionne

Visceral Pain, edited by Gerald F. Gebhart

Reflex Sympathetic Dystrophy: A Reappraisal, edited by Wilfrid Jänig and Michael Stanton-Hicks

Pain Treatment Centers at a Crossroads: A Practical and Conceptual Reappraisal, edited by Mitchell J.M. Cohen and James N. Campbell

Proceedings of the 8th World Congress on Pain, edited by Troels S. Jensen, Judith A. Turner, and Zsuzsanna Wiesenfeld-Hallin

Molecular Neurobiology of Pain, edited by David Borsook

Measurement of Pain in Infants and Children, edited by G. Allen Finley and Patrick J. McGrath

Sickle Cell Pain, by Samir K. Ballas

Assessment and Treatment of Cancer Pain, edited by Richard Payne, Richard B. Patt, and C. Stratton Hill.

Chronic and Recurrent Pain in Children and Adolescents, edited by Patrick J. McGrath and G. Allen Finley

Progress in Pain Research and Management
Volume 14

Opioid Sensitivity
of Chronic Noncancer Pain

Editors

Eija Kalso, MD, DMedSci

*Department of Anesthesia, Helsinki University
Central Hospital, Helsinki, Finland*

Henry J. McQuay, DM

*Pain Relief Unit, Nuffield Department of Anaesthetics,
University of Oxford, Oxford, United Kingdom*

Zsuzsanna Wiesenfeld-Hallin, PhD

*Department of Medical Laboratory Sciences and Technology,
Division of Clinical Neuropathology, Karolinska Institute,
Huddinge University Hospital, Huddinge, Sweden*

IASP PRESS® • **SEATTLE**

Timely topics in pain research and treatment have been selected for publication, but the information provided and opinions expressed have not involved any verification of the findings, conclusions, and opinions by IASP®. Thus, opinions expressed in *Opioid Sensitivity of Chronic Noncancer Pain* do not necessarily reflect those of IASP or of the Officers and Councillors.

No responsibility is assumed by IASP for any injury and/or damage to persons or property as a matter of product liability, negligence, or from any use of any methods, products, instruction, or ideas contained in the material herein. Because of the rapid advances in the medical sciences, the publisher recommends that there should be independent verification of diagnoses and drug dosages.

Library of Congress Cataloging-in-Publication Data

Opioid sensitivity of chronic noncancer pain / editors, Eija Kalso,
    Henry J. McQuay, Zsuzsanna Wiesenfeld-Hallin.
        p.   cm. — (Progress in pain research and management ; v.   14)
        Includes bibliographical references and index.
        ISBN 0-931092-28-0 (alk. paper)
        1. Opioids—Therapeutic use Congresses.   2. Chronic pain—Chemotherapy
Congresses. 3. Opioid receptors—Receptors Congresses.   I. Kalso, Eija, 1955–
II. McQuay, H. J. (Henry J.) III. International Association for the Study of Pain.
Research Symposium (1st : 1998 : Helsinki, Finland) IV. Series.
        [DNLM: 1. Pain—drug therapy Congresses.   2. Analgesics, Opioid—
therapeutic use Congresses.   3. Chronic Disease—drug therapy
Congresses.   4.   Receptors, Opioid—physiology Congresses. Wl
PR677BL v. 14 1999]
RM666.025065   1999
615'.783—dc21
DNLM/DLC
for Library of Congress   99-35762
                                                                                                CIP

Published by:

IASP Press
International Association for the Study of Pain
909 NE 43rd St., Suite 306
Seattle, WA 98105 USA
Fax: 206-547-1703

Printed in the United States of America

Contents

Contributing Authors

Pawel Alster, PhD *Department of Medical Laboratory Sciences and Technology, Division of Clinical Neurophysiology, Karolinska Institute, Huddinge University Hospital, Huddinge, Sweden*

Flemming Bach, MD, PhD *Department of Neurology and Danish Pain Research Center, Aarhus University Hospital, Aarhus, Denmark*

Gary J. Bennett, PhD *Department of Neurology, MCP Hahnemann University, Philadelphia, Pennsylvania, USA*

Vahri Beaumont, PhD *Department of Pharmacology, University of Bristol, Bristol, United Kingdom; currently Neurobiology Division, Department of Molecular and Cell Biology, University of California at Berkeley, Berkeley, California, USA*

Waltraud Binder, PhD *Clinic for Anesthesia and Critical Care Medicine, Benjamin Franklin University Hospital, Free University of Berlin, Berlin, Germany*

Sandra R. Chaplan, MD *Department of Anesthesiology, University of California, La Jolla, California, USA*

J.-G. Cui, MD *Department of Clinical Neuroscience, Section of Neurosurgery, Karolinska Hospital, Stockholm, Sweden*

Roman Dertwinkel, MD *Department of Anesthesiology, Intensive Care, and Pain Therapy, Bergmannsheil University Hospital, Ruhr University of Bochum, Bochum, Germany*

Anthony H. Dickenson, PhD *Department of Pharmacology, University College, London, United Kingdom*

Barbara Donner, MD *Department of Anesthesiology, Intensive Care, and Pain Therapy, Bergmannsheil University Hospital, Ruhr University of Bochum, Bochum, Germany*

Andy Dray, PhD *Department of Pharmacology, AstraZeneca R&D Montreal, St. Laurent, Quebec, Canada*

Robert Elde, PhD *Department of Neuroscience, University of Minnesota, Minneapolis, Minnesota, USA*

Peter J.D. Evans, FRCA *Pain Management Centre, Charing Cross Hospital, London, United Kingdom*

Gerald F. Gebhart, PhD *Department of Pharmacology, University of Iowa, Iowa City, Iowa, USA*

Geoffrey Gourlay, BPharm, PhD *Pain Management Unit, Flinders Medical Centre, Bedford Park, South Australia, Australia*

Gisèle Guilbaud, MD, DSc *Research Unit on the Physiopharmacology of the Nervous System, INSERM, Paris, France*

Gunnar Grant, MD *Department of Neuroscience, Karolinska Institute, Stockholm, Sweden*

Stefan Grass, MD *Department of Medical Laboratory Sciences and Technology, Division of Clinical Neurophysiology, Karolinska Institute, Huddinge University Hospital, Huddinge, Sweden*

Jing-Xia Hao, MD, DMSc *Department of Medical Laboratory Sciences and Technology, Division of Clinical Neurophysiology, Karolinska Institute, Huddinge University Hospital, Huddinge, Sweden*

Graeme Henderson, PhD *Department of Pharmacology, School of Medical Sciences, Bristol, United Kingdom*

Orsolya Hoffmann, MD, DMSc *Department of Medical Laboratory Sciences and Technology, Division of Clinical Neurophysiology, Karolinska Institute, Huddinge University Hospital, Huddinge, Sweden*

Tomas Hökfelt, MD *Department of Neuroscience, Karolinska Institute, Stockholm, Sweden*

Shailen Joshi, BSPharm *Department of Pharmacology, University of Iowa, Iowa City, Iowa, USA*

Gong Ju, MD *Department of Neurobiology, Institute of Neurosciences, The Fourth Military Medical University, Xi'an, P.R. China*

Eija Kalso, MD, DMedSci *Department of Anesthesia, Helsinki University Central Hospital, Helsinki, Finland; currently Department of Anesthesia and Intensive Care, Karolinska Institute, Huddinge University Hospital, Huddinge, Sweden*

Valérie Kayser, BPharm, DSc *Research Unit on the Physiopharmacology of the Nervous System, INSERM, Paris, France*

H. Keita, MD *Research Unit on the Physiopharmacology of the Nervous System, INSERM, Paris, France*

Ian Kitchen, PhD *Pharmacology Research Group, School of Biological Sciences, University of Surrey, Guildford, Surrey, United Kingdom*

Josephine Lai, PhD *Department of Pharmacology, Health Sciences Center, University of Arizona, Tucson, Arizona, USA*

Bengt Linderoth, MD, PhD *Department of Clinical Neuroscience, Section of Neurosurgery, Karolinska Hospital, Stockholm, Sweden*

Guilherme de Araújo Lucas, MD, PhD *Department of Medical Laboratory Sciences and Technology, Division of Clinical Neurophysiology, Karolinska Institute, Huddinge University Hospital, Huddinge, Sweden*

Halina Machelska, PhD *Clinic for Anesthesia and Operative and Intensive Medicine, Benjamin Franklin University Clinic, Free University of Berlin, Berlin, Germany*

T. Philip Malan, Jr., MD, PhD *Departments of Pharmacology and Anesthesiology, Health Sciences Center, University of Arizona, Tucson, Arizona, USA*

Henry J. McQuay, DM *Pain Relief Unit, Nuffield Department of Anaesthetics, University of Oxford, Oxford, United Kingdom*

Björn Meyerson, MD, PhD *Department of Clinical Neuroscience, Section of Neurosurgery, Karolinska Hospital, Stockholm, Sweden*

Michael H. Ossipov, PhD *Department of Pharmacology, Health Sciences Center, University of Arizona, Tucson, Arizona, USA*

N. Ozaki, MD, PhD *Department of Pharmacology, College of Medicine, University of Iowa, Iowa City, Iowa, USA*

Gavril W. Pasternak, MD, PhD *The Cotzias Laboratory of Neuro-Oncology, Memorial Sloan-Kettering Cancer Center, New York, New York, USA*

Serge Perrot, MD *Research Unit on the Physiopharmacology of the Nervous System, INSERM, Paris, France*

Jan Persson, MD, PhD *Pain Section, Department of Anesthesia and Intensive Care, Huddinge University Hospital, Huddinge, Sweden*

Aida Plesan, MD *Department of Medical Laboratory Sciences and Technology, Division of Clinical Neurophysiology, Karolinska Institute, Huddinge University Hospital, Huddinge, Sweden*

Frank Porreca, PhD *Departments of Pharmacology and Anesthesiology, Health Sciences Center, University of Arizona, Tucson, Arizona, USA*

Maureen Riedl, PhD *Department of Neuroscience, University of Minnesota, Minneapolis, Minnesota, USA*

Michael Rowbotham, MD *Pain Clinical Research Center and Mount Zion Pain Management Center, University of California, San Francisco, California, USA*

Michael Schäfer, MD *Clinic for Anesthesia and Critical Care Medicine, Benjamin Franklin University Hospital, Free University of Berlin, Berlin, Germany*

J.N. Sengupta, PhD *Department of Pharmacology, University of Iowa, Iowa City, Iowa, USA; currently Gastrointestinal Pharmacology, Astra Hassle, Molendal, Sweden*

Tiejun Sten Shi, MD *Department of Neuroscience, Karolinska Institute, Stockholm, Sweden*

Samuel Shuster, PhD *Department of Neuroscience, University of Minnesota, Minneapolis, Minnesota, USA*

Christoph Stein, MD *Clinic for Anesthesia and Operative and Intensive Medicine, Benjamin Franklin University Clinic, Free University of Berlin, Berlin, Germany*

Michael Strumpf, MD *Department of Anesthesiology, Intensive Care, and Pain Therapy, Bergmannsheil University Hospital, Ruhr University of Bochum, Bochum, Germany*

Xin Su, MD *Department of Pharmacology, University of Iowa, Iowa City, Iowa, USA*

Rie Suzuki, BSc *Department of Pharmacology, University College, London, United Kingdom*

Yong-Guang Tong, MD, DMSc *Department of Neurobiology, Institute of Neurosciences, The Fourth Military Medical University, Xi'an, P.R. China*

Hui Fredrik Wang Department of Neuroscience, Karolinska Institute, Stockholm, Sweden

Zsuzsanna Wiesenfeld-Hallin, PhD *Department of Medical Laboratory Sciences and Technology, Division of Clinical Neurophysiology, Karolinska Institute, Huddinge University Hospital, Huddinge, Sweden*

Xiao-Jun Xu, MD, DMSc *Department of Medical Laboratory Sciences and Technology, Division of Clinical Neurophysiology, Karolinska Institute, Huddinge University Hospital, Huddinge, Sweden*

Zhi-Qing David Xu, MD, DMSc *Department of Neuroscience, Karolinska Institute, Stockholm, Sweden*

Wei Yu, MD *Department of Medical Laboratory Sciences and Technology, Division of Clinical Neurophysiology, Karolinska Institute, Huddinge University Hospital, Huddinge, Sweden*

Michael Zenz, MD *Department of Anesthesiology, Intensive Care, and Pain Therapy, Bergmannsheil University Hospital, Ruhr University of Bochum, Bochum, Germany*

Xu Zhang, MD, DMSc *Department of Neurobiology, Institute of Neurosciences, The Fourth Military Medical University, Xi'an, P.R. China*

Foreword

This book is based on the first international research symposium of the International Association for the Study of Pain (IASP), held in Helsinki, Finland, from November 30 to December 1, 1998. A suggestion made by Dr. F. Cervero, chair of the IASP Committee on Research, prompted the IASP Council, at its meeting in October 1997, to agree to organize an annual research symposium, with the exception of the years of the IASP World Congress. The first symposium convened in 1998, the year we celebrated IASP's 25th anniversary.

The symposium, organized by Drs. E. Kalso, H.J. McQuay, and Z. Wiesenfeld-Hallin, was entitled "Opioid Sensitivity of Chronic Noncancer Pain," a subject similar to the mission of the Task Force on Opioid Sensitivity of Different Chronic Noncancer Pain States, chaired by Dr. Kalso, that I established in 1997. I am very keen that the conclusions from the meeting should serve as a reference point for future developments of the task force. I also hope that both the symposium and this book will initiate further, more systematic clinical studies that will lead to better therapeutic approaches to the control of chronic noncancer pain.

I am sure some of you may say that another book on opioids is excessive. This is not my point of view, however, as many chapters cover new aspects of the mechanisms of action, therapeutic evaluation, and clinical use of opioids. Since the identification of the opioid receptors in 1973, followed by the discovery of the enkephalins in 1975, aspects of this subject area have been oversimplified, so much so that we have often been overly naïve. The receptors were not isolated and cloned until 20 years later, and even now many questions in the opioid field are still unanswered. By way of example, classical pharmacological approaches have supported the idea of subtypes of opioid receptors, but molecular biologists have not yet clearly identified these subtypes. Research in the field of opioid receptors is still very active, and many laboratories are investigating the production of increasingly specific agonists designed either to cross or remain outside the blood–brain barrier.

The studies based on the use of morphine in cancer pain are well known, and when the guidelines on opioid prescribing are respected, many patients experience relief of their pain. Unfortunately, in this clinical area we must still overcome a certain amount of resistance, which in most cases arises from a lack of information, but alas, also from economic problems in the developing nations.

Furthermore, some patients suffering from chronic noncancer pain, often with extremely intense pain, transitory or persistent, could benefit from morphine treatment. This is the case with inflammatory, ischemic, visceral, and musculoskeletal pain. Controlled clinical studies in this area would allow the development of therapeutic guidelines and treatment regimes and allow the use of morphine in treating many patients who suffer particularly intense pain from noncancer origins.

Finally, much of this book is dedicated to noncancer pain of neuropathic origins, another field where ideas are well developed. About 15 years ago, neuropathic pains were considered completely insensitive to morphine. This point of view became a dogma, although it was based on clinical studies that were often anecdotal or lacked a rigorous systematic approach. Today, many clinical research groups are involved in the study of the effects of opioids on neuropathic pain. Although it appears that pain from central origins (brainstem and cerebral lesions) often responds poorly to opioids, this is not the case for many patients with peripheral neuropathies, who gain significant relief of their pain with morphine. This is perhaps not surprising, because neuropathic pain embraces a diverse set of symptoms and syndromes. Only systematic clinical studies will allow dissection of these various components, which are likely to have different physiopathological bases. Note also that basic scientists use many different experimental models of neuropathic pain. Although these models may seem to be a far cry from the human clinical situation, they are providing increasingly important data fundamental to our understanding of the mechanisms that underlie neuropathic pain. I have no doubt that a better understanding of the physiological, pharmacological, and pathological fundamentals will lead to an improvement in the pharmacological treatment of neuropathic pain, which at present is far from satisfactory for both patients and doctors.

JEAN-MARIE BESSON, PharmD, DSc
President of IASP
INSERM, Paris, France

Preface

For centuries, opioids have been the target of heated discussions and even the cause of political crises. The clinical debate has long been focused on the safety of opioids in both acute and chronic pain. After much hard work it is now generally accepted that opioids do not cause significant respiratory depression if the dose is titrated against the patient's pain. It is also widely accepted that the need for postoperative opioids varies significantly between individuals. Opioid responsiveness of various acute pain conditions has not, however, been seriously debated. One explanation may be that other methods, such as regional analgesia, can be effectively used in severe postoperative pain.

Medicine has accepted the use of opioids in chronic cancer pain. Unfortunately, opioids are still not available for all cancer patients who could benefit from them. Over the last decade the discussion has turned to the use of opioids in chronic noncancer pain. Legal considerations and adverse effects in long-term use remain major issues, and attitudes in different countries vary significantly. The question that has excited both clinicians and basic researchers, however, is whether all pains can been relieved by opioids. In this context the opioid responsiveness of neuropathic pain has been a focus for debate.

The current president of the International Association for the Study of Pain, Jean-Marie Besson, set up a task force committee to work on this problem. When Fernando Cervero, chair of the IASP Research Committee, proposed a series of research symposia, he provided an opportunity to invite researchers to discuss this question of high clinical relevance.

The 1st IASP Research Symposium was held in Helsinki, Finland, in 1998. This was 10 years after the publication of an article by S. Arnér and B.A. Meyerson ("Lack of analgesic effect of opioids on neuropathic and idiopathic forms of pain." *Pain* 1988; 33:11–23) that initiated the heated discussion about opioid sensitivity of neuropathic pain. That study is one of the most frequently cited papers in pain research, and is heavily cited in this volume. Over the past 10 years our knowledge about opioid receptors and their function in various pathophysiological conditions has increased considerably. Experimental models have been developed to represent various chronic pain conditions. Cloning of the opioid receptors and the production of gene-manipulated animals have engendered a whole new area of research.

Compared with 10 years ago, can we now predict which patient will benefit from opioids and which will not? Basic research has taught us that acute inflammatory pain responds better to opioids than do other types of acute pain (simulated by electrical stimulation, noxious heat, and pinch). The clinical utility of this knowledge has not been tested sufficiently, perhaps because nonopioid drugs are also effective in inflammatory pain.

Most basic and clinical research has focused on opioid responsiveness of neuropathic pain. Most studies indicate that peripheral neuropathies respond to opioids, but that different models differ significantly in responsiveness. These variations will, we hope, help to explain why different clinical neuropathies also vary in response to opioids. Well-controlled clinical studies indicate that opioids, after both intravenous and oral administration, do relieve pain due to peripheral neuropathies. No controlled clinical studies on opioids are available on neuropathic pains of central origin (e.g., central post-stroke pain, pain following spinal cord injury), but the clinical impression is that these conditions do not respond even to high doses of opioids. This clinical experience is supported by results from basic research.

Opioid responsiveness of other chronic "nociceptive" pain conditions has not been studied systematically. Interestingly, chronic ischemic pain seems to be fairly unresponsive to opioids (see Chapter 21). The best controlled study on long-term use of opioids in musculoskeletal pain did not show high opioid sensitivity (D.E. Moulin, A. Iezzi, R. Amireh, W.K.J. Sharpe, and H. Merskey. "Randomised trial of morphine for chronic non-cancer pain." *Lancet* 1996; 347:143–147). The argument against poor opioid responsiveness in neuropathic pain has been that the dose-response curve is shifted to the right. We do not know whether this would be the case in chronic nociceptive pain.

Studies have not addressed the influence of duration or severity of chronic pain on opioid sensitivity. Evidence now suggests that long-lasting pain may induce phenotypic changes in expression of many neuroactive substances and receptors in the dorsal root ganglia, which could render previously opioid-sensitive pains insensitive.

Differential efficacy in chronic pain syndromes is not only a characteristic of opioids, but is also apparent with other drug classes such as tricyclic antidepressants. Nevertheless, the debate has focused on opioids because of their huge medical and political importance, and little attention has been paid to demonstrating of the phenomenon with other drug classes. We would like to believe that the debate about differential opioid efficacy will lead to constructive science that will illuminate the fundamental biological mechanisms of chronic pain. The debate could, of course, become redundant if new, effective remedies emerge. Such serendipity might be more probable if we knew the mechanisms. Meanwhile, a key reason for holding the symposium was to establish the evidence of opioid efficacy in chronic pain, and we must defend the right of patients to receive opioids when they are indicated and effective. The symposium thus had two motives: the hope that study of opioid responsiveness of different pain syndromes might lead to better understanding, and the hope that reviewing opioid efficacy might reveal the uses most likely to benefit patients.

EIJA KALSO, HENRY J. MCQUAY, AND
ZSUZSANNA WIESENFELD-HALLIN

Acknowledgments

The organizers wish to thank the following pharmaceutical companies that sponsored the 1st IASP Research Symposium, 30 November–1 December, in Helsinki, Finland:

ASTRA PAIN CONTROL
FAULDING
GRÜNENTHAL
JANSSEN-CILAG
NAPP
NYCOMED AMERSHAM
UPSA

Part I

Function and Dysfunction
of Opioid Receptors

Opioid Sensitivity of Chronic Noncancer Pain,
Progress in Pain Research and Management,
Vol. 14, edited by Eija Kalso, Henry J. McQuay,
and Zsuzsanna Wiesenfeld-Hallin, IASP Press,
Seattle, © 1999.

1

Targeting of Opioid Receptors to Presynaptic Sites

Maureen Riedl, Samuel Shuster, and Robert Elde

Department of Neuroscience, University of Minnesota, Minneapolis, Minnesota, USA

The sensitivity of a pain state to pharmacological treatment can depend on a variety of factors. In general, the responsiveness or tone of neural circuits is a regulated variable that is altered in pathological conditions. For example, injury can disrupt normal neural pathways and thus decrease neuronal activation or inhibition. Tissue damage can also lead to release of various chemical modulators that can affect neurons at the site of injury. Alterations in the synthesis of receptors and neurotransmitters, in the production of second messengers, and in the availability of receptors for occupancy by ligands all can alter the sensitivity of a pain state to pharmacological treatment.

One mechanism by which a cell may alter the availability of a presynaptic receptor for occupancy by a ligand is stimulus-dependent translocation of the receptor to the plasma membrane. Recent evidence from in vitro studies has shown that some proteins—particularly a neuronal glutamate transporter (Davis et al. 1998), a glucose transporter, GLUT-4 (James 1994), and a GABA transporter, GAT1 (Quick et al. 1997)—are redistributed from intracellular stores to the plasma membrane in response to stimulation. More recently, studies have demonstrated stimulus-dependent translocation of the G-protein-coupled dopamine D1 receptor in cell culture (Brismar et al. 1998) and translocation of the type A GABA receptor to postsynaptic membranes in central nervous system (CNS) neurons (Wan et al. 1997).

We have found that some presynaptic opioid receptors undergo stimulus-dependent translocation from the membrane of a pool of storage vesicles to the plasma membrane of the nerve terminal. Activation of presynaptic opioid receptors leads to an inhibition of transmitter release, most likely through inactivation of calcium channels or activation of potassium channels (for review, see North 1993). Thus, stimulus-dependent translocation of opioid receptors in nerve terminals provides a mechanism by which a neuron may rapidly increase its vulnerability to presynaptic inhibition and cause a rapid decrease in transmitter release.

PRESYNAPTIC VERSUS POSTSYNAPTIC TARGETING OF OPIOID RECEPTORS

Three members of the opioid receptor family were cloned in the early 1990s, beginning with the mouse δ-opioid receptor (DOR1) in 1992 (Evans et al. 1992; Kieffer et al. 1992). Cloning of the rat μ-opioid receptor (MOR1) (Chen et al. 1993; Fukuda et al. 1993; Thompson et al. 1993) and κ-opioid receptor (KOR1) (Li et al. 1993; Meng et al. 1993; Minami et al. 1993; Nishi et al. 1993) soon followed. These three receptors belong to the family of seven-transmembrane G-protein-coupled receptors and are highly homologous. The greatest amount of divergence in the amino acid sequence of these receptors occurs within the amino terminus (N-terminus), the first extracellular loop, and the carboxy terminus. We therefore used amino acid sequences from these regions to make antipeptide antisera to the opioid receptors. We obtained immunocytochemically useful antisera from regions of the N-terminus (regions I, II), the first extracellular loop (region III), and the carboxy terminus (region IV) of the rat DOR1 sequence and from carboxy terminus (region IV) of both the rat KOR1 and MOR1 sequences (Fig. 1).

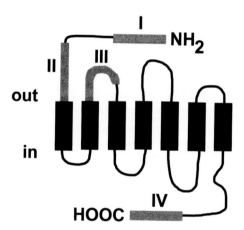

Fig. 1. Schematic diagram of an opioid receptor that shows seven membrane-spanning regions. Antipeptide antisera were raised to region I (amino acids 3–17) of DOR1, region II (amino acids 30–46) of DOR1, region III (amino acids 103–120) of DOR1, and region IV of DOR1, MOR1, and KOR1.

Results from immunohistochemical experiments in the rat CNS revealed that MOR1 immunoreactivity (ir) is localized primarily in or near postsynaptic structures (Arvidsson et al. 1995b). MOR1-immunoreactive puncta outline the membrane of cell bodies and dendrites of neurons in many regions of the CNS, including the spinal cord (Fig. 2A). Electron microscope studies show that MOR1-ir is associated predominantly with

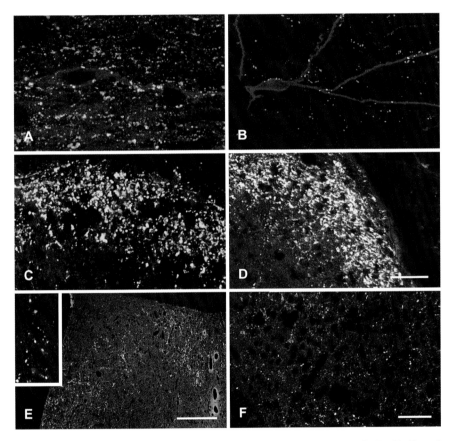

Fig. 2. Two-color immunofluorescent confocal images from rat (A, C, D, E, F) and guinea pig (B) brain and spinal cord. (A) MOR1 immunoreactivity (MOR1-ir) (red) outlines the soma and dendrites of a neuron in the superficial dorsal horn of the spinal cord. Enkephalin-ir (green) is seen in nearby puncta. (B) KOR1-ir (red) outlines the soma and dendrites of a brainstem neuron. Immunoreactivity for prodynorphin is shown in green. (C) DOR1-ir (red) and CGRP-ir (green) are co-localized (yellow) in fibers in the superficial dorsal horn of the spinal cord. Note the beaded appearance of DOR1 immunoreactive fibers. (D) DOR1-ir (red) and SP-ir (green) are extensively co-localized in the superficial dorsal horn of the spinal cord. (E) The high degree of co-localization between DOR1-ir and SP-ir is also apparent in the septum. (F) One brain region that does not show extensive co-localization of DOR1-ir and SP-ir is the suprachiasmatic nucleus. Scale bars: D = 50 μm, E = 200 μm, F = 50 μm.

extrasynaptic sites in postsynaptic plasma membranes (Cheng et al. 1996, 1997; Svingos et al. 1996; Wang et al. 1996, 1998; Gracy et al. 1997), although MOR1 also occurs within axons (Ding et al. 1995a,b; see also Arvidsson et al. 1995b).

KOR1-ir is also localized primarily on or near postsynaptic structures throughout much of the CNS (Arvidsson et al. 1995c). Fig. 2B shows KOR1-ir associated with the soma and dendrites of a neuron from guinea pig brainstem. Puncta of prodynorphin-ir can be seen nearby. Ultrastructural studies confirm the localization of KOR1-ir to postsynaptic membranes (Svingos et al. 1999), although it has also been found in presynaptic structures (Drake et al. 1996, 1997; Shuster et al. 1999; Svingos et al. 1999).

In contrast to KOR1-ir and MOR1-ir, DOR1-ir is associated primarily with presynaptic structures (Dado et al. 1993; Arvidsson et al. 1995a). The immunohistochemical morphology of DOR1-ir is similar to that of a neuropeptide, with the characteristic beaded appearance of fine axons. In fact, DOR1-ir is often co-localized with calcitonin gene-related peptide (CGRP) in primary afferent fibers (Fig. 2C). Electron microscope studies have confirmed the presynaptic localization of DOR1-ir in the spinal cord and dorsal root ganglia (DRG) (Cheng et al. 1995; Zhang et al. 1998).

DOR1 SHOWS A HIGH DEGREE OF CO-LOCALIZATION WITH SUBSTANCE P

In examining the presynaptic distribution of DOR1-ir and comparing its distribution with that of many neuropeptides, we were struck by the high degree of co-localization between DOR1-ir and immunoreactivity for the neuropeptide substance P (SP-ir) throughout the brain and spinal cord and within the periphery. The co-localization of DOR1-ir and SP-ir is shown in the superficial dorsal horn of the spinal cord (Fig. 2D) and the septum (Fig. 2E); we found a similar pattern in most other CNS tissues (Table I). In fact, the only brain area examined that did not show a high degree of co-localization of DOR1-ir and SP-ir was the suprachiasmatic nucleus. We examined many species, including the rat, mouse, guinea pig, and monkey. In the rat, immunoreactivity for both DOR1 and SP occurred in the suprachiasmatic nucleus, yet labeling was localized in spatially separated structures (Fig. 2F).

Such a high degree of co-localization raised the specter of cross-reactivity, so we performed extensive control experiments to eliminate this possibility. First, we eliminated staining with DOR1 antisera by preabsorbing the antisera with the peptide against which the antisera were raised (Arvidsson

Table I
Regions of the central nervous system in which
co-localization of DOR1 and substance P
immunoreactivity has been detected

Amygdaloid nuclei
Arcuate nucleus
Bed nucleus of the stria terminalis
Brainstem reticular formation
Entopeduncular nucleus
Hypothalamic areas
Interpeduncular nuclei
Islands of Calleja
Lateral habenular nucleus
Lateral spinal nucleus of the spinal cord
Nucleus accumbens
Nucleus of the solitary tract
Parabrachial nuclei
Paraventricular hypothalamic nucleus
Paraventricular thalamic nucleus
Periaqueductal gray
Raphe nuclei
Spinal cord, lamina X
Spinal cord, superficial dorsal horn
Spinal cord, ventral horn
Spinal tract of nerve V
Striatum
Substantia nigra
Ventral pallidum

et al. 1995a; Dado et al. 1993). Second, we demonstrated that RIN-r1046-38 cells, a rat insulinoma cell line that has been proven by radioimmunoassay, high-performance liquid chromatography, and Northern blot analysis to contain SP (McGregor et al. 1993), were not stained by antisera to DOR1. This result confirms that DOR1 antisera do not recognize SP. Finally, we injected antisense oligonucleotides from the DOR1 sequence intrathecally in mice, which resulted in a knockdown of DOR1-ir in the superficial dorsal horn that was not seen in animals that had received injections of vehicle or mismatch antisense (Lai et al. 1996). These findings suggest that the DOR1 antisera recognized the cloned δ-opioid receptor.

Electron microscope studies in the superficial dorsal horn of the spinal cord and locus ceruleus have shown DOR1-ir associated with the presynaptic plasma membrane and with the membrane of several classes of vesicles (Cheng et al. 1995; van Bockstaele et al. 1997; Zhang et al. 1998). These studies report that DOR1-ir is sometimes associated with the plasma membrane, but is even more often associated with vesicles within the axon terminal. While a portion of this intracellular DOR1-ir may represent internalized receptors, some is associated with large, dense-core vesicles. DOR1 internalization is known to occur in response to ligand binding (Trapaidze et al. 1996; Chu et al. 1997; Cvejic and Devi 1997; Gaudriault et al. 1997; Afify et al. 1998) and most likely occurs via endocytosis into small vesicles. In contrast, the existence of DOR-ir on large, dense-core vesicles suggests that these vesicles have not yet had access to the plasma membrane. Indeed, DOR1-ir in DRG neurons is associated predominantly with large, dense-core vesicles (Zhang et al. 1998).

Large, dense-core vesicles are subcellular organelles that contain neuropeptides. Given the high degree of co-localization between DOR1 and SP, it is likely that SP is one of the neuropeptides contained within the lumen of DOR1-positive, large, dense-core vesicles. The release of neuropeptides is known to be the result of a sustained depolarization. It is therefore possible that DOR1 is inserted into the plasma membrane as a consequence of the fusion of large, dense-core vesicles with the plasma membrane. Such fusion would result in the release of SP and the exteriorization of DOR1. Thus, access of the receptor to ligand could be increased by an initial depolarizing stimulus. We decided to examine the effect of a depolarizing stimulus on δ-opioid-receptor binding in rat synaptosome preparations.

STIMULUS-DEPENDENT TRANSLOCATION OF DELTA-OPIOID-RECEPTOR BINDING SITES

In preliminary studies, we used [³H]-deltorphin II to measure the amount of δ-opioid receptor available for ligand binding. Deltorphin II specifically binds to the δ-opioid receptor, and since it is a hydrophilic ligand it is unlikely to cross the plasma membrane and be sequestered within the synaptosomes (Staehelin and Hertel 1983). One group of synaptosomes received fresh buffer with normal potassium concentrations, while the experimental group received buffer with a high concentration of potassium for 1 minute. In a saturating concentration of [³H]-deltorphin II, an average 30% increase in [³H]-deltorphin II binding occurred after stimulation. The statistical significance of this increase was determined using a paired Student's t test. This increase in [³H]-deltorphin II binding could represent a significant increase in the number of DOR1 receptors on the surface of the synaptosome.

The same experiments were performed under calcium-free conditions. A small (5%), but statistically significant decrease in [^{3}H]-deltorphin II binding was seen. Fusion of large, dense-core vesicles with the plasma membrane is a calcium-dependent event. These data suggest that a stimulus sufficient to result in neuropeptide release also resulted in a statistically significant increase in δ-opioid-receptor binding at the plasma membrane.

These preliminary data suggest a stimulus-dependent translocation of DOR1 from internal, large, dense-core vesicle stores, to the plasma membrane (Fig. 3) and indicate that the availability of DOR1 for occupancy by either an endogenous or exogenous ligand can depend on the excitability of the nerve terminal. Stimulus-dependent translocation appears to be a rapid mechanism by which a neuron can regulate its sensitivity to pharmacological treatment.

PRESYNAPTIC KOR1 IN THE HYPOTHALAMO-NEUROHYPOPHYSIAL SYSTEM

A similar phenomenon has been demonstrated with KOR1 in the hypothalamo-neurohypophysial system (Shuster et al. 1999). This system is

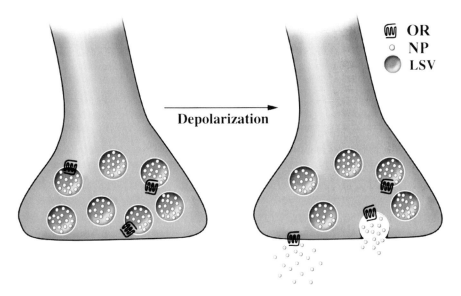

Fig. 3. Schematic diagram of stimulus-dependent translocation of presynaptic opioid receptors (OR). Opioid receptors are associated with the membrane of neuropeptide (NP)-containing large secretory vesicles (LSV). Following depolarization, peptide-containing vesicles fuse with the plasma membrane, causing peptide release and insertion of the opioid receptor into the plasma membrane.

composed of the magnocellular neuronal cell bodies in the paraventricular and supraoptic nuclei of the hypothalamus and the axonal projections of these neurons to the posterior lobe of the pituitary. Neuropeptides released from nerve terminals in the posterior pituitary are delivered directly into the bloodstream via fenestrated capillaries. Magnocellular neurons of the paraventricular and supraoptic nuclei produce two principal signaling peptides: vasopressin, which is involved in maintaining fluid balance, and

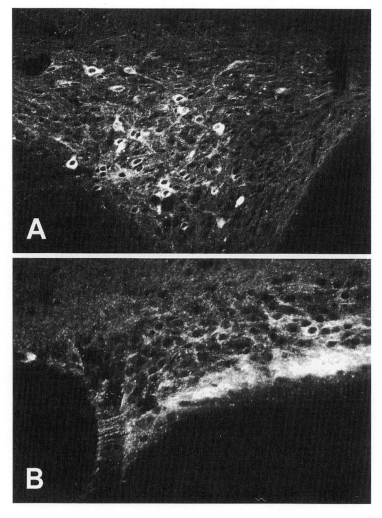

Fig. 4. Immunofluorescent confocal images of (A) the paraventricular nucleus and (B) the supraoptic nucleus of the rat. KOR1-ir is associated with cell bodies in these regions, and in several cases, KOR1-ir is associated with more than one process from a single neuron, which suggests that KOR1-ir is associated with dendrites of these neurons.

oxytocin, which is involved in uterine contractions and milk ejection. In this system, KOR1-ir is associated with the cell bodies and dendrites of neurons in the paraventricular and supraoptic nuclei (Fig. 4) and in the nerve terminals in the posterior pituitary. Therefore, in this system, KOR1 appears to be transported to both postsynaptic membranes and presynaptic nerve terminals.

Ultrastructural studies of the posterior lobe of the pituitary show that $62.5 \pm 1.8\%$ of the KOR1-ir found within nerve terminals is associated with large secretory vesicles (Fig. 5A). In contrast, $10.8 \pm 1.2\%$ of the KOR1-ir found within nerve terminals is associated with the plasma membrane (Fig. 5B). The remaining KOR1-ir within nerve terminals is associated with either small, clear vesicles or unidentifiable structures within the cytoplasm of the nerve terminal. These data suggest that most of the KOR1-ir in nerve terminals of the posterior pituitary is associated with the membrane of large secretory vesicles and is not exposed to the extracellular space; it is therefore not available for occupancy by ligands.

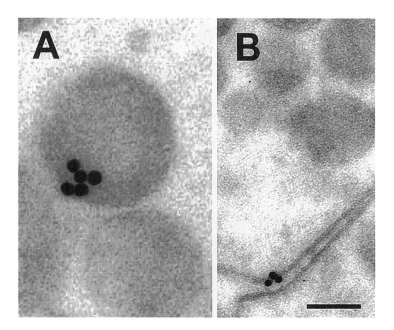

Fig. 5. Electron microscope images of KOR1-ir associated with the membrane of a large secretory vesicle in the posterior lobe of the pituitary. (A) $62.5 \pm 1.8\%$ of KOR1-ir in nerve terminals of the posterior pituitary was associated with the membrane of large secretory vesicles. (B) $10.8 \pm 1.2\%$ of KOR1-ir in nerve terminals of the posterior pituitary is associated with the plasma membrane. Scale bar = 100 nm.

STIMULUS-DEPENDENT TRANSLOCATION
OF KOR1-IR

Adjacent sections of the same vesicle stained with antiserum to KOR1 and a monoclonal antibody to the precursor of vasopressin are shown in Fig. 6. Because the precursor of vasopressin is processed within the vesicle, these data suggest that one of the neuropeptides contained within KOR1-positive large secretory vesicles is the neuropeptide vasopressin. Dehydration causes vasopressin release (Bourque et al. 1994), and can be mimicked by acute and chronic salt loading (Shoji et al. 1994). We examined the posterior pituitary of rats 15 and 60 minutes after salt loading with an intraperitoneal injection of 0.9 mol/L saline (Fig. 7). In animals that had received a sham injection (injection of needle but no fluid delivery), 58.2 ± 3.6% of the KOR1-ir in nerve terminals was associated with large secretory vesicles. Fifteen minutes after salt loading, 42.1 ± 1.0% of KOR1-ir in nerve terminals was associated with large secretory vesicles. This decrease in KOR1-ir associated with large secretory vesicles was accompanied by a 178% increase in KOR1-ir associated with the plasma membrane. Within 1 hour of salt loading, the amount of KOR1-ir associated with both large secretory vesicles and the plasma membrane returned to normal levels. These data

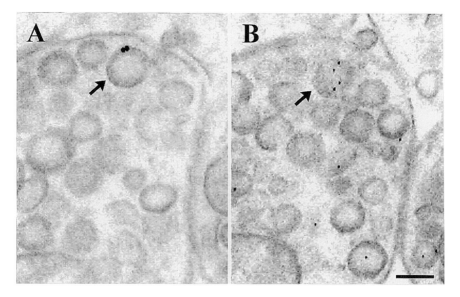

Fig. 6. Electron microscope images of (A) KOR1-ir and (B) immunoreactivity for vasopressin neurophysin in the posterior lobe of the pituitary. Adjacent sections of the same vesicle show KOR1-ir and vasopressin neurophysin-ir associated with the same large secretory vesicle. Scale bar = 250 nm.

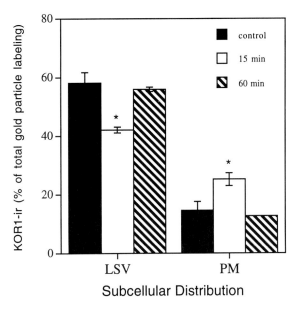

Subcellular Distribution

Fig. 7. Graph showing translocation of KOR1-ir (labeled with gold particles) from large secretory vesicles (LSV) to the plasma membrane (PM) in response to stimulation. A statistically significant decrease in KOR1-ir associated with the membrane of large secretory vesicles (LSV) was seen 15 minutes after saline injection ($P < 0.05$). A corresponding increase in KOR1-ir associated with the plasma membrane (PM) occurred. One hour after salt loading, KOR1-ir was returned to control levels.

suggest that KOR1 can be transiently translocated from internal stores of large secretory vesicles to the plasma membrane in response to depolarizing physiological stimuli.

CONCLUSIONS

It appears that all three opioid receptors are transported to axon terminals. Two of these presynaptic opioid receptors—DOR1 throughout much of the central and peripheral nervous system and KOR1 in at least the hypothalamo-neurohypophysial system—are associated with the membrane of large, dense-core vesicles. In the case of DOR1, the neuropeptide contents of such vesicles are likely to include SP, whereas in the case of KOR1, the contents of such vesicles in the posterior pituitary include vasopressin. In response to stimulation, these receptors are translocated from their location on large, peptide-containing vesicles to the plasma membrane. The results of translocation are an increased number of receptors on the cell surface and neuropeptide release. These presynaptic opioid receptors, once inserted into the plasma membrane, are available for occupancy by ligands and are likely to be functional, although this has not yet been directly examined.

These studies suggest that stimulus-dependent translocation of presynaptic opioid receptors may be a mechanism by which neurons modulate their responsiveness to opioid peptides. Data from several studies suggest that this process may be particularly relevant in increasing opioid effectiveness during inflammation. Opioid agonists, including morphine, can exhibit a greater antinociceptive potency under experimentally produced inflammatory conditions than under control conditions. This increase in antinociceptive potency can be blocked by the addition of a δ-opioid-receptor antagonist (Ossipov et al. 1995). Furthermore, inflammation results in an increase in SP transported in the sciatic nerve and an increase in both SP and CGRP release in the periphery and in spinal cord dorsal horn (Nanayama et al. 1989; Donnerer et al. 1992, 1993; Garry and Hargreaves 1992; Abbadie et al. 1997; Allen et al. 1999). These results have been attributed to a variety of factors, including a decrease in neuropeptides, an increase in nerve growth factor, and infiltration of immune cells; however, stimulus-dependent translocation could be one regulatory mechanism at work in this system to increase opioid antinociceptive potency.

ACKNOWLEDGMENTS

The authors thank Dr. Ulf Arvidsson, Dr. Jang-Hern Lee, Dr. Laura Stone, Dr. Lucy Vulchanova, and Dr. Martin Wessendorf for their knowledge and expertise during the early phases of these projects. We also wish to thank Galina Kalyuzhnaya, Xinren Li, and Jianlin Wang for their able technical assistance, and acknowledge the financial support provided by grants from the National Institutes on Drug Abuse.

REFERENCES

Abbadie C, Trafton J, Liu H, Mantyh PW, Basbaum AI. Inflammation increases the distribution of dorsal horn neurons that internalize the neurokinin-1 receptor in response to noxious and non-noxious stimulation. *J Neurosci* 1997; 17:8049–8060.

Afify EA, Law PY, Riedl M, Elde R, Loh HH. Role of carboxyl terminus of mu-and delta-opioid receptor in agonist-induced down-regulation. *Brain Res Mol Brain Res* 1998; 54:24–34.

Allen BJ, Li J, Menning PM, et al. Primary afferent fibers that contribute to increased substance P receptor internalization in the spinal cord after injury. *J Neurophysiol* 1999; 81:1379–1390.

Arvidsson U, Dado RJ, Law P-Y, et al. Delta (δ)-opioid receptor immunoreactivity: distribution in brain stem and spinal cord and relationship to biogenic amines and enkephalin. *J Neurosci* 1995a; 15:1215–1235.

Arvidsson U, Riedl M, Chakrabarti S, et al. Distribution and targeting of a μ-opioid receptor (MOR1) in brain and spinal cord. *J Neurosci* 1995b; 15:3328–3341.

Arvidsson U, Riedl M, Chakrabarti S, et al. The κ-opioid receptor (KOR1) is primarily postsynaptic: combined immunohistochemical localization of the receptor and endogenous opioids. *Proc Natl Acad Sci USA* 1995c; 92:5062–5066.

Bourque CW, Oliet SH, Richard D. Osmoreceptors, osmoreception, and osmoregulation. *Front Neuroendocrinol* 1994; 15:231–274.

Brismar H, Asghar M, Carey RM, Greengard P, Aperia A. Dopamine-induced recruitment of dopamine D1 receptors to the plasma membrane. *Proc Natl Acad Sci USA* 1998; 95:5573–5578.

Chen Y, Mestek A, Liu J, Hurley JA, Yu L. Molecular cloning and functional expression of a mu-opioid receptor from rat brain. *Mol Pharmacol* 1993; 44:8–12.

Cheng PY, Svingos AL, Wang H, et al. Ultrastructural immunolabeling shows prominent presynaptic vesicular localization of delta-opioid receptor within both enkephalin- and nonenkephalin-containing axon terminals in the superficial layers of the rat cervical spinal cord. *J Neurosci* 1995; 15:5976–5988.

Cheng PY, Moriwaki A, Wang JB, Uhl GR, Pickel VM. Ultrastructural localization of mu-opioid receptors in the superficial layers of the rat cervical spinal cord: extrasynaptic localization and proximity to Leu5-enkephalin. *Brain Res* 1996; 731:141–154.

Cheng PY, Liu-Chen LY, Pickel VM. Dual ultrastructural immunocytochemical labeling of mu and delta opioid receptors in the superficial layers of the rat cervical spinal cord. *Brain Res* 1997; 778:367–380.

Chu P, Murray S, Lissin D, von Zastrow M. Delta and kappa opioid receptors are differentially regulated by dynamin-dependent endocytosis when activated by the same alkaloid agonist. *J Biol Chem* 1997; 272:27124–27130.

Cvejic S, Devi LA. Dimerization of the delta opioid receptor: implication for a role in receptor internalization. *J Biol Chem* 1997; 272:26959–26964.

Dado RJ, Law PY, Loh HH, Elde R. Immunofluorescent identification of a delta (δ)-opioid receptor on primary afferent nerve terminals. *Neuroreport* 1993; 5:341–344.

Davis KE, Straff DJ, Weinstein EA, et al. Multiple signaling pathways regulate cell surface expression and activity of the excitatory amino acid carrier 1 subtype of Glu transporter in C6 glioma. *J Neurosci* 1998; 18:2475–2485.

Ding YQ, Nomura S, Kaneko T, Mizuno N. Co-localization of mu-opioid receptor-like and substance P-like immunoreactivities in axon terminals within the superficial layers of the medullary and spinal dorsal horns of the rat. *Neurosci Lett* 1995a; 198:45–48.

Ding YQ, Nomura S, Kaneko T, Mizuno N. Presynaptic localization of mu-opioid receptor-like immunoreactivity in retinal axon terminals within the terminal nuclei of the accessory optic tract: a light and electron microscope study in the rat. *Neurosci Lett* 1995b; 199:139–142.

Donnerer J, Schuligoi R, Stein C. Increased content and transport of substance P and calcitonin gene-related peptide in sensory nerves innervating inflamed tissue: evidence for a regulatory function of nerve growth factor in vivo. *Neuroscience* 1992; 49:693–698.

Donnerer J, Schuligoi R, Stein C, Amann R. Upregulation, release and axonal transport of substance P and calcitonin gene-related peptide in adjuvant inflammation and regulatory function of nerve growth factor. *Regul Pept* 1993; 46:150–154.

Drake CT, Patterson TA, Simmons ML, Chavkin C, Milner TA. Kappa opioid receptor-like immunoreactivity in guinea pig brain: ultrastructural localization in presynaptic terminals in hippocampal formation. *J Comp Neurol* 1996; 370:377–395.

Drake CT, Chavkin C, Milner TA. Kappa opioid receptor-like immunoreactivity is present in substance P-containing subcortical afferents in guinea pig dentate gyrus. *Hippocampus* 1997; 7:36–47.

Evans CJ, Keith DJ Jr, Morrison H, Magendzo K, Edwards RH. Cloning of a delta opioid receptor by functional expression. *Science* 1992; 258:1952–1955.

Fukuda K, Kato S, Mori K, Nishi M, Takeshima H. Primary structures and expression from cDNAs of rat opioid receptor delta- and mu-subtypes. *FEBS Lett* 1993; 327:311–314.

Garry MG, Hargreaves KM. Enhanced release of immunoreactive CGRP and substance P from spinal dorsal horn slices occurs during carrageenan inflammation. *Brain Res* 1992; 582:139–142.

Gaudriault G, Nouel D, Dal Farra C, Beaudet A, Vincent JP. Receptor-induced internalization of selective peptidic mu and delta opioid ligands. *J Biol Chem* 1997; 272:2880–2888.

Gracy KN, Svingos AL, Pickel VM. Dual ultrastructural localization of mu-opioid receptors and NMDA-type glutamate receptors in the shell of the rat nucleus accumbens. *J Neurosci* 1997; 17:4839–4848.

James DE. Targeting of the insulin-regulatable glucose transporter (GLUT-4). *Biochem Soc Trans* 1994; 22:668–670.

Kieffer BL, Befort K, Gaveriaux RC, Hirth CG. The delta-opioid receptor: isolation of a cDNA by expression cloning and pharmacological characterization. *Proc Natl Acad Sci USA* 1992; 89:12048–12052.

Lai J, Riedl M, Stone LS, et al. Immunofluorescence analysis of antisense oligodeoxynucleotide-mediated 'knock-down' of the mouse delta opioid receptor in vitro and in vivo. *Neurosci Lett* 1996; 213:205–208.

Li S, Zhu J, Chen C, et al. Molecular cloning and expression of a rat kappa opioid receptor. *Biochem J* 1993; 295:629–633.

McGregor GP, Fehmann C, Hartel R, et al. Investigations of the expression and post-translational processing of the preprotachykinin-I (PPT-I) gene by rat pancreatic, insulin-producing tumor cell-lines. *Regul Pept* 1993; 46:444–446.

Meng F, Xie GX, Thompson RC, et al. Cloning and pharmacological characterization of a rat kappa opioid receptor. *Proc Natl Acad Sci USA* 1993; 90:9954–9958.

Minami M, Toya T, Katao Y, et al. Cloning and expression of a cDNA for the rat kappa-opioid receptor. *FEBS Lett* 1993; 329:291–295.

Nanayama T, Kuraishi Y, Ohno H, Satoh M. Capsaicin-induced release of calcitonin gene-related peptide from dorsal horn slices is enhanced in adjuvant arthritic rats. *Neurosci Res* 1989; 6:569–572.

Nishi M, Takeshima H, Fukuda K, Kato S, Mori K. cDNA cloning and pharmacological characterization of an opioid receptor with high affinities for kappa-subtype-selective ligands. *FEBS Lett* 1993; 330:77–80.

North RA. Opioid actions on membrane ion channels. In: Herz (Ed). *Handbook of Experimental Pharmacology: Opioids I*. Berlin: Springer-Verlag, 1993, pp 773–797.

Ossipov MH, Kovelowski CJ, Porreca F. The increase in morphine antinociceptive potency produced by carrageenan-induced hindpaw inflammation is blocked by naltrindole, a selective delta-opioid antagonist. *Neurosci Lett* 1995; 184:173–176.

Quick MW, Corey JL, Davidson N, Lester HA. Second messengers, trafficking-related proteins, and amino acid residues that contribute to the functional regulation of the rat brain GABA transporter GAT1. *J Neurosci* 1997; 17:2967–2979.

Shoji M, Kimura T, Kawarabayasi Y, et al. Effects of acute salt loading on vasopressin mRNA level in the rat brain. *Am J Physiol* 1994; 266:R1591–R1595.

Shuster SJ, Riedl M, Li X, Vulchanova L, Elde R. Stimulus-dependent translocation of kappa opioid receptors to the plasma membrane. *J Neurosci* 1999; 19:2658–2664.

Staehelin M, Hertel C. [³H]CGP-12177, a beta-adrenergic ligand suitable for measuring cell surface receptors. *J Recept Res* 1983; 3:35–43.

Svingos AL, Moriwaki A, Wang JB, Uhl GR, Pickel VM. Ultrastructural immunocytochemical localization of mu-opioid receptors in rat nucleus accumbens: extrasynaptic plasmalemmal distribution and association with Leu5-enkephalin. *J Neurosci* 1996; 16:4162–4173.

Svingos AL, Colago EE, Pickel VM. Cellular sites for dynorphin activation of kappa-opioid receptors in the rat nucleus accumbens shell. *J Neurosci* 1999; 19:1804–1813.

Thompson RC, Mansour A, Akil H, Watson SJ. Cloning and pharmacological characterization of a rat mu opioid receptor. *Neuron* 1993; 11:903–913.

Trapaidze N, Keith DE, Cvejic S, Evans CJ, Devi LA. Sequestration of the delta opioid receptor. Role of the C terminus in agonist-mediated internalization. *J Biol Chem* 1996; 271:29279–29285.

van Bockstaele EJ, Commons K, Pickel VM. Delta-opioid receptor is present in presynaptic axon terminals in the rat nucleus locus coeruleus: relationships with methionine5-enkephalin. *J Comp Neurol* 1997; 388:575–586.

Wan Q, Xiong ZG, Man HY, et al. Recruitment of functional GABA(A) receptors to postsynaptic domains by insulin. *Nature* 1997; 388:686–690.

Wang H, Moriwaki A, Wang JB, Uhl GR, Pickel VM. Ultrastructural immunocytochemical localization of mu opioid receptors and Leu5-enkephalin in the patch compartment of the rat caudate-putamen nucleus. *J Comp Neurol* 1996; 375:659–674.

Wang QP, Ochiai H, Guan JL, Nakai Y. Ultrastructural localization of mu-1 opioid receptor in the dorsal raphe nucleus of the rat. *Synapse* 1998; 29:240–247.

Zhang X, Bao L, Arvidsson U, Elde R, Hokfelt T. Localization and regulation of the delta-opioid receptor in dorsal root ganglia and spinal cord of the rat and monkey: evidence for association with the membrane of large dense-core vesicles. *Neuroscience* 1998; 82:1225–1242.

Correspondence to: Maureen Riedl, PhD, Department of Neuroscience, University of Minnesota, 4-270 Basic Sciences and Biomedical Engineering, 312 Church Street SE, Minneapolis, MN 55455, USA. Tel: 612-624-4436; Fax: 612-624-8118; email: maureen@med.umn.edu.

Opioid Sensitivity of Chronic Noncancer Pain,
Progress in Pain Research and Management,
Vol. 14, edited by Eija Kalso, Henry J. McQuay,
and Zsuzsanna Wiesenfeld-Hallin, IASP Press,
Seattle, © 1999.

2

Function and Dysfunction of Opioid Receptors in the Spinal Cord

Anthony H. Dickenson and Rie Suzuki

Department of Pharmacology, University College, London, United Kingdom

The use of opium as a drug dates back thousands of years. In more recent times, in the 17th century, Johann Daniel Major and Johann Sigismund Elsholtz administered an intravenous solution of opium to a hunting dog. They noted that the animal did not respond to pin-prick and also refused to hunt. This is probably one of the earliest experiments on the analgesic effects of opium. Morphine, the main active agent in opioid, has become the "gold standard" analgesic to which all other opioids are compared. The isolation and characterization of the three main, or "classical" opioid receptors, mu (μ), delta (δ), and kappa (κ), and the continuing development of different agonists and antagonists for these receptors have allowed many studies on the physiological roles of the opioid receptors (see Uhl et al. 1994; Kieffer 1997). However, the development of novel analgesics acting on δ and κ receptors, which potentially may lack the typical μ-receptor-mediated side effects, has not yet been achieved. Nevertheless, studies over the last decade have revealed that morphine and other opioids may not always produce the same degree of analgesia in all conditions. Thus, opioid analgesia can be altered by inflammation and also by nerve damage. This chapter examines current knowledge on the mechanisms of action of opioids at the spinal cord level relevant to the relief of pain, reports data on the mechanisms for altering opioid controls in different pain states, and attempts to relate this basic research to opioid therapy.

OPIOIDS AND OPIOID RECEPTORS

The discovery of opioid receptors, closely followed by the isolation and identification of the endogenous opioid peptides, the natural transmitters for

17

the receptors (Hughes et al. 1975; Kosterlitz 1985), and then the isolation of the receptors were undoubtedly major breakthroughs in understanding the actions of opioids. Opioids act by binding to and activating the μ-, δ-, and κ-opioid receptors (Table I). The endogenous opioid peptides, the endomorphin, enkephalin, and dynorphin family of closely related endogenous opioids, are not completely specific for any one receptor (Kosterlitz 1985). Thus, a degree of confusion characterizes the literature on the roles of the endogenous opioids, but it is likely that the physiological release of each of the opioid peptides in the spinal cord leads to activation of a single receptor.

Anatomical studies using immunohistochemical stains for the mRNA for the propeptides, and the generation of antibodies to sequences of amino acids comprising the receptors, have allowed a high degree of resolution in localizing the neurons containing the different opioids and their receptors (Anton et al. 1996; Riedl et al. 1996; Zhang et al. 1998). Quantitative autoradiographic studies enable measurement of the number of opioid receptors and also estimation of the influence of pathological factors on the number of receptors in the spinal cord (Besse et al. 1990, 1992; Jia et al. 1998; Rahman et al. 1998). Thus, studies have demonstrated alterations in opioid peptide synthesis and opioid receptor number in animal models of different pain states. The levels of dynorphin in the spinal cord during inflammation are increased enormously due to the induction of the gene for the synthesis of the parent propeptide, and the number of opioid receptors in the spinal cord is dramatically reduced by dorsal root section (Dubner and Ruda 1992). The actions of opioids are also subject to physiological modulation by activity in other pharmacological systems situated in spinal cord circuitry (see Dickenson 1994). These changes in opioid actions offer a rationale for some clinical observations on opioid effectiveness and strong support for combination therapy with opioids.

Table I
Opioid receptors and their ligands

Opioid Receptor	Endogenous Agonist Ligands	Synthetic Agonist Ligands	Antagonists
μ	β-Endorphin Endomorphins	Morphine DAMGO	Naloxone β-FNA
δ	Met-enkephalin Leu-enkephalin	DPDPE SNC-80 DSTBULET	Naltrindole Naloxone
κ	Dynorphin $A_{(1-13)}$ Dynorphin $A_{(1-8)}$ Dynorphin B	U50488H Bremazocine Pentazocine	Naloxone Nor-BNI
ORL1	Nociceptin/OFQ	None so far	$[\text{Phe}^1\Psi(\text{CH}_2\text{NH})\text{Gly}^2]\text{NC}_{(1-13)}\text{NH}_2$

An unexpected consequence of the cloning of the opioid receptors was the finding of a fourth receptor. In 1992 the amino acid sequence of the δ-opioid receptor was determined by expression cloning, which made it possible to clone the μ and κ receptors, given their expected homology to the cloned δ receptor (Evans et al. 1992; Kieffer et al. 1992; Chen et al. 1993; Uhl et al. 1994). This approach was extended to search for further novel members of the opioid receptor gene family, and the cDNA encoding a previously unrecognized receptor protein was identified in humans, rats, and mice (Wick et al. 1994; Peluso et al. 1998). This new receptor, the hORL1 (human opioid receptor-like 1), exhibited substantial sequence identities with the other three opioid receptors. The endogenous ligand for the ORL1 receptor was then isolated and named nociceptin or orphanin FQ (Meunier et al. 1995; Reinscheid et al. 1995). The peptide consists of 17 amino acid residues and so falls into the same general size range as the other endogenous opioid peptides. Naloxone, the universal opioid-receptor antagonist, has low affinity for the ORL1 receptor. Therefore, previous functional studies that probed the physiological roles of endogenous opioids by using naloxone or other selective antagonists probably failed to manipulate the nociceptin system. The functional roles of nociceptin are now being extensively studied, and early results appear rather contradictory, although the receptor, when activated, produces typical inhibitory effects on neurons (Connor et al. 1996; Vaughan and Christie 1996).

The recent isolation and cloning of the opioid receptors was a major step forward in understanding the molecular basis of opioid actions, and anatomical probes based on the receptor sequence have been of great value in localizing particular receptors. In addition to the discovery of the ORL1 receptor, these molecular studies have revealed a further puzzling issue. With all transmitter systems, the greater the number of receptors, the greater is the potential for highly selective agents acting on one particular receptor. These conditions may enable the desirable effects of broader spectrum drugs to be separated from their unwanted effects if different receptors mediate both sets of actions. Research suggests that the μ, δ, and κ receptors consist of subtypes: two μ subtypes (μ_1 and μ_2), two δ subtypes, and three κ subtypes (Pasternak and Wood 1986; Traynor 1989; Jiang et al. 1991). This theory is based on pharmacological and physiological studies, but has not yet been confirmed by molecular approaches. Thus, all opioid receptors isolated to date, irrespective of the species and tissue, consist of a single receptor type (Uhl et al. 1994; Kieffer 1997). Perhaps alternative splicing might produce the subtypes, or local neuronal tissue environments might allow the subtypes to be expressed; also, the cell lines used to date may underestimate the variability within the opioid receptor family, and potential subtypes may yet emerge. What is known, however, is that the rat and mouse opioid receptors are apparently identical in structure and pharmacology to the human receptors (Kieffer 1997), so that comparative studies are justified. Other problems that have been overcome are the high susceptibility of the endogenous opioids to rapid degradation by peptidases and the very poor ability of peptides to penetrate membranes. The enkephalins can be protected from breakdown by systemically active peptidase inhibitors (Roques et al. 1993). Also, the synthesis of more stable analogues of endogenous opioids, and most usefully, the production of nonpeptide agonists at the opioid receptors, have generated very useful agents that may in turn lead to novel clinical drugs.

All the opioid receptors and their endogenous peptides are found in the spinal cord. The receptors are located both on the terminals of fine afferent fibers and on spinal cord neurons, whereas the opioid peptides only originate from spinal neurons. The spinal actions of morphine were first demonstrated in animals in 1974 (Besson and Chaouch 1987), and a plethora of further studies using behavioral and electrophysiological approaches have centered on the spinal effects of opioids (see Yaksh and Nouiehed 1985; Dickenson 1994). This chapter focuses on the actions of morphine at the μ receptor. This drug has high affinity for the μ receptor, with relative affinity of at least 50 times less for the δ receptor and minimal affinity for the κ or ORL1 receptors (Kosterlitz 1985; Wick et al. 1994; Kieffer 1997). When very high doses such as those achieved in vitro have been used, some non-μ effects of morphine have been reported. However, in vivo, the inhibitory effects of doses of spinal morphine that are sufficient to abolish the C-fiber-evoked responses of dorsal horn nociceptive neurons are not reversed by naltrindole, a δ-receptor antagonist. Likewise, there is no evidence for μ–δ cross-tolerance (Kalso et al. 1993). Thus, morphine produces most of its physiological effects by actions at the μ receptor. This characteristic opens the door for the consideration of nonpeptide opioid-receptor agonists with good affinity for the δ, κ, or ORL1 receptors as potential analgesics with a profile that differs from that of the most commonly used morphine-like drugs.

MECHANISMS OF OPIOID ANALGESIA

The opioid receptors are part of the superfamily of G-protein-coupled receptors that spans seven transmembranes. Binding of an opioid to the extracellular domain elicits a conformational change in the receptor that leads to intracellular changes which result in inhibition. The three mechanisms of action of opioids discussed in this section simply relate to the location of the receptors on neuronal circuitry. These primary events by which opioids reduce the transmission of pain are identical to the mechanisms by which opioids on non-pain-related cells cause their unwanted effects.

PRESYNAPTIC ACTIONS OF OPIOIDS

Opioids predominantly exert a presynaptic action on the terminals of neurons. Autoradiographic studies using labeled selective ligands for the opioid receptors and immunohistochemical methods with antisera to the receptor protein reveal a high level of opioid receptors in the spinal cord around the C-fiber terminal zones in lamina I and the substantia gelatinosa, with lower levels found in deeper layers (Besse et al. 1990; Rahman et al. 1998; Zhang et al. 1998). Opioid receptors are synthesized in the cell bodies of small afferent fibers in the dorsal root ganglion (DRG) and then transported within the nerves to the peripheral and central terminals of the fibers. The bulk of the receptors are located on the presynaptic terminals of C fibers as they enter the spinal cord; interestingly, δ receptors are found on the membranes of vesicles in terminals in the afferents, a highly strategic position for the modulation of transmitter release (Zhang et al. 1998). The manufacture of opioid receptors in afferent sensory nerves means that they can be vulnerable to pathological damage to a peripheral nerve. Thus, nerve section (rhizotomy) leads to a dramatic drop in opioid receptors at the spinal level, with about 70% lost due to failure of transport (Besse et al. 1990). Less severe neuropathy may also lead to reduced numbers of functional receptors, although early increases can occur in some models after partial nerve damage (Stevens et al. 1991; Besse et al. 1992). Inhibition of a terminal following the activation of opioid receptors will cause a reduction in the release of transmitters from the afferent nerve. This presynaptic action, in common with all inhibitory effects of opioids at other sites, results from an opening of potassium channels (μ, δ, and ORL1 receptors) or a closing of calcium channels (κ receptor) (Duggan and North 1984; Connor et al. 1996; Vaughan and Christie 1996). The hyperpolarization of the terminal resulting from the opening of potassium channels will lead to a decrease in the opening of calcium channels as action potentials invade the terminal. Kappa opioids will directly reduce this calcium influx, resulting in decreased transmitter release. C fibers release a number of multiple transmitters including the tachykinins, excitatory amino acids, and various other excitatory peptides that act on multiple excitatory receptors located on spinal cord neurons. Thus, the large numbers of opioid receptors in the dorsal horn on the terminals of thin afferent fibers, when activated, will reduce the release of all transmitters contained in the fibers. Consequently, by this presynaptic action, opioids can potentially abolish transmitter release from fine afferent fibers and prevent the activation of multiple postsynaptic receptors (see Dickenson 1994).

The peripheral receptors have no function in normal tissue because opioids do not influence peripheral nerve function under resting conditions, but they become accessible after inflammation. This may result from the actions of inflammatory mediators and other agents at the sites of tissue damage, which render the perineurium of the C fibers leaky so that opioids can gain access to the peripheral opioid receptors. As a consequence, peripheral effects of opioids, although somewhat weak, can be demonstrated in animals and humans after inflammation (Stein 1994; Antonijevic et al. 1995) and also after peripheral nerve damage (Kayser et al. 1995). This peripheral action may be useful in inflammatory sites since it could avoid some of the central side effects of opioids.

Overall, the evidence supports an effectiveness of μ-, δ-, and κ-receptor agonists as peripheral analgesics in models of inflammation. Interestingly, the same models show clear parallel increases in the spinal effects of opioids (Hylden et al. 1991; Stanfa et al. 1992), which will be discussed below. However, in contrast to the three original opioid receptors, the activation of the ORL1 receptor appears to generate nociception at peripheral levels via the release of substance P (Inoue et al. 1998), although other studies report the opposite (Helyes et al. 1997).

However, the predominant actions of opioids in the production of analgesia are in the central nervous system (CNS), at spinal and at supraspinal sites. Although studies have been somewhat contradictory on the relative proportions of opioid receptors, some have not used the most selective ligands for the receptors and so may not represent the true relative distribution of the receptors. The most likely distribution is that the μ receptor forms about 70%, the δ receptor 20–30%, and the κ receptor 5–10% of the total opioid sites in the rat spinal cord (Besse et al. 1990; Rahman et al. 1998).

Dorsal root rhizotomy results in the degeneration of primary afferents and leads to a loss of the presynaptic opioid receptors that normally would be transported from the DRG cell body to the central terminals. This experimental approach allows the relative numbers of pre- and postsynaptic receptors to be calculated. The proportion of presynaptic sites in the spinal cord varies for each receptor and ranges from 0% to 70%. The most prevalent presynaptic receptors are μ receptors, with over 70% of the total μ receptor sites localized on afferent terminals; a similar case exists for the δ receptor

(Besse et al. 1990). ORL1 receptors are also found in the superficial dorsal horn and appear to be at least partly presynaptic (Wick et al. 1994); a rapid induction of these receptors occurs after peripheral inflammation (Jia et al. 1998). Direct evidence for the presynaptic action of μ and δ opioids comes from neurochemical studies that show an opioid inhibition of C-fiber-evoked transmitter release (substance P and glutamate) (Hirota et al. 1985; Kangra and Randic 1991). Furthermore, both in vitro and in vivo electrophysiological studies have shown that spontaneous and evoked activity is reduced by opioids in a manner indicative of presynaptic actions (Dickenson and Sullivan 1986; North 1989; Hori et al. 1992). The synthesis of opioid receptors in C fibers, but not the largest low-threshold A fibers, is the major reason for the selective effects of spinal opioids on noxious evoked activity, sparing low-threshold responses (Dickenson and Sullivan 1986).

In addition to their inhibitory effects, opioids can have facilitatory effects on C-fiber transmission at low doses; a characteristic of all μ-receptor agonists is that the lowest doses of the agents enhance C-fiber activity. As the dose is increased, inhibitions then predominate (Dickenson et al. 1987; Crain and Shen 1990; Stanfa et al. 1992). These low-dose effects may be the one exception to findings that the primary actions of opioids are solely inhibitory.

POSTSYNAPTIC ACTIONS OF OPIOIDS

A second action of opioids at the spinal level is via a postsynaptic hyperpolarization that reduces evoked activity in the neuronal pathways. Only 25% of μ and δ receptors are found on spinal neurons (Besse et al. 1990). Functional data from electrophysiological and behavioral studies support opioid actions at postsynaptic receptors; opioids were shown to reduce the pronociceptive actions of glutamate and substance P, which act on directly on spinal neurons (Hylden and Wilcox 1983; Lombard and Besson 1989; Magnuson and Dickenson 1991). Postsynaptic hyperpolarizations of neurons arise from the same ionic mechanisms, either through the opening of potassium ion channels or the closing of calcium channels. The postsynaptic opioid receptors may be located on the dendrites of projection neurons, on interneurons, or on the cell body of projection cells. At the first two sites the action of the opioids would be selective for noxious transmission. However, opioid receptors on output neurons would be able to reduce A-fiber-evoked activity, and a small reduction in this type of response is observed after administration of spinal opioids. However, maximal 30% reductions of low-threshold activity occur with opioid doses that abolish C-fiber activity. Thus, minor inhibitions of low-threshold inputs by opioids are likely to account for the weak effects of opioids on allodynias. Electrophysiological evidence from comparative studies in animals with and without presynaptic opioid receptors indicates that the postsynaptic actions of opioids require higher doses of systemic morphine compared to presynaptic effects (Lombard and Besson 1989). Thus, the predicted loss of presynaptic receptors after nerve section and the subsequent contribution to the reduced opioid sensitivity of postamputation pain could be partly overcome by dose escalation.

The final action of opioids involves an indirect postsynaptic action. This opioid disinhibitory effect appears to be produced via γ-aminobutyric acid (GABA) and enkephalin neurons in the substantia gelatinosa. Opioid receptors seem to inhibit an inhibitory neuron, which in turn leads to increased activity of another inhibitory neuron in the circuit. This release from inhibition of the second neuron produces a depression of activity of output neurons. Both morphological and electrophysiological evidence supports this action (Magnuson and Dickenson 1991).

SPINAL ANALGESIA

The spinal action of opioids is an excellent example of how basic research in animals can lead to improvements in the clinical relief of pain. The knowledge gained from basic animal studies showing an opioid inhibition of nociceptive spinal neurons and the direct analgesia following epidural and intrathecal opioids was soon applied to humans (Yaksh and Nouiehed 1985; Besson and Chaouch 1987). Considerable attention has been focused on opioid receptor subtypes in the spinal cord, using both electrophysiological and behavioral approaches. This volume covers the effects of opioids in several pain states. Importantly, the use of various different models of clinical pain states has led to animal studies addressing the extent and mechanisms of plasticity in opioid spinal function, since pathological and physiological/pharmacological events can alter the degree of opioid antinociception (see Dickenson 1994).

Many electrophysiological and behavioral studies have shown that μ-, δ-, and κ-receptor agonists and nociceptin acting at the ORL1 receptor cause antinociception and inhibition of spinal nociceptive neurons after intrathecal (i.t.) application (Yaksh and Nouiehed 1985; Dickenson 1994; Stanfa et al. 1996). These mechanisms have been discussed in the preceding sections. In broad terms, the most potent opioids are the μ-receptor ligands, which presumably reflects the fact that μ-opioid sites are the most numerous in the spinal cord. Another important factor is the inverse relationship between lipophilicity and potency for a range of synthetic opioids acting at the μ receptor (McQuay et al. 1989; Dickenson et al. 1990). According to this study, the opioid with the highest potency was morphine, which is the least lipophilic. Drugs with high systemic potency due to their lipophilicity, such as fentanyl, were relatively ineffective after spinal application, probably because of nonspecific binding of the lipophilic opioids in the lipid-rich fiber tracts capping the cord, or because vascular redistribution reduced the dose of opioid reaching the receptors in the gelatinosa.

The spinal cord has high levels of opioid receptors and endogenous opioids. Nociceptin-like immunoreactivity and ORL1 receptors are located in the dorsal horn of the spinal cord and in midbrain and brain stem sites, in some cases alongside the enkephalins, dynorphins, and endomorphins. Nociceptin has been identified in the spinal cord in areas adjacent to but mostly separate from the location of the other endogenous opioids. Rhizotomy does not alter spinal level of the opioid peptides, which indicates that they are all derived from intrinsic spinal neurons or descending pathways from the brain (Riedl et al. 1996). The enkephalins and endorphins are inhibitory, as are μ and δ synthetic opioids (except for low-dose μ facilitations), but dynorphin, the endogenous κ-opioid receptor agonist, differs in several of its effects. When applied spinally, it facilitates activity of some neurons and inhibits other nociceptive neurons (Knox and Dickenson 1987); a spinal application of a κ-receptor antagonist both increases and decreases individual neuronal activity in normal animals, but is considerably more effective in animals with inflammation (Stanfa and Dickenson 1994a). The consequences for pain transmission are not understood. The functions of nociceptin in the processing of noxious events are also controversial (Henderson and McKnight 1997; Dartland et al. 1998; Taylor and Dickenson 1998), although the discrepancies may be resolved on the basis of the differential spinal and supraspinal actions of the peptide. In general, when administered into supraspinal sites, nociceptin produces hyperalgesia, whereas spinal administration clearly is inhibitory and produces analgesia (Dartland et al. 1998; Taylor and Dickenson 1998). These spinal antinociceptive effects of the peptide are observed in behavioral and in vivo and in vitro electrophysiological studies. Thus, nociceptin suppresses spinal reflexes and dorsal horn neuronal activity, and i.t. nociceptin is also antinociceptive in the tail-flick test at doses that do not induce motor deficits or sedation (Dartland et al. 1998; Taylor and Dickenson 1998).

All electrophysiological studies on the effector mechanism of the ORL1 receptor would support the concept that the receptor is inhibitory, as receptor activation opens potassium channels and closes calcium channels in a manner identical to that of μ, δ, and κ opioids. Nociceptin inhibits voltage-dependent Ca^{2+} channels in a human neuroblastoma cell line (Connor et al. 1996) and opens an inwardly rectifying potassium conductance at the ORL1 receptor in the dorsal raphe nucleus and in hippocampal neurons (Vaughan and Christie 1996). Similar to other members of the opioid receptor super-family, nociceptin inhibits the release of both glutamate and GABA from nerve terminals in the CNS (Henderson and McKnight 1997). Furthermore, in vitro studies have shown that nociceptin reduces postsynaptic currents via presynaptic actions, whilst postsynaptic activity is not altered (Wick et al. 1994). However, what appear to be marked postsynaptic effects can be clearly demonstrated in vivo (Stanfa et al. 1996).

The supraspinal hyperalgesia seen in behavioral studies with nociceptin (Dartland et al. 1998; Taylor and Dickenson 1998) may be reconciled with the location of the inhibitory receptor on inhibitory neurons at supraspinal sites; the net effect of ORL1-receptor activation would thus be disinhibition. In accordance with this idea, the hyperalgesia seen supraspinally may, in fact, be due to an "anti-opioid' action in that nociceptin can reverse systemic and supraspinal morphine antinociception and also opioid-mediated, stress-induced antinociception. The idea that nociceptin can act as a functional anti-opioid peptide is restricted to the brain since no such effect is seen at spinal levels (see Taylor and Dickenson 1998).

Most studies have failed to reverse the antinociceptive effects of nociceptin, although high doses of naloxone are able to antagonize some actions. This lack of a specific and potent antagonist has hampered functional studies, so the recent description of a selective competitive antagonist, [Phe$^1\Psi$(CH$_2$NH)Gly^2]NC$_{(1-13)}$NH$_2$, was a major step forward (Guerrini et al. 1998). However, although this compound is an antagonist at peripheral sites, when given spinally it behaves as a full and potent agonist (Carpenter et al. 1998). This action suggests the existence of multiple receptors for nociceptin. Work with transgenic mice lacking the ORL1 receptor is also a major development in the elucidation of the physiological roles of the receptor system; studies to date report no change in nociceptive threshold in these animals, which suggests little endogenous tone in the nociceptin system, similar to observations in mice lacking other opioid systems (see Mogil and Grisel 1998). However, more detailed tests with a wide range of stimuli are needed.

CHANGES IN OPIOID SYSTEMS

Considerable clinical and animal data indicate that the analgesic effects of opioids will vary depending on the particular pain state. Obviously, the key area of clinical interest is the treatment of pain when opioid sensitivity is reduced. Neuropathic pain states frequently fall into this category, although the extreme view that they are unresponsive to opioids (Arnér and Meyerson 1988) has been replaced by the idea that increasing the dose may result in adequate pain control (Portenoy et al. 1990). Side effects may, however, preclude sufficient increase in dose. Furthermore, within a group of patients with neuropathic pain, some will show a good response, although most will not (Jadad et al. 1992). Likewise, some patients with neuropathic pain have responded to morphine (Rowbotham et al. 1991). It is imperative that clinical studies address the issue of whether the various symptoms and types of neuropathic pain syndromes have differential sensitivity to morphine. Contrary to the situation with nerve injury, much animal evidence indicates that inflammatory pain is accompanied by an increased sensitivity to opioids, although no clinical data are available, except on the peripheral actions of opioids in inflammation (see Chapter 20). Several factors may explain changes in opioid actions, and a better understanding of these potential systems will greatly benefit the treatment of difficult pains.

LOSS OF OPIOID RECEPTORS

Section of a peripheral nerve will lead to the loss of up to 70% of μ-opioid receptors on the presynaptic terminals of C fibers in the spinal cord (Besse et al. 1990). In animals with rhizotomy, both electrophysiological (Lombard and Besson 1989) and behavioral studies (Xu et al. 1993) show that higher doses of morphine are required to produce antinociception compared to normal animals. Thus, a loss of opioid receptors due to either peripheral or central lesions will lead to a reduction in opioid actions that potentially could be countered by dose escalation.

ACTIONS OF ANTI-OPIOID PEPTIDES

FLFQPQRFamide and cholecystokinin (CCK) are nonopioid peptides found within the spinal cord and elsewhere in the brain; when given spinally they prevented μ- but not δ-mediated neuronal inhibitions and reduced i.t. morphine analgesia in behavioral studies (Wang and Han 1990; Stanfa et al. 1994). They are also able to reduce supraspinal opioid analgesia elicited by μ opioids, and so may have general wide controls on morphine analgesia. Thus, an increase in the levels or release of these peptides would limit the effects of morphine independently of any change in opioid receptor number. Preventing the actions of the peptides with antagonists or antibodies both potentiates the analgesic effects of morphine and reduces tolerance (Baber et al. 1989; Dourish et al. 1990; Xu et al. 1993).

NMDA-RECEPTOR-MEDIATED ACTIVITY

The NMDA receptor, one of the receptors for the excitatory amino acid glutamate, both induces and maintains persistent enhancements of the excitability of dorsal horn neurons to prolonged stimulation (McMahon et al. 1993; Dickenson 1997). Wind-up is a key spinal mechanism requiring activation of the NMDA receptor that both amplifies and prolongs the firing produced by repeated C-fiber stimulation (Dickenson 1990). As a result, wind-up may be one of the events underlying prolonged or chronic pain and the production of so-called central hypersensitive states. Evidence from animal studies indicates that this mechanism is involved in the induction and maintenance of hyperalgesia in models of inflammatory, ischemic, and neuropathic pain (Dickenson 1997).

Neuropathic pains are at least partly mediated by the NMDA receptor, which may relate to changes in opioid sensitivity. All opioids reduce, or with high doses block the C-fiber inputs onto the deeper dorsal horn nociceptive neurons, probably via activation of the presynaptic opioid receptors to prevent the release of primary afferent transmitters and so prevent C-fiber activity from activating spinal neurons (Dickenson 1994). However, if the peripheral stimulation continues, wind-up overcomes the inhibitions of input and the neurons commence firing. As wind-up increases the activity of neurons, a higher dose of opioid will be required to block the increased excitability. Thus, at moderate doses, opioids delay wind-up without inhibiting the process itself. In contrast, NMDA antagonists abolish wind-up (Dickenson 1990). Thus, threshold doses of morphine combined with low doses of NMDA antagonists are able to elicit dramatic inhibitory effects (Chapman and Dickenson 1992), a synergism that suggests low probability of side effects. Importantly, in a model of neuropathic pain where morphine is inoperative, the co-application of an NMDA antagonist restored the ability of morphine to inhibit the response (Yamamoto and Yaksh 1992).

A-FIBER ALLODYNIA

Doses of morphine that abolish C-fiber activity in normal animals have only minor effects on A-fiber activity. Thus, the allodynia transmitted via A-fiber afferents may well have a weak sensitivity to opioids because presynaptic opioid receptors are only associated with C fibers (Dickenson 1994), and the only mechanism by which opioids could reduce A-fiber activity would be through the smaller number of postsynaptic receptors.

MORPHINE ANALGESIA IN INFLAMMATION

The effects of systemic opioids in models of inflammatory nociception have been studied in detail, including models of generalized arthritis (Kayser and Guilbaud 1983; Neil et al. 1986; Millan et al. 1987), and those producing more localized inflammation (Joris et al. 1990; Kayser et al. 1991; Ossipov et al. 1995a) and unilateral inflammation (Stein et al. 1988). Generally, the antinociceptive potency of opioids is greater in models of inflammation than with acute noxious stimuli in normal animals. Contributing to the enhanced potency of systemic opioids in inflammation are opioid actions at sites in the inflamed peripheral tissue; naloxone administered directly into an inflamed paw is able to antagonize the actions of systemically administered opioids (Stein et al. 1988; Kayser et al. 1991). However, as with normal animals, central sites make a major contribution to the increased ability of opioids to produce analgesia. Thus, the development of inflammation in the periphery induces changes in the ability of opioids acting at sites in the spinal cord to modulate nociceptive transmission.

Behavioral (Hylden et al. 1991) and electrophysiological studies (Stanfa et al. 1992) show that within a few hours of the induction of peripheral inflammation, spinal opioid-receptor agonists have enhanced potency against noxious stimuli. The inflammation-induced enhancement in the spinal potency of agonists acting at μ, δ, and κ receptors is not uniform, and morphine exhibits a far greater increase in spinal potency than do δ or κ opioids, which show only relatively modest increases in potency. This non-uniform enhancement in the potency of opioids acting at the different receptors was also observed in the behavioral study of Hylden et al. (1991), where μ-agonist actions were enhanced more than those of the δ agonist [D-Pen^2,D-Pen^5]enkephalin (DPDPE). Thus, the enhancement in opioid potency in inflammation at spinal sites predominates for the μ receptor. Although less studied, nociceptin is effective against both the early and late phases of the formalin inflammatory response, akin to other opioids, and the i.t. administration of the peptide resulted in an attenuation of thermal hyperalgesia following peripheral inflammation (Taylor and Dickenson 1998). Interestingly, the mRNA for the nociceptin precursor can be detected in the DRG within 30 minutes of inflammation (Andoh et al. 1997), whereas it is almost absent in normal animals. Furthermore, an inflammation-induced upregulation of the receptor occurs in the superficial spinal cord (Jia et al. 1998). This response suggests that the release of de novo nociceptin from the afferents following inflammation would act as a simultaneous auto- and heteroreceptor control of the release of nociceptin and of the excitatory amino acids and peptides in small afferents. The consequences for pain transmission are complex.

Several important factors must be considered when addressing the basis for the alterations in potency of opioids in inflammation. The enhancement in the spinal potency of the exogenously administered opioids occurs rapidly (Hylden et al. 1991; Stanfa et al. 1992), with a substantial enhancement in morphine potency within 1 hour (Stanfa et al. 1992). The changes are unilateral and not generalized. There is a preferential enhancement in the spinal potency of μ opioids such as morphine compared with the δ- and κ-opioid agonists tested.

Inflammation induces highly specific changes in spinal systems that are primarily directed against the μ-opioid receptor, and so broad alterations in transmitter release from peripheral nerves, levels of neuronal activity, or other global changes are unlikely as they would be expected to produce equivalent changes in the potency of agonists at all three opioid receptors. This altered potency of spinal opioids in inflammation could arise from a change in either the number or affinity of spinal opioid receptors, but there is little evidence for any marked change in spinal opioid receptors, even after weeks of inflammation (see Stanfa and Dickenson 1993).

A selective increase in μ-opioid potency could be predicted if release of the "anti-opioid" peptides, cholecystokinin (CCK) and FLFQPQRFamide, were depleted or reduced in the inflammatory state. The other possible mechanism is that the development of inflammation leads to increased activity of descending noradrenergic systems that can also interact with spinal events. Alpha-2-adrenoceptor agonists such as clonidine, dexmedetomidine, and noradrenaline potentiate the antinociceptive effects of μ agonists such as morphine (Yaksh and Reddy 1981; Hylden and Wilcox 1983; Sullivan et al. 1987, 1992a,b; Wilcox et al. 1987; Loomis et al. 1988; Ossipov et al. 1990; Plummer et al. 1992), but do not enhance the effects of δ agonists (Sullivan et al. 1992b), with no evidence for a strong interaction between α_2-adrenoceptor agonists and κ-opioid agonists. Hence, an increased spinal release of noradrenaline in the inflamed state could potentiate the actions of μ-opioid agonists.

Considerable evidence indicates that CCK may play an important role in modulating CNS opioid mechanisms, based partly on the finding that small doses of CCK reduce morphine analgesia in the rat tail-flick test (Faris et al. 1983). In addition, the weak CCK-receptor antagonist, proglumide, was shown to enhance opioid analgesia (Watkins et al. 1984). Strong evidence from studies using exogenous CCK and CCK-receptor antagonists reveals that in the normal animal, physiological levels of CCK in the spinal cord can interfere with the actions of μ-opioid agonists such as morphine (Watkins et al. 1984; Magnuson et al. 1990; Stanfa and Dickenson 1993; Zhou et al. 1993). Although less extensively studied, this negative modulation of opioid actions by CCK does not appear to extend to opioids acting at δ- (Magnuson et al. 1990; Wang and Han 1990) or κ-opioid receptors (Barbaz et al. 1989; but see Wang and Han 1990). This supports the finding that spinal μ-opioid agonists show a far greater enhancement in antinociceptive potency after inflammation than do either δ- or κ-selective opioid agonists.

The CCK receptors in the rat spinal cord are mainly of the CCK_B type (Baber et al. 1989; Hill and Woodruff 1990) and are located primarily in laminae I and II, both presynaptic (approximately 50–60%) and postsynaptic to the primary afferent fibers (Ghilardi et al. 1992). This distribution pattern mirrors that of the μ-opioid receptor in the rat spinal cord. The mechanism by which CCK diminishes the antinociceptive effect of μ opioids is unknown, but CCK might alter the binding of opioid agonists to their respective receptors through an allosteric interaction (Wang and Han 1990), although not all studies have found this effect (Slaninova et al. 1991). CCK is capable of mobilizing calcium from intracellular stores via postreceptor mechanisms, which would lead to the physiological antagonism of the suppression of calcium entry into nerve terminals following opioid receptor activation (Wang et al. 1992). A further suggested mechanism is that CCK, acting on the CCK_B receptor, decreases the availability of the enkephalins. Other evidence suggests that enkephalins can synergize with morphine in the production of analgesia and that CCK reduces enkephalin levels, with a negative effect on morphine analgesia (Ossipov et al. 1994; Vanderah et al. 1994).

In normal animals, endogenous CCK negatively modulates the antinociceptive actions of μ opioids in the spinal cord. When this interaction is studied in animals with carrageenan inflammation, CCK_B-receptor antagonism no longer increases the potency of spinal morphine, in direct contrast to the situation in normal animals (Stanfa and Dickenson 1993). That endogenous CCK can no longer antagonize morphine in these animals suggests reduced levels of the peptide, a theory supported by the finding that exogenous CCK is still able to attenuate the antinociceptive effects of i.t. morphine (Stanfa and Dickenson 1993). Thus, the receptors and effector mechanisms must still be intact, so a decreased availability of CCK within the spinal cord following carrageenan inflammation (either due to a decreased release of CCK or depleted levels of the peptide within the dorsal horn) most likely explains the lack of effect of the CCK antagonist in these animals. It appears that the availability of CCK within the spinal cord, and consequently its ability to modify opioid analgesia, is not fixed but can be modified; furthermore, different pain states appear to alter its availability.

Spinal noradrenaline, released from descending pathways, can control nociception in the dorsal horn of the spinal cord. Noradrenergic axons and terminals occur in the dorsal horn of the spinal cord in all laminae, although they are particularly dense in the superficial dorsal horn (Westlund 1992). In a several species, including humans, activation of spinal α_2 adrenoceptors leads to analgesia (Headley et al. 1978; Fleetwood-Walker 1985; Yaksh 1985; Sullivan et al. 1987, 1992a); in addition, threshold doses of α_2-adrenoceptor agonists potentiated the antinociceptive effects of spinal opioids in both behavioral and electrophysiological studies. Inflammation-induced increases in noradrenaline levels could contribute to the observed increased actions of opioids. In fact, an increase in the turnover of noradrenaline in the spinal cord has been reported in arthritic rats (Weil-Fugazza et al. 1986), and unspecified tonic descending inhibition of dorsal horn neurons is enhanced following the development of acute inflammation (Cervero et al. 1991; Schaible et al. 1991).

Alpha-2-adrenergic antagonists have been used to gauge the tonic control of spinal nociceptive transmission by descending noradrenergic controls in both normal animals and following the development of inflammation. In normal animals, descending noradrenergic controls have no major role in the tonic control of spinal nociceptive processing, but following carrageenan inflammation, nociceptive responses may be subject to enhanced α_2-adrenergic controls (Green et al. 1998). However, this mechanism is not likely to interact with morphine analgesia as high spinal doses of two α_2-adrenoceptor antagonists (idazoxan and atipamezole) administered in conjunction with morphine did not alter the potency of i.t. morphine (Stanfa and Dickenson 1994b). Thus, spinal synergism with noradrenaline acting at α_2 adrenoceptors is unlikely to be responsible for the enhancement in opioid effects on the inflamed side.

Finally, inflammation increases the levels of the κ-opioid peptide dynorphin (Dubner and Ruda 1992), and studies with nor-binaltorphimine (nor-BNI) show increases in κ-opioid-mediated effects at spinal sites in inflammation (Stanfa and Dickenson 1994a). Naloxone also produces complex bidirectional effects on nociception. It has not yet been possible to clearly equate these effects of the opioid antagonist naloxone to the functioning of particular opioid receptors. In particular, the functional consequences of the upregulation of dynorphin and κ-opioid controls are unclear because administration of the peptide and activation of the receptor both enhance and reduce the transmission of nociceptive information at the spinal level.

The functional consequences of the enhanced effects of exogenous opioid actions in inflammation are far more clear-cut. In the spinal cord, the inhibitory actions of μ-receptor agonists such as morphine are preferentially and rapidly enhanced within the first hours after the induction of inflammation.

Although increases in descending inhibitory controls involving the α_2 adrenoceptor could be responsible, via their ability to potentiate the effect of morphine, it appears unlikely that this mechanism occurs in the spinal cord. The key factor in this increased potency is a reduction in the spinal levels or release of the peptide CCK. This reduced functional role of CCK removes an endogenous brake on morphine analgesia. The exact sequence of events that follow peripheral inflammation and lead to these spinal changes remains unclear.

These findings emphasize that opioid analgesia should not be regarded as fixed but can be altered by the level of activity in local spinal transmitter systems (Dickenson 1994), some of which have been described here. This plasticity of opioid function in the inflammatory state where both spinal and peripheral opioid controls are enhanced results in augmented opioid analgesia. Possibly, these increased opioid controls represent an adaptation to compensate for the enhanced nociceptive transmission produced by inflammation. In contrast, nerve section can lead to marked reductions in opioid analgesia (Lombard and Besson 1989). If these findings, based on extensive animal studies with several models of inflammation, are applicable to humans, the enhanced effects of μ opioids in inflammation provides a rationale for using very low doses of opioids such as codeine or morphine (with consequent low side-effect liability) to treat pain of inflammatory origins.

MORPHINE ANALGESIA AND NEUROPATHIC PAIN

Neuropathic pain arising from peripheral nerve injury is a clinical disorder characterized by combinations of spontaneous burning pain, sensory loss, hyperalgesia, and allodynia. The mechanisms underlying neuropathic pain are complex and appear to involve various peripheral and central components of sensory systems (see references in Fields and Rowbotham 1994). The treatment of pain arising from nerve injury can be difficult, and the opioid sensitivity of neuropathic pain remains debatable. A recent series of clinical studies have reported that morphine lacks full analgesic efficacy in neuropathic pain states. However, there is no real consensus from these studies; one reported that opioids were ineffective (Arnér and Meyerson 1988), whereas another maintained that dose escalation produced good analgesia (Portenoy et al. 1990). Further studies showed that, in general, morphine could be effective in a group of patients with neuropathy (Rowbotham et al. 1991), although the analgesia attained was less than that achieved in a group with nociceptive pain (Jadad et al. 1992). Resolution of this problem has important clinical implications.

To further our understanding of the mechanisms underlying neuropathic pain, several animal models have been developed that replicate some of the symptoms of human neuropathic pain conditions (Bennett and Xie 1988; Seltzer et al. 1990; Kim and Chung 1992). Assessment of the antinociceptive potency and efficacy of morphine in these animal models has often led to contradicting results. It appears that the efficacy of morphine in attenuating allodynia or hyperalgesia in these behavioral studies is largely dependent on the animal model, the measure, and more importantly, the route of administration of the drug. However, no clear pattern emerges. Although many behavioral studies have been conducted on animal models of neuropathic pain, little attention has been paid to the electrophysiological changes that occur in the spinal cord following nerve injury. Such electrophysiological studies would provide an important link between the previously described behavioral data and the neuronal plasticity in the spinal cord following nerve injury.

A recent electrophysiological study assessed and compared the effects of administration of systemic and i.t. morphine on dorsal horn neuronal responses in the selective spinal nerve ligation (SNL) model of nerve injury (Suzuki et al. 1999). In general, the results demonstrated that the i.t. route of morphine administration more effectively inhibited the evoked neuronal responses (electrical, mechanical, and thermal stimuli) of spinal-nerve-ligated rats than did the systemic route. The spinal neurons of spinal-nerve-ligated rats exhibited a reduced sensitivity to systemic morphine as compared to normal and sham-operated rats. The systemic route produced marked side effects (e.g., respiratory depression) in the anesthetized animals, which limited dose escalation. Interestingly, i.t. morphine administration produced a greater inhibitory effect in spinal-nerve-ligated rats as compared to normal or sham-operated rats, which contradicts several previous behavioral studies (Lee et al. 1995; Mao et al. 1995). Thus, current electrophysiological findings and the results of some previous behavioral studies appear to be somewhat discrepant.

The wide-dynamic-range or convergent neurons recorded in the electrophysiological studies are involved in both ascending pathways and reflex circuitries (Schouenborg and Sjolund 1983; see references in Dubner 1997). Many of the behavioral studies assessed changes in withdrawal thresholds as measures of allodynia and morphine efficacy (Lee et al. 1995; Wegert et al. 1997). This method clearly contrasts with electrophysiological approaches that are based on the ability of morphine to produce inhibitions of the overall evoked neuronal responses to electrical, mechanical, or thermal stimuli. It is possible that morphine may not exert an effect on the withdrawal thresholds to mechanical and thermal stimuli, while it still inhibits the suprathreshold firing of spinal neurons. Although reductions in neuronal responses were observed after morphine administration, which most likely represents a reduced sensory response to the stimulus, the level of activity in spinal circuitry may still exceed levels required to elicit a withdrawal reflex.

These route-dependent differences in opioid effectiveness may reflect the locally achieved tissue concentration of morphine. It may be envisaged that i.t. administration produces a higher spinal concentration of morphine compared to that achieved with the systemic route and thus leads to greater spinal opioid-receptor occupancy (Matos et al. 1995). Autoradiographic studies have shown a significant early (2–5 days postoperative) increase in the ipsilateral μ-opioid-receptor binding in the chronic constriction injury (CCI) model of nerve injury, which later declines to control levels (Stevens et al. 1991; Besse et al. 1992). Previous behavioral studies of the SNL model have shown i.t. morphine to be less effective than systemic morphine in reducing mechanical allodynia (Bian et al. 1995; Lee et al. 1995) and thermal hyperalgesia (Wegert et al. 1997). In addition, i.t. morphine is effective but with a decreased efficacy against thermal hyperalgesia in spinal-nerve-ligated rats as compared to sham-operated rats (Ossipov et al. 1995a,b). In the CCI model of nerve injury, studies have shown a reduced sensitivity of thermal hyperalgesia of CCI rats to i.t. morphine, as compared to normal (Yamamoto and Yaksh 1991) and sham-operated rats (Mao et al. 1995). However, systemic morphine was partially effective in reversing allodynia (Hedley et al. 1995; Koch et al. 1996), thermal hyperalgesia (Lee et al. 1994; Backonja et al. 1995; Hedley et al. 1995), and spontaneous pain behavior (Jazat and Guilbaud 1991) in CCI rats. Indeed, one study demonstrated that systemic morphine exerts an augmented analgesic potency in reversing the mechanical allodynia of the nerve-injured paw as compared to the contralateral sham-operated paw (Kayser et al. 1991).

While neuropathic pain has been reported to be resistant to the analgesic effects of morphine (Arnér and Meyerson 1988), it is now generally acknowledged that neuropathic pain is not opioid resistant but exhibits a reduced sensitivity to systemic opioids (Portenoy et al. 1990; Jadad et al. 1992). Evidence now demonstrates that opioids are not totally ineffective in reducing neuronal responses related to symptoms of neuropathic pain. The extent to which morphine can alter these responses appears to be dependent on the route of administration.

The mechanisms underlying the reduced antinociceptive efficacy of morphine are complex and involve various components. There is ample evidence for the localization of μ-opioid receptor mRNA and μ-binding sites in small-diameter DRG and the presence of μ-opioid receptors on C-fiber afferents that terminate in the superficial dorsal horn of the spinal cord together with a smaller proportion of postsynaptic sites (Besse et al. 1990; Mansour et al. 1994). However, evidence for the presence of opioid receptors on large-diameter Aβ afferents is lacking. Hence although morphine exerts presynaptic inhibitory effects on C-fiber-evoked activity, it has minor effects on large-diameter-fiber terminals (see references in Dickenson 1994). Paradoxically, this characteristic is beneficial in non-neuropathic pain states because it allows the preservation of tactile sensitivity, yet it may be responsible for the poor sensitivity of Aβ-fiber-evoked mechanical allodynia in neuropathic pain states. In addition, substantial evidence points to an increased spinal CCK level following peripheral nerve injury, which interferes with the action of opioid drugs (see references in Stanfa et al. 1994; Nichols et al. 1995). Previous studies have shown that the diminished morphine responsiveness of rats with sciatic nerve section and SNL results from increased levels of CCK, which physiologically antagonizes morphine-induced antinociception (Xu et al. 1993; Nichols et al. 1995). A recent study by Xu et al. (1993) also suggests that an increase in spinal CCK (due to novel synthesis of the peptide in primary afferent fibers; Verge et al. 1993) reduces the potency of spinal morphine in a rat model of neuropathic pain. In addition, the authors suggested that an upregulation of CCK may account for the relative opioid insensitivity of neuropathic pain in humans (Xu et al. 1993). This study in neuropathic animals is an example of changes in spinal CCK systems contrary to those suggested in inflammatory models. A sufficiently high local concentration of morphine delivered to the spinal cord by i.t. administration may overcome this physiological antagonism of morphine analgesia. Systemic administration may not achieve the required local spinal concentration of morphine (Matos et al. 1995) in the absence of adverse side effects (such as respiratory depression, sedation, vomiting, and constipation), which can prevent full dose escalation under neuropathic conditions (Portenoy et al. 1990).

The problem of opioid responsiveness in neuropathic pain states may not simply be that of a reduced opioid sensitivity but, rather, the failure to deliver a sufficiently high concentration of the systemic opioid to the spinal cord in the absence of adverse side effects. Trials of the effectiveness of spinal opioids in neuropathic patients may resolve this issue. Spinal opioids may be a useful approach to pain control in neuropathic pain states where systemic routes produce inadequate analgesia. The lack of consensus among the animal studies on the effect of morphine in several different models of neuropathic pain may be due to varying opioid sensitivities of the different types and symptoms of neuropathic pain. The timing of treatment relative to the duration of the neuropathy is another important consideration, and early opioid intervention may prove to be beneficial.

Although findings have been inconsistent. opioids have exhibited reduced effectiveness following peripheral nerve injury. Nociceptin has reversed thermal hyperalgesia in CCI rats, which suggests a possible therapeutic role in treating neuropathic pain states (see Taylor and Dickenson 1998).

CONCLUSIONS

It is apparent how the concomitant activation of other transmitter systems such as the NMDA and CCK can reduce opioid actions and the potential for blocking this interference with the use of antagonists. However, the activation of nonopioid controls can be harnessed to increase opioid analgesia. Reduction of excitability with local anesthetics in the presence of opioids also leads to a marked potentiation (Dickenson 1994). In addition, considerable evidence indicates that the co-administration of drugs acting at the α_2 adrenoceptor with opioid-receptor agonists can produce supra-additive or synergistic effects (Dickenson and Sullivan 1993).

To conclude, the recent advances in our understanding of opioid function and dysfunction and a clearer understanding of the factors that can influence the efficacy of opioids form a basis for improving clinical outcome. Opioids and their receptors are part of the integrated functional pharmacological repertoire of neurons so that alteration in the status of opioid receptors and the activation of other transmitter systems will interact to modulate the function of the CNS. This knowledge can be harnessed through combination therapy, and the clinical use of these drugs can be improved by recognizing the potential of plasticity in opioid actions.

ACKNOWLEDGMENTS

This work in the authors' laboratory was funded by the European Community Biomed II programs BMH4-CT95-0172 and CT97 2317, The Wellcome Trust, and the Medical Research Council. Rie Suzuki has an Overseas Research Scholarship at University College, London.

REFERENCES

Andoh T, Itoh M, Kuraishi Y. Nociception gene expression in rat dorsal root ganglia induced by peripheral inflammation. *Neuroreport* 1997; 8:2793–2796.
Anton B, Fein J, To T, et al. Immunohistochemical localization of ORL-1 in the central nervous system of the rat. *J Comp Neurol* 1996; 368:229–251.

Antonijevic I, Mousa SA, Schäfer M, Stein C. Perineurial defect and peripheral opioid analgesia in inflammation. *J Neurosci* 1995; 15:165–172.

Arnér S, Meyerson BA. Lack of analgesic effect of opioids on neuropathic and idiopathic forms of pain. *Pain* 1988; 33:11–23.

Baber NS, Dourish CT, Hill DR. The role of CCK, caerulein, and CCK antagonists in nociception. *Pain* 1989; 39:307–328.

Backonja M-M, Miletic G, Miletic V. The effect of continuous morphine analgesia on chronic thermal hyperalgesia due to sciatic constriction injury in rats. *Neurosci Lett* 1995; 196:61–64.

Barbaz BS, Hall NR, Liebman JM. Antagonism of morphine analgesia by CCK-8-S does not extend to all assays nor all opiate analgesics. *Peptides* 1989; 9:1295–1300.

Bennett GJ, Xie YK. A peripheral mononeuropathy in the rat that produces disorders of pain sensation like those seen in man *Pain* 1988; 33:87–107.

Besse D, Lombard MC, Zakac JM, Roques BP, Besson JM. Pre- and postsynaptic distribution of mu, delta and kappa opioid receptors in the superficial layers of the cervical dorsal horn of the rat spinal cord. *Brain Res* 1990; 521:15–22.

Besse D, Lombard MC, Perrot S, Besson JM. Regulation of opioid binding sites in the superficial dorsal horn of the rat spinal cord following loose ligation of the sciatic nerve: comparison with sciatic nerve section and lumbar dorsal rhizotomy. *Neuroscience* 1992; 50:921–933.

Besson JM, Chaouch A. Peripheral and spinal mechanisms of nociception. *Physiol Rev* 1987; 67:67–186.

Bian D, Nichols ML, Ossipov MH, Lai J, Porreca F. Characterization of the antiallodynic efficacy of morphine in a model of neuropathic pain in rats. *Neuroreport* 1995; 6:1981–1984.

Carpenter KC, Dickenson AH. Evidence that [Phe1 (CH2-NH)Gly2] nociceptin (1–13), a peripheral ORL-1 receptor antagonist, acts as an agonist in the rat spinal cord. *Br J Pharm* 1998; 125:949–951.

Cervero F, Schaible HG, Schmidt RF. Tonic descending inhibition of spinal cord neurones driven by joint afferents in normal cats and in cats with an inflamed knee joint. *Exp Brain Res* 1991; 83:675–678.

Chapman V, Dickenson AH. The combination of NMDA antagonism and morphine produces profound antinociception in the rat dorsal horn. *Brain Res* 1992; 573:321–323.

Chen Y, Mestek A, Liu J, Hurley JA, Yu L. Molecular cloning and functional expression of a μ-opioid receptor from rat brain. *Mol Pharm* 1993; 44:8–12.

Connor M, Yeo A, Henderson G. The effect of nociceptin on Ca^{2+} channel current and intracellular Ca^{2+} in the SH-SY5Y human neuroblastoma cell line. *Br J Pharmacol* 1996; 118:205–207.

Crain SM, Shen KF. Opioids can evoke direct receptor mediated excitatory effects on sensory neurones. *Trends Pharmacol Sci* 1990; 11:77–81.

Dartland T, Heinricher MM, Grandy DK. Orphanin FQ/nociceptin: a role in pain and analgesia, but so much more. *Trends Neurosci* 1998; 21:215–221.

Dickenson AH. A cure for wind-up: NMDA receptor antagonists as potential analgesics. *Trends Pharm Sci* 1990; 11:307–330.

Dickenson AH. Where and how do opioids act? In: Gebhart GF, Hammond DL, Jensen TS (Eds). *Proceedings of the 7th World Congress on Pain*, Progress in Pain Research and Management, Vol. 2. Seattle: IASP Press, 1994, pp 525–552.

Dickenson AH. Mechanisms of central hypersensitivity: excitatory amino acid mechanisms and their control. In: Dickenson AH, Besson JM (Eds). *The Pharmacology of Pain*, Handbook of Experimental Pharmacology, Vol. 130. Berlin: Springer-Verlag, 1997, pp 167–210.

Dickenson AH, Sullivan AF. Electrophysiological studies on the effects of the effects of intrathecal morphine on nociceptive neurones in the rat dorsal horn. *Pain* 1986; 24:211–222.

Dickenson AH, Sullivan AF. Combination therapy in analgesia; seeking synergy. *Curr Opin Anaesthesiol* 1993; 6:861–865.

Dickenson AH, Sullivan AF, Knox RJ, Zajac Z, Roques BP. Opioid receptor types in the rat spinal cord: electrophysiological studies with μ and δ opioid receptor agonists in the control of nociception. *Brain Res* 1987; 413:649–652.

Dickenson AH, Sullivan AF, McQuay HJ. Intrathecal etorphine, fentanyl and buprenorphine on spinal nociceptive neurones in the rat. *Pain* 1990; 42:227–234.

Dourish CT, O'Neill MF, Coughlan J, et al. The selective CCK-B receptor antagonist L-365,260 enhances morphine analgesia and prevents morphine tolerance in the rat. *Eur J Pharmacol* 1990; 176:35–44.

Dubner R. Neural basis of persistent pain: sensory specialization, sensory modulation, and neuronal plasticity. In: Jensen TS, Turner JA, Wiesenfeld-Hallin Z (Eds). *Proceedings of the 8th World Congress on Pain,* Progress in Pain Research and Management, Vol. 8. Seattle: IASP Press, 1997, pp 243–257.

Dubner R, Ruda MA. Activity dependent neuronal plasticity following tissue injury and inflammation. *Trends Neurosci* 1992; 15:96–103.

Duggan AW, North RA. Electrophysiology of opioids. *Pharmacol Rev* 1984; 35:219–281.

Evans CJ, Keith DE, Morrisson H, Magendzo K, Edwards RH. Cloning of a delta receptor by functional expression. *Science* 1992; 258:1952–1955.

Faris PL, Komisaruk BR, Watkins LR, Mayer DJ. Evidence for the neuropeptide cholecystokinin as an antagonist of opiate analgesia. *Science* 1983; 219:310–312.

Fields HL, Rowbotham MC. Multiple mechanisms of neuropathic pain: a clinical perspective. In: Gebhart GF, Hammond DL, Jensen TS (Eds). *Proceedings of the 7th World Congress on Pain,* Progress in Pain Research and Management, Vol. 2. Seattle: IASP Press, 1994, pp 437–454.

Fleetwood-Walker SM, Mitchell R, Hope PJ, Molony V, Iggo A. An α2 receptor mediates the selective inhibition by noradrenaline of nociceptive responses of identified dorsal horn neurones. *Brain Res* 1985; 334:243–254.

Ghilardi JR, Allen CJ, Vigna SR, McVey DC, Mantyh PW. Trigeminal and dorsal root ganglion neurons express CCK receptor binding sites in the rat, rabbit, and monkey: possible site of opiate-CCK analgesic interactions. *J Neurosci* 1992; 12:4854–4866.

Green M, Lyons L, Dickenson AH. α2 adrenoceptor antagonists enhance responses of dorsal horn neurones to formalin induced inflammation. *Eur J Pharmacol* 1998; 347:201–204.

Guerrini R, Calo G, Rizzi A, et al. A new selective antagonist of the nociceptin receptor. *Br J Pharmacol* 1998; 123:163–165.

Headley PM, Duggan AW, Griersmith BT. Selective reduction by noradrenaline and 5-hydroxytryptamine of nociceptive responses of cat dorsal horn neurones. *Brain Res* 1978; 145:185–189.

Hedley LR, Martin B, Waterbury LD, Clarke DE, Hunter JC. A comparison of the action of mexiletine and morphine in rodent models of acute and chronic pain. *Proc West Pharmacol Soc* 1995; 38:103–104.

Helyes Z, Nemeth J, Pinter E, Szolcsanyi L. Inhibition by nociceptin of neurogenic inflammation and release of SP and CGRP from sensory nerve terminals. *Br J Pharmacol* 1997; 121:613–661.

Henderson G, McKnight AT. The orphan opioid receptor and its endogenous ligand—nociceptin/orphanin FQ. *Trends Pharmacol Sci* 1997; 18:293–300.

Hill DR, Woodruff GN. Differentiation of central cholecystokinin receptor binding sites using the non-peptide antagonists MK-329 and L-365,260. *Brain Res* 1990; 526:276–283.

Hirota N, Kuraishi Y, Hino Y, Satoh M, Takagi H. Met-enkephalin and morphine but not dynorphin inhibit noxious stimuli induced release of substance P from rabbit dorsal horn in situ. *Neuropharmacology* 1985; 24:567–570.

Hori Y, Endo K, Takahashi T. Presynaptic inhibitory action of enkephalin on excitatory transmission in superficial dorsal horn of rat spinal cord. *J Physiol* 1992; 450:673–685.

Hughes J, Smith TW, Kosterlitz HW, et al. Identification of two related pentapeptides from the brain with potent opiate agonist activity. *Nature* 1975; 258:577–579.

Hylden JLK, Wilcox GL. Pharmacological characterization of substance P induced nociception in mice: modulation by opioid and noradrenergic agonists at the spinal level. *J Pharmacol Exp Ther* 1983; 226:398–404.

Hylden JLK, Thomas DA, Iadorola MJ, Nahin RL, Dubner R. Spinal opioid analgesic effects are enhanced in a model of unilateral inflammation/hyperalgesia: possible involvement of noradrenergic mechanisms. *Eur J Pharm* 1991; 194:135–143.

Inoue M, Kobayashi M, Kozaki S, Zimmer A, Ueda H. Nociceptin/orphanin FQ-induced nociceptive responses through substance P release from peripheral nerve endings in mice. *Proc Natl Acad Sci USA* 1998; 95:10949–10953.

Jadad AR, Carroll D, Glynn CJ, Moore RA, McQuay HJ. Morphine responsiveness of chronic pain: double-blind randomized crossover study with patient-controlled analgesia. *Lancet* 1992; 339:1367–1371.

Jazat F, Guilbaud G. The 'tonic' pain-related behaviour seen in mononeuropathic rats is modulated by morphine and naloxone. *Pain* 1991; 44:97–102.

Jia YP, Linden D, Serie J, Seybold V. Nociceptin/orphanin FQ binding increases in superficial laminae of the rat spinal cord during persistent peripheral inflammation. *Neurosci Lett* 1998; 250:21–24.

Jiang QAE, Takemori AE, Sultana M, et al. Differential antagonism of opioid delta antinociception by [D-Ala2, Leu5, Cys6] enkephalin and naltrindole 5'-isothiocyanate: evidence for delta receptor subtypes. *J Pharmacol Exp Ther* 1991; 257:1069–1077.

Joris J, Costello A, Dubner R, Hargreaves KM. Opiates suppress carrageenan-induced edema and hyperthermia at doses that inhibit hyperalgesia. *Pain* 1990; 43:95–103.

Kalso EA, Sullivan AF, McQuay HJ, Dickenson AH, Roques BP. Cross-tolerance between mu opioid and alpha-2 adrenergic receptors, but not between mu and delta opioid receptors in the spinal cord of the rat. *J Pharmacol Exp Ther* 1993; 265:551–558.

Kangra I, Randic M. Outflow of endogenous aspartate and glutamate from the rat spinal dorsal horn in vitro by activation of low- and high-threshold primary afferent fibres. Modulation by μ opioids. *Brain Res* 1991; 553:347–352.

Kayser V, Guilbaud G. The analgesic effects of morphine, but not those of the enkephalinase inhibitor thiorphan, are enhanced in arthritic rats. *Brain Res* 1983; 267:131–138.

Kayser V, Chen YL, Guilbaud G. Behavioural evidence for a peripheral component in the enhanced antinociceptive effect of a low dose of systemic morphine in carrageenin-induced hyperalgesic rats. *Brain Res* 1991; 560:237–244.

Kayser V, Lee SH, Guilbaud G. Evidence for a peripheral component in the enhanced antinociceptive effect of a low dose of systemic morphine in rats with peripheral mononeuropathy. *Neuroscience* 1995; 64:537–545.

Kieffer BL. Molecular aspect of opioid receptors. In: Dickenson AH, Besson JM (Eds). *The Pharmacology of Pain,* Handbook of Experimental Pharmacology, Vol. 130. Berlin: Springer-Verlag, 1997, pp 281–304.

Kieffer BL, Befort C, Gavieraux C, Hirth CG. The δ-opioid receptor: isolation of a cDNA by expression cloning and pharmacological characterization. *Proc Natl Acad Sci USA* 1992; 89:12048–12052.

Kim SH, Chung JM. An experimental model for peripheral neuropathy produced by segmental spinal nerve ligation in the rat. *Pain* 1992; 50:355–363.

Knox RJ, Dickenson AH. Effects of selective and non-selective κ opioid agonists on cutaneous C-fibre evoked responses of rat dorsal horn neurones. *Brain Res* 1987; 415:21–29.

Koch BD, Faurot GF, McGuirk JR Clarke DE, Hunter JC. Modulation of mechano-hyperalgesia by clinically effective analgesics in rats with a peripheral mononeuropathy. *Analgesia* 1996; 2:157–164.

Kosterlitz HW. Opioid peptides and their receptors. *Proc R Soc Lond B Biol Sci* 1985; 225:27–40.

Lee SH, Kayser V, Desmeules J, Guilbaud G. Differential action of morphine and various opioid agonists on thermal allodynia and hyperalgesia in mononeuropathic rats. *Pain* 1994; 57:233–240.

Lee Y-W, Chaplan SR, Yaksh T L. Systemic and supraspinal, but not spinal, opiates suppress allodynia in a rat neuropathic pain model. *Neurosci Lett* 1995; 186:111–114.

Lombard MC, Besson JM. Attempts to gauge the relative importance of pre-and postsynaptic effects of morphine on the transmission of noxious messages in the dorsal horn of the rat spinal cord. *Pain* 1989; 37:335–346.

Loomis CW, Milne B, Cervenko FW. A study of the interaction between clonidine and morphine on analgesia and blood pressure during continuous intrathecal infusion in the rat. *Neuropharmacology* 1988; 27:191–199.

Magnuson DSK, Dickenson AH. Lamina-specific effects of morphine and naloxone in dorsal horn of rat spinal cord in vitro. *J Neurophysiol* 1991; 66:1941–1950.

Magnuson DSK, Sullivan AF, Simmonet G, Roques BP, Dickenson AH. Differential interactions of cholecystokinin and FLFQPQRFamide with μ and δ opioid antinociception in rat spinal cord. *Neuropeptides* 1990; 16:213–218.

Mansour A, Fox CA, Thompson RC, Akil H, Watson SJ. Mu-opioid receptor mRNA expression in the rat CNS: comparison to mu-receptor binding. *Brain Res* 1994; 643:245–265.

Mao J, Price DD, Mayer DJ. Experimental mononeuropathy reduces the antinociceptive effects of morphine: implications for common intracellular mechanisms involved in morphine tolerance and neuropathic pain. *Pain* 1995; 61:353–364.

Matos FF, Rollema H, Taiwo YO, Levine JD, Basbaum AI. Relationship between analgesia and extracellular morphine in brain and spinal cord in awake rats. *Brain Res* 1995; 693:187–195.

McMahon SB, Lewin GR, Wall PD. Central excitability triggered by noxious inputs. *Curr Opin Neurobiol* 1993; 3:602–610.

McQuay HJ, Sullivan AF, Smallman K, Dickenson AH. Intrathecal opioids, potency and lipophilicity. *Pain* 1989; 36:111–115.

Meunier J-C, Mollereau C, Toll L, et al. Isolation and structure of the endogenous agonist of opioid receptor-like ORL1 receptor. *Nature* 1995; 377:532–535.

Millan MJ, Czlonkowski A, Pilcher CWT, et al. A model of chronic pain in the rat: functional correlates of alterations in the activity of opioid systems. *J Neurosci* 1987; 7:77–87.

Mogil JS, Grisel JE. Transgenic studies of pain. *Pain* 1998; 77:107–128.

Neil A, Kayser V, Gacel G, Besson J-M, Guilbaud G. Opioid receptor types and antinociceptive activity in chronic inflammation: both κ- and μ-opiate agonists are enhanced in arthritic rats. *Eur J Pharmacol* 1986; 130:203–208.

Nichols ML, Bian D, Ossipov MH, Lai J, Porreca F. Regulation of antiallodynic efficacy by CCK in a model of neuropathic pain in rats. *J Pharmacol Exp Ther* 1995; 275:1339–1345.

North RA. Drug receptors and the inhibition of nerve cells. *Br J Pharmacol* 1989; 98:13–28.

Ossipov MH, Harris S, Lloyd P, Messineo E. An isobolographic analysis of the antinociceptive effect of systemically and intrathecally administered combinations of clonidine and opiates. *J Pharmacol Exp Ther* 1990; 255:1107–1116.

Ossipov MH, Kovelowski CJ, Vanderah T, Porreca F. Naltrindole, an opioid δ antagonist, blocks the enhancement of morphine-antinociception induced by a CCKB antagonist in the rat. *Neurosci Lett* 1994; 181:9–12.

Ossipov MH, Lopez Y, Nichols ML, Bian D, Porreca F. The loss of antinociceptive efficacy of spinal morphine in rats with nerve ligation injury is prevented by reducing spinal afferent drive. *Neurosci Lett* 1995a; 199:87–90.

Ossipov MH, Lopez Y, Nichols ML, Bian D, Porreca, F. Inhibition by spinal morphine of the tail-flick response is attenuated in rats with nerve ligation injury. *Neurosci Lett* 1995b; 199:83–86.

Pasternak GW, Wood PJ. Multiple opioid receptors. *Life Sci* 1986; 28:1889–1893.

Peluso J, LaForge KS, Matthes HW, et al. Distribution of nociceptin/orphanin FQ receptor transcript in human central nervous system and immune cells. *J Neuroimmunol* 1998; 81:184–192.

Plummer JL, Cmielewski PL, Gourlay GK, Owen H, Cousins MJ. Antinociceptive and motor effects of intrathecal morphine combined with intrathecal clonidine, noradrenaline, carbachol or midazolam in rats. *Pain* 1992; 49:145–152.

Portenoy RK, Foley KM, Inturrisi CE. The nature of opioid responsiveness and its implications for neuropathic pain: new hypotheses derived from studies of opioid infusions. *Pain* 1990; 43:273–286.

Rahman W, Dashwood M, Fitzgerald MC, et al. Postnatal development of multiple opioid receptors in the spinal cord and the development of spinal morphine analgesia. *Dev Brain Res* 1998; 108:239–254.

Reinscheid RK, Nothacker H-P, Bourson A, et al. Orphanin FQ: a neuropeptide that activates an opioidlike G protein-coupled receptor. *Science* 1995; 270:792–794.

Riedl M, Shuster S, Vulchanova L, et al. Orphanin FQ/nociceptin immunoreactive nerve fibers parallel those containing endogenous opioids in rat spinal cord. *Neuroreport* 1996; 7:1369–1372.

Roques BP, Noble F, Dauge V, Fournie-Zaluski MC, Beaumont A. Neutral endopeptidase 24.11: structure, inhibition and experimental and clinical pharmacology. *Pharmacol Rev* 1993; 45:88–146.

Rowbotham MC, Reisner LM, Fields HL. Both intravenous lidocaine and morphine reduce the pain of post-herpetic neuralgia. *Neurology* 1991; 41:1024–1028.

Schaible HG, Neugebauer V, Cervero F, Schmidt RF. Changes in tonic descending inhibition of spinal neurones with articular input during the development of acute arthritis in the cat. *J Neurophysiol* 1991; 66:1021–1032.

Schouenborg J, Sjolund BH. Activity evoked by A- and C-afferent fibres in rat dorsal horn and its relation to a flexion reflex. *J Neurophysiol* 1983; 50:1108–1121.

Seltzer Z, Dubner R, Shir Y. A novel model of neuropathic pain disorders produced in rats by partial sciatic nerve injury. *Pain* 1990; 43:205–218.

Slaninova J, Knapp RJ, Wu J, et al. Opioid receptor binding properties of analgesic analogues of cholecystokinin octapeptide. *Eur J Pharmacol* 1991; 200:195–198.

Stanfa LC, Dickenson AH. Cholecystokinin as a factor in the enhanced potency of spinal morphine following carrageenan inflammation. *Br J Pharmacol* 1993; 108:967–973.

Stanfa LC, Dickenson AH. Electrophysiological studies on the spinal roles of endogenous opioids in carrageenan inflammation. *Pain* 1994a; 56:185–191.

Stanfa LC, Dickenson AH. Enhanced alpha-2 adrenergic controls and spinal morphine potency in inflammation. *NeuroReport* 1994b; 5:469–472.

Stanfa LC, Sullivan AF, Dickenson AH. Alterations in neuronal excitability and the potency of spinal mu, delta and kappa opioids after carrageenan-induced inflammation. *Pain* 1992; 50:345–354.

Stanfa L, Dickenson AH, Xu X-J, Wiesenfeld-Hallin Z. CCK and morphine analgesia. *Trends Pharmacol Sci* 1994; 15:65–66.

Stanfa LC, Chapman V, Dickenson AH. Inhibitory action of nociceptin on spinal dorsal horn neurones of the rat, in vivo. *Br J Pharmacol* 1996; 118:1875–1877.

Stein C. Interaction of immune-competent cells and nociceptors. In: Gebhart GF, Hammond DL, Jensen TS (Eds) *Proceedings of the 7th World Congress on Pain.* Progress in Pain Research and Management, Vol. 2. Seattle: IASP Press, 1994, pp 285–297.

Stein C, Millan MJ, Yassouridis A, Hertz A. Antinociceptive effects of μ- and κ-agonists in inflammation are enhanced by a peripheral opioid receptor-specific mechanism. *Eur J Pharmacol* 1988; 155:255–264.

Stevens CW, Kajander KC, Bennett GJ, Seybold VS. Bilateral and differential changes in spinal mu, delta and kappa opioid binding in rats with a painful, unilateral neuropathy. *Pain* 1991; 46:315–326.

Sullivan AF, Dashwood MR, Dickenson AH. α2-Adrenoceptor modulation of nociception in rat spinal cord: location, effects and interactions with morphine. *Eur J Pharmacol* 1987; 138:169–177.

Sullivan AF, Kalso EA, McQuay HJ, Dickenson AH. The antinociceptive actions of dexmedetomidine on dorsal horn neuronal responses in the anaesthetized rat. *Eur J Pharmacol* 1992a; 215:127–133.

Sullivan AF, Kalso EA, McQuay HJ, Dickenson AH. Evidence for the involvement of the m but not d opioid receptor subtype in the synergistic interaction between opioid and α2 adrenergic antinociception in the rat spinal cord. *Neurosci Lett* 1992b; 139:65–68.

Suzuki R, Chapman V, Dickenson AH. The effectiveness of spinal and systemic morphine on rat dorsal horn neuronal responses in the spinal nerve ligation model of neuropathic pain. *Pain* 1999; 80:215–228.

Taylor F, Dickenson AH. Nociceptin/orphanin FQ: new opioid, new analgesic? *Neuroreport* 1998; 9:R65–70.

Traynor J. Subtypes of the κ opioid receptor: fact or fiction? *Trends Pharmacol Sci* 1989; 10:52–53.

Uhl GR, Childers S, Pasternak G. An opiate receptor gene family reunion. *Trends Neurosci* 1994; 17:89–93.

Vanderah T, Lai J, Yamamura HI, Porreca F. Antisense oligodeoxynucleotide to the CCKB receptor produces naltrindole- and [Leu5]enkephalin antiserum-sensitive enhancement of morphine antinociception. *Neuroreport* 1994; 5:2601–2605.

Vaughan CW, Christie MJ. Increase by the ORL1 receptor (opioid receptor-like1) ligand, nociceptin, of inwardly rectifying K conductance in dorsal raphe nucleus neurones. *Br J Pharmacol* 1996; 117:1609–1611.

Verge VMK, Wiesenfeld-Hallin Z, Hökfelt T. Cholecystokinin in mammalian primary sensory neurons and spinal cord: in situ hybridization studies in rat and monkey. *Eur J Neurosci* 1993; 5:240–250.

Wang X-J, Han J-S. Modification by cholecystokinin octapeptide of the binding of μ, δ, and κ-opioid receptors. *J Neurochem* 1990; 55:1379–1382.

Wang J, Ren M, Han J. Mobilization of calcium from intracellular stores as one of the mechanisms underlying the antiopioid effect of cholecystokinin octapeptide. *Peptides* 1992; 13:947–951.

Watkins LR, Kinscheck IB, Mayer DJ. Potentiation of opiate analgesia and apparent reversal of morphine tolerance by proglumide. *Science* 1984; 224:395–396.

Wegert S, Ossipov MH, Nichols ML, et al. Differential activities of intrathecal MK-801 or morphine to alter responses to thermal and mechanical stimuli in normal or nerve-injured rats. *Pain* 1997; 71:57–64.

Weil-Fugazza J, Godefroy F, Manceau V, Besson JM. Increased norepinephrin and uric acid levels in the spinal cord of arthritic rats. *Brain Res* 1986; 374:190–194.

Westlund KN. Anatomy of noradrenergic pathways modulating pain. In: Besson JM, Guilbaud G (Eds). *Towards the Use of Noradrenergic Agonists for the Treatment of Pain.* Excerpta Medica. Amsterdam: Elsevier, 1992, pp 91–118.

Wick MJ, Minnerath SR, Lin X, et al. Isolation of a novel cDNA encoding a putative membrane receptor with high homology to the cloned μ, δ and κ opioid receptors. *Mol Brain Res* 1994; 27:37–44.

Wilcox GL, Carlsson K-H, Jochim A, Jurna I. Mutual potentiation of antinociceptive effects of morphine and clonidine on motor and sensory responses in rat spinal cord. *Brain Res* 1987; 405:84–93.

Xu XJ, Puke MJC, Verge VMK, et al. Up-regulation of cholecystokinin in primary sensory neurons is associated with morphine insensitivity in experimental neuropathic pain in the rat. *Neurosci Lett* 1993; 152:129–132.

Yaksh TL. Pharmacology of spinal adrenergic systems which modulate spinal nociceptive processing. *Pharmacol Biochem Behav* 1985; 22:845–858.

Yaksh TL, Nouiehed R. Physiology and pharmacology of spinal opiates. *Ann Rev Pharmacol Toxicol* 1985; 25:433–462.

Yaksh TL, Reddy SVR. Studies in the primate on the analgetic affects associated with intrathecal actions of opiates, α-adrenergic agonists and baclofen. *Anesthesiology* 1981; 54:451–467.

Yamamoto T, Yaksh TL. Spinal pharmacology of thermal hyperesthesia induced by incomplete ligation of sciatic nerve. I. Opioid and nonopioid receptor. *Anesthesiology* 1991; 75:817–826.

Yamamoto, T, Yaksh TL. Studies on the spinal interaction of morphine and the NMDA antagonist MK-801 on the hyperesthesia observed in a rat model of sciatic mononeuropathy. *Neurosci Lett* 1992; 135:67–70.

Zhang X, Bao L, Arvidsson U, Eldes R, Hokfelt T. Localization and regulation of the delta-opioid receptor in dorsal root ganglia and spinal cord of the rat and monkey: evidence for association with the membrane of large dense-core vesicles. *Neuroscience* 1998; 82:1225–1242.

Zhou Y, Sun Y-H, Zhang Z-W, Han JS. Increased release of immunoreactive cholecystokinin octapeptide by morphine and potentiation of m-opioid analgesia by CCKB receptor antagonist L-365,260 in rat spinal cord. *Eur J Pharmacol* 1993; 234:147–154.

Correspondence to: Anthony H. Dickenson, Department of Pharmacology, University College, Gower Street, London WC1E 6BT, United Kingdom. Tel: 44-171-419-3742; Fax: 44-171-380-7298; email: anthony.dickenson@ucl.ac.uk.

Opioid Sensitivity of Chronic Noncancer Pain,
Progress in Pain Research and Management,
Vol. 14, edited by Eija Kalso, Henry J. McQuay,
and Zsuzsanna Wiesenfeld-Hallin, IASP Press,
Seattle, © 1999.

3

Opioid Receptors in the Periphery

Halina Machelska, Waltraud Binder, and Christoph Stein

Department of Anesthesiology and Critical Care Medicine, Benjamin Franklin University Hospital, Free University of Berlin, Berlin, Germany

All types of opioid receptors (μ, δ, and κ) are expressed in primary sensory neurons of animals and humans. These receptors are synthesized in the dorsal root ganglia (DRG) and transported toward the central and peripheral nerve endings. The peripheral axonal transport is upregulated during inflammation. Experimental and clinical studies of the functional significance of these receptors have shown potent analgesic (antinociceptive) effects after the peripheral administration of low, centrally inactive doses of opioid receptor agonists. Endogenous opioid peptides also elicit such effects and are synthesized in immune cells that migrate preferentially to injured sites under pathological conditions. Under environmentally stressful stimuli or in response to exogenous releasing agents (e.g., corticotropin-releasing factor [CRF] and cytokines), these cells secrete opioids. Analgesic effects can result from a decreased excitability of the nerves or from a diminished release of excitatory, pronociceptive neuropeptides. An increasing body of evidence also suggests a role of opioids in the modulation of inflammation. The local administration of small doses of opioids or the use of compounds with limited access to the central nervous system (CNS) can produce potent opioid-receptor-specific anti-inflammatory effects, which can result from an attenuated release of proinflammatory neuropeptides or of cytokines from immune cells. This chapter will summarize the discoveries on peripheral analgesic and anti-inflammatory actions of opioids.

PERIPHERAL OPIOID RECEPTORS

Anatomical (LaMotte et al. 1976; Stein et al. 1990; Hassan et al. 1993; Jeanjean et al. 1995; Ji et al. 1995; Stein et al. 1996; Coggeshall et al. 1997), molecular (Mansour et al. 1995), and electrophysiological studies (Moises et al. 1994) have shown that all three opioid receptors are expressed within sensory neurons. They have been found on cell bodies in the DRG (Ji et al. 1995; Mansour et al. 1995; Zhang et al. 1998) and on central (LaMotte et al. 1976) and peripheral terminals of primary afferent neurons in animals (Stein et al. 1990; Hassan et al. 1993; Coggeshall et al. 1997) and humans (Stein et al. 1996). In line with these results, a recent study found that both the peripheral antinociceptive effects of μ-, δ-, and κ-selective agonists and the immunoreactivity of all three receptors in the DRG were diminished by pretreatment with capsaicin, a selective neurotoxin of primary afferent neurons (Zhou et al. 1998). Saturation and competition experiments indicate that the pharmacological characteristics of these peripheral receptors are similar to those in the brain (Hassan et al. 1993).

Activation of such neuronal opioid receptors results in antinociception. Possible mechanisms include increased potassium and decreased calcium currents in DRG neurons through interactions with G proteins (G_i and/or G_o) (Kanjhan 1995), the inhibition of a tetrodotoxin-resistant sodium current (Gold and Levine 1996), and an attenuation of the excitability of peripheral nociceptive terminals and of the propagation of action potentials (Andreev et al. 1994; Schaible and Schmidt 1996). Similar to their effects at the soma and at central terminals, opioids inhibit the calcium-dependent release of pronociceptive, proinflammatory compounds (e.g., substance P) from peripheral sensory nerve endings (Yaksh 1988; Yonehara et al. 1992).

PERIPHERAL OPIOID RECEPTORS IN INFLAMMATION

Studies using antisera-recognizing unique epitopes of the cloned μ-, δ-, and κ-opioid receptors have shown that peripheral inflammation can influence the expression of opioid receptors in peripheral sensory neurons (Ji et al. 1995; Zhang et al. 1998). Although the levels of opioid receptor mRNAs in the DRG do not vary significantly (Schäfer et al. 1995), changes in the number of opioid receptors have been observed. Thus, while μ receptors are upregulated, δ and κ receptors are downregulated in the DRG (Zhang et al. 1998). This finding suggests that inflammation may cause an increased transport of receptors toward the nerve endings. Indeed, studies show that the axonal transport of opioid receptors in fibers of the sciatic nerve is greatly enhanced under inflammatory conditions (Hassan et al. 1993; Jeanjean et al. 1995). Subsequently, the density of opioid receptors on cutaneous nerve fibers in the inflamed tissue increases, an effect abolished by ligating the sciatic nerve (Hassan et al. 1993). These findings indicate that the enhanced peripherally directed axonal transport leads to receptor upregulation on peripheral nerve terminals.

In addition, pre-existing, but possibly inactive neuronal opioid receptors may be altered by the specific milieu (e.g., low pH) of inflamed tissue, and thus rendered active. Indeed, low pH increases opioid agonist efficacy in vitro by altering the interaction of opioid receptors with G proteins in neuronal membranes (Selley et al. 1993). Furthermore, the ability of opioids to decrease the excitability of primary afferent neurons (via inhibition of adenylyl cyclase and subsequent inhibition of cation currents) is much more pronounced when neuronal cyclic adenosine monophosphate levels are increased, a common scenario in inflammation (Ingram and Williams 1994).

Inflammation also increases the number of peripheral sensory nerve terminals (a process known as "sprouting") (Hassan et al. 1992) and entails a disruption of the perineurium (Antonijevic et al. 1995). Under normal circumstances, tight intercellular contacts at the innermost layer of the perineurium act as a diffusion barrier for substances like peptides that have high molecular weight or are hydrophilic (Olsson 1990). This barrier preserves homeostasis in the endoneurial tissue and continues up to the peripheral endings of afferent somatic and autonomic nerve fibers (Olsson 1990). An exception are noncorpuscular nerve endings, a subgroup of somatic afferents that terminate either within the perineurium or just outside it (Kruger and Halata 1996). Opioid receptors are located not only at the tips but also more proximally along the axon (Frank 1985; Stein et al. 1990, 1996; Hassan et al. 1993). These loci are clearly ensheathed by perineurium (Olsson 1990) and are potential sites of action for opioids. Inflammatory conditions lead to a deficiency of the perineurial barrier and an enhanced permeability of endoneurial capillaries (Olsson 1990). Recent studies have shown that peripheral opioid analgesia and perineurial disruption coincide during the earliest stages of an inflammatory reaction and that both can be induced by increasing the osmolarity in normal subcutaneous tissue (Antonijevic et al. 1995). Moreover, disruption of the perineurium, which can be caused by inflammation or artificially induced by the extraneural application of hyperosmolar solutions, greatly facilitates the passage of opioid peptides and other macromolecules to sensory neurons (Antonijevic et al. 1995). These observations indicate an unrestricted transperineurial passage of peptides in inflammation, which is integral for the direct interaction of opioids with sensory nerves.

It has been suggested that opioid receptors are also located on sympathetic postganglionic neuron terminals (Wüster et al. 1981; Berzetei et al. 1987, 1988) and that they may contribute to peripheral opioid antinociception in bradykinin hyperalgesia (Taiwo and Levine 1991). However, some reports argue against the involvement of sympathetic neurons in the latter model (Koltzenburg and Reeh 1992; Schuligoi et al. 1994). Also, studies attempting the direct demonstration of opioid receptor mRNA in sympathetic ganglia have produced negative results (Schäfer et al. 1994). Moreover, chemical sympathectomy with 6-hydroxydopamine does not change the expression of opioid receptors in DRG or the peripheral antinociceptive effects of μ-, δ-, and κ-opioid agonists in Freund's adjuvant-induced inflammation (Zhou et al. 1998).

Finally, opioid-binding sites and the expression of opioid receptor transcripts have been demonstrated in immune cells (Hassan et al. 1993; Sharp et al. 1998). Opioid-mediated modulation of the proliferation of these cells and several of their functions (e.g., chemotaxis, superoxide and cytokine production, and mast cell degranulation) has been reported (Bryant and Holaday 1993; Panerai and Sacerdote 1997). These immunomodulatory actions can be stimulatory or inhibitory (Heijnen et al. 1991; Panerai and Sacerdote 1997) and have been ascribed to the activation of opioid receptors (Sharp et al. 1998). However, the significance of those effects for nociception has not yet been investigated.

PERIPHERAL EXOGENOUS OPIOID ANALGESIA

Activation of opioid receptors on peripheral sensory nerve endings results in potent analgesia. These effects have been observed under pathological conditions such as neuropathic pain (Kayser et al. 1995), colorectal distention (Burton and Gebhart 1998), bone damage (Houghton et al. 1998), and inflammation (by Freund's adjuvant, formalin, carrageenan, prostaglandin, or from neurogenic causes) of subcutaneous tissue, viscera, or joints (reviewed in Barber and Gottschlich 1992, 1997; Stein 1993). Opioid-mediated peripheral analgesia is greatly enhanced in inflammation, perhaps due to the mechanisms discussed above (see "Peripheral opioid receptors in inflammation"). In addition, a decreased functional activity of the endogenous anti-opioid peptide cholecystokinin (CCK) might play a role. CCK mRNA, CCK peptide, and CCK receptors have been found in the DRG (references in Schäfer et al. 1998). Intraplantar application of CCK dose-dependently inhibits peripheral μ-opioid analgesia. This effect seems to be mediated by CCK_B receptors and protein kinase C. However, endogenous CCK is probably not tonically active (Schäfer et al. 1998).

Central effects typically associated with opioids, such as tolerance, dependence, and respiratory depression, can be avoided by the peripheral application of small, systemically inactive doses of agents (Stein 1993). One strategy to improve the side-effect profile of opioid analgesics is to restrict their access to the CNS. One method is the incorporation of highly polar hydrophilic substituents (Barber and Gottschlich 1992; Giardina et al. 1995). However, this leads to a reduction of the biological activity of such compounds (Barber and Gottschlich 1992). Another strategy is to introduce one or more moderately hydrophilic groups (Giardina et al. 1995). Recently, a new approach based on the inclusion of both hydrophilic and hydrophobic portions in molecules preserved both peripheral selectivity and high potency at opioid receptors (Barber and Gottschlich 1997). Potent peripheral analgesic effects of such compounds have been widely described (for review see Giardina et al. 1995; Barber and Gottschlich 1997).

Rigorous criteria such as reversibility by opioid-receptor antagonists (e.g., naloxone), dose-dependency, and stereospecificity have been applied to demonstrate the opioid-receptor specificity of these peripheral effects. The comparison of agonists with differing affinities for the three types of opioid receptors has shown that ligands with a preference for μ receptors are generally most potent, but δ and κ ligands are active as well. Considering the different characteristics of the various models, it is conceivable that, depending on the nature and stage of the inflammatory reaction, different types of opioid receptors may become active (Barber and Gottschlich 1992; Stein 1993).

Peripheral opioid actions on nociceptors are of clinical relevance. Opioid receptors have been identified in peripheral nerve terminals in human synovia (Stein et al. 1996), and intra-articular morphine produces naloxone-reversible analgesia in humans (Stein et al. 1991). A sizable body of clinical literature has now confirmed the analgesic efficacy of exogenous opioids outside the CNS (reviewed in Stein et al. 1997; see also Chapter 20 of this volume).

PERIPHERAL ENDOGENOUS OPIOID ANALGESIA

Potent peripheral analgesia can also be induced by the interaction of peripheral opioid receptors with opioid peptides released from immune cells under inflammatory conditions (Stein 1995). A study using a rat model of unilateral localized paw inflammation found mRNAs encoding proopiomelanocortin (POMC) and proenkephalin (PENK) and the respective opioid peptide products β-endorphin (END) and enkephalin (ENK) within T and B lymphocytes, monocytes, and macrophages (Stein et al. 1990, 1996; Przewlocki et al. 1992; Cabot et al. 1997). Small amounts of dynorphin (DYN) are also detectable by immunocytochemistry (Hassan et al. 1992). Opioids derived from the adrenals and the pituitary have been excluded as sources for opioid ligands at peripheral receptors (Parsons et al. 1990).

Recent studies indicate that END-producing lymphocytes migrate to inflamed tissue, where they secrete the opioid to inhibit pain. Then, depleted of the peptide, they travel to the regional lymph nodes (Cabot et al. 1997). This migratory pattern is reminiscent of memory-type T cells. The trafficking of these cells is not random; such lymphocytes are specifically directed to sites of antigenic or microbial invasion (e.g., inflammatory lesions of the skin) (Butcher and Picker 1996). Consistent with this notion, END was indeed found mostly in memory-type T cells (Cabot et al. 1997). These findings suggest that local signals not only stimulate the synthesis of opioid peptides in resident inflammatory cells, but also attract opioid-containing cells from the circulation to the site of tissue injury to reduce pain.

What are the mechanisms underlying the migration of opioid-containing immunocytes to inflamed tissue? Studies during the last 10 years have revealed that extravasation of immune cells is a multistep process involving the sequential activation of various adhesion molecules on immune cells and the vascular endothelium. Initially, circulating leukocytes are captured and roll on the endothelium of vessels, a process mediated by selectins on leukocytes (L-selectin) and endothelial cells (P- and E-selectin) and by their carbohydrate ligands. The rolling leukocytes can then be activated by chemoattractants. This process leads to upregulation and increased avidity of integrins, which mediate the firm adhesion of leukocytes to endothelial cells by binding to immunoglobulin ligands. Finally, the leukocytes transmigrate through the endothelial wall and are directed to the sites of inflammation. Interruption of the leukocyte–endothelial cell cascade (e.g., by monoclonal antibodies against adhesion molecules or by blocking agents like polysaccharides) blocks immune cell extravasation (Springer 1994; Butcher and Picker 1996). Recent studies have shown that this treatment can influence endogenous pain control in inflammation. Pretreatment of rats with a selectin blocker, fucoidin (Ley et al. 1993), abolishes peripheral opioid analgesia (Machelska et al. 1998) by preventing the infiltration of END-containing immunocytes and the consequent decrease of the END content in the inflamed tissue (Machelska et al. 1998). These findings indicate that the immune system uses mechanisms of cell migration not only to fight pathogens but also to control pain within injured tissue. Thus, pain may be exacerbated by measures inhibiting the immigration of opioid-producing cells, or conversely, analgesia may be conveyed by adhesive interactions that recruit those cells to injured tissue.

Once immune cells reach the site of inflammation, they must secrete opioids to produce pain relief. Endogenous opioid peptides are released by different kinds of stress. Forcing rats to swim in cold water selectively produces potent analgesia in tissue inflamed with Freund's adjuvant (reviewed in Stein 1995). CRF and cytokine receptors are present and upregulated on immune cells within inflamed tissue. The local application of small, systemically inactive doses of CRF, interleukin-1 (IL-1), and other cytokines produces potent antinociceptive effects in inflamed, but not in noninflamed tissue (reviewed in Schäfer et al. 1997). Both stress- and CRF-induced peripheral analgesia are blocked by opioid-receptor antagonists, by antibodies against opioid peptides, by immunosuppression, and by blocking the selectin-mediated extravasation of opioid-containing immune cells (Stein et al. 1990; Przewlocki et al. 1992; Schäfer et al. 1997; Machelska et al. 1998). Furthermore, CRF and IL-1 can release END from immune cell suspensions prepared from lymph nodes in vitro (Cabot et al. 1997; Schäfer et al. 1997). This release is specific to CRF and IL-1 receptors, is calcium dependent, and is mimicked by elevated extracellular concentrations of potassium. This process is consistent with a regulated pathway of release from secretory vesicles, as in neurons and endocrine cells (Cabot et al. 1997). In summary, these findings indicate that CRF and cytokines can cause secretion of opioids from immune cells, which subsequently activate opioid receptors on sensory nerves to inhibit pain. The most important endogenous secretagogue appears to be locally produced CRF, since endogenous analgesia is abolished when the synthesis of CRF is inhibited by antisense oligodeoxynucleotides or when CRF antagonists are administered locally (Schäfer et al. 1996).

The clinical relevance of endogenous opioids mediating peripheral analgesia is evident in patients undergoing knee surgery. Blocking of intra-articular opioid receptors by local administration of the opioid antagonist naloxone resulted in significantly increased postoperative pain (Stein et al. 1993). This finding implies that in a stressful (e.g., postoperative) situation, opioids are tonically released from inflamed tissue and activate peripheral opioid receptors to attenuate pain. Importantly, these endogenous opioids do not interfere with exogenous morphine, i.e., intra-articular morphine is an equally potent analgesic in patients with and without opioid-producing inflammatory synovial cells (Stein et al. 1996). Thus, in contrast to the rapid development of opioid tolerance in the CNS, immune-cell-derived opioids do not seem to produce cross-tolerance to morphine at peripheral opioid receptors.

PERIPHERAL ANTI-INFLAMMATORY EFFECTS OF OPIOIDS

Evidence is conclusive that opioid agonists are able to modulate the inflammatory response, although controversy still exists regarding the receptor types involved. Russell and colleagues (1985) have shown that the κ-opioid agonists U50,488H and trifluadom can inhibit carrageenan-induced paw swelling in the rat, and Gyires et al. (1985) observed the same effect with morphine. Moreover, the effects of morphine were dose-dependent (ED_{50} = 1.6 mg/kg) and partially antagonized by naloxone. Morphine also significantly reduces the neurogenic edema response to saphenous nerve stimulation, an effect that is antagonized by naloxone, and reduces the plasma extravasation induced in the knee joint by capsaicin (Green and Levine 1992). This plasma extravasation is also attenuated by specific δ and κ agonists (Green and Levine 1992). In addition, opioid peptides such as dynorphin A and hemorphin-7 have also been shown to modulate inflammation (Wie et al. 1998; Sanderson et al. 1998).

In the formalin-induced extravasation model, opioids administered directly into the inflamed site can have either pro- or anti-inflammatory effects (Hong and Abbott 1995). In this model, μ and δ agonists attenuated plasma extravasation in both the early and late phases after formalin, while κ agonists enhanced extravasation, but only in the early phase. All these effects were blocked by a peripherally selective opioid antagonist (Hong and Abbott 1995). This study also found that the δ agonist [D-Pen^2,D-Pen^5]enkephalin (DPDPE) inhibited plasma extravasation in formalin-induced inflammation, while few peripheral effects at δ receptors had been reported previously.

In the adjuvant arthritis model, naloxone inhibited the contralateral spread of inflammation when administered at high doses, an effect attributed to an agonist action (Millan and Colpaert 1991). Most studies indicate that opioid agonists rather than antagonists attenuate experimental arthritis. Kappa-opioid agonists appear to be the most successful; they attenuate the severity of adjuvant arthritis in a dose-dependent, stereoselective, and antagonist-reversible manner (Wilson et al. 1996; Binder and Walker 1998). High doses of morphine are also able to attenuate arthritis in animals (Levine et al. 1985; Walker et al. 1996).

The κ-opioid agonist U50,488H has a greater anti-inflammatory effect when administered locally rather than centrally in adjuvant arthritis. When administered directly into an inflamed paw, at a dose that produces no systemic effects, it has potent anti-inflammatory action; to achieve the same result with systemic administration requires at least four times the dosage, with concomitant systemic effects (Wilson et al. 1996). This indicates that

U50,488H produces its anti-inflammatory effects in the periphery, a hypothesis confirmed by use of the peripherally selective κ agonist asimadoline (EMD61,753). This agonist includes hydrophilic and hydrophobic groups and has very limited ability to cross the blood–brain barrier. It inhibits the plasma extravasation evoked by electrical stimulation of the saphenous nerve, an anti-inflammatory action that is reversible by the local administration of the κ antagonist nor-binaltorphimine (Barber et al. 1994). Importantly, asimadoline is a potent anti-inflammatory and antiarthritic compound that reduces the severity of adjuvant arthritis in rats by up to 80%. These effects are dose-dependent and reversible by specific opioid antagonists (Binder et al. 1998).

Although the mechanisms by which opioids act to inhibit inflammation are still a matter of speculation, both neuronal and immune mechanisms have been implicated (for review see Walker et al. 1997). Indeed, the close spatial and functional association between nerves and immune cells is indicative of a neuronal–immune system interaction (Schaible and Grubb 1993).

Synovial joints are extensively innervated by afferent fibers that show immunoreactivity for neuropeptides, such as substance P (SP) and calcitonin gene-related peptide (CGRP) (Ahmed et al. 1994). Furthermore, substantial evidence suggests that the nervous system may facilitate the bilateral spread of such inflammatory diseases as arthritis (Levine et al. 1985). Joints that have previously been denervated, either by hemiplegia, poliomyelitis (Glick 1967), or experimental administration of the neurotoxin capsaicin (Inman et al. 1989), do not develop arthritic disease. Distal joints such as the hands and feet, which are the most common sites of rheumatoid arthritis (Levine et al. 1985), are more densely innervated by sensory nerves that show immunoreactivity for neuropeptides such as SP and CGRP (Ahmed et al. 1994; Schaible and Grubb 1993). SP and CGRP are also found at higher levels in DRG that innervate distal joints than in those which innervate proximal joints (Smith et al. 1993). These observations suggest that neuropeptides and the nervous system play an important role in inflammation.

Opioids can regulate the release of neurotransmitters such as acetylcholine, noradrenaline, dopamine, and SP in the central and peripheral nervous systems (for review, see Sarne et al. 1996). The actions of opioids on SP release are especially relevant in inflammation (Hökfelt et al. 1980; Schaible and Grubb 1993). The latter neuropeptide, released from the peripheral terminals of primary afferent neurons, generates peripheral signs of inflammation, especially increased vascular permeability (Heller et al. 1994). Its release may be inhibited by opioids (Jessell and Iverson 1977; Yaksh 1988), although the proposed mechanisms are complex (for review, see Walker et al. 1997). High doses of the κ-opioid agonist U50,488H inhibited SP release while low doses facilitated its release; conversely, low doses of morphine inhibited but high doses enhanced SP release (Suarez-Roca and Maixner 1993).

Immune mechanisms are also likely to be involved in the anti-inflammatory effects of opioids; in particular, opioid receptors are located on immune cells and have similar characteristics to those found on neurons (Bidlack et al. 1992, Walker et al. 1997). For example, in vivo and in vitro exposure to morphine results in variable immunomodulatory actions such as increased production of the cytokine IL-6, and suppression of T-lymphocyte function (Thomas et al. 1995). Opioid peptides may relieve inflammation by inhibiting either the release or synthesis of cytokines from immune cells (Bryant et al. 1993). Because immuno-hyperactivity might be an important aspect of arthritis, opioid modulation of the immune system could be an important component of the attenuation of inflammation by these drugs. The role of the nervous system (particularly opioid transmitters) and its interaction with the immune system in the development and maintenance of inflammation is thus of great potential significance in inflammatory diseases. Peripherally selective opioids that are able to modulate both these systems may therefore be a promising novel drug therapy.

CONCLUSIONS

Many experimental and clinical trials have demonstrated the analgesic and anti-inflammatory efficacy of small, systemically inactive doses of exogenous opioids, administered in the vicinity of peripheral nerve terminals. Opioid receptors are present on those terminals, and endogenous opioid peptides are detectable in inflamed tissue in animals and humans. Opioid peptides, found in the cells of the immune system, produce endogenous inhibition of pain. The effects of opioids on the release or actions of proinflammatory neuropeptides and cytokines from immune cells can account for their peripheral anti-inflammatory effects. The local application of systemically inactive doses of opioids or compounds with limited access to the CNS provides a new perspective for pain management by producing analgesia or anti-inflammatory effects without central side effects such as dysphoria, respiratory depression, sedation, or addiction. The prominence of local opioid actions in inflamed tissue is an advantage, considering that most subacute or chronic painful conditions are associated with inflammation (e.g., postoperative pain, cancer pain, and arthritis). In addition to their immunological functions, immunocytes are involved in intrinsic pain inhibition. This role provides new insights into pain associated with a compromised immune system, as in AIDS and cancer. Furthermore, the activation of opioid production and release from immune cells may be a novel approach to the development of peripherally acting analgesics.

REFERENCES

Ahmed M, Bjurholm A, Srinivasan GR, Theodorsson E, Kreicbergs A. Extraction of neuropeptides from joint tissue for quantification by radioimmunoassay: a study in the rat. *Peptides* 1994; 15:317–322.

Andreev N, Urban L, Dray A. Opioids suppress spontaneous activity of polymodal nociceptors in rat paw skin induced by ultraviolet irradiation. *Neuroscience* 1994; 58:793–798.

Antonijevic I, Mousa SA, Schäfer M, Stein C. Perineural defect and peripheral opioid analgesia in inflammation. *Neuroscience* 1995; 15:165–172.

Barber A, Gottschlich R. Opioid agonists and antagonists: an evaluation of their peripheral actions in inflammation. *Med Res Rev* 1992; 12:525–562.

Barber A, Gottschlich R. Central and peripheral nervous system: novel developments with selective, non-peptidic kappa-opioid receptor agonists. *Expert Opin Invest Drugs* 1997; 6:1351–1368.

Barber A, Bartoszyk GD, Bender HM, et al. A pharmacological profile of the novel, peripherally-selective kappa-opioid receptor agonist, EMD 61753. *Br J Pharmacol* 1994; 113:1317–1327.

Berzetei PI, Yamamura HI, Duckles SP. Characterization of rabbit ear artery opioid receptors using a δ-selective agonist and antagonist. *Eur J Pharmacol* 1987; 139:61–66.

Berzetei PI, Fong A, Yamamura HI, Duckles SP. Characterization of kappa opioid receptors in the rabbit ear artery. *Eur J Pharmacol* 1988; 151:449–455.

Bidlack JM, Saripalli LD, Lawrence DM. Kappa-opioid binding sites on a murine lymphoma cell line. *Eur J Pharmacol* 1992; 227:257–265.

Binder W, Walker JS. The peripherally selective kappa-opioid agonist, asimadoline, attenuates adjuvant arthritis. *Br J Pharmacol* 1998; 124:647–654.

Bryant HU, Holaday JW. Opioids in immunologic processes. In: Herz A (Ed). *Handbook of Experimental Pharmacology: Opioids II*. Berlin: Springer-Verlag, 1993, pp 361–392.

Burton MB, Gebhart GF. Effects of kappa-opioid receptor agonists on responses to colorectal distension in rats with and without acute colonic inflammation. *J Pharmacol Exp Ther* 1998; 285:707–715.

Butcher EC, Picker LJ. Lymphocyte homing homeostasis. *Science* 1996; 272:60–66.

Cabot PJ, Carter L, Gaiddon C, et al. Immune cell-derived beta-endorphin: production, release, and control of inflammatory pain in rats. *J Clin Invest* 1997; 100:142–148.

Coggeshall RE, Zhou S, Carlton SM. Opioid receptors on peripheral sensory axons. *Brain Res* 1997; 764:126–132.

Frank GB. Stereospecific opioid receptors on excitable cell membranes. *Can J Physiol Pharmacol* 1985; 63:1023–1032.

Giardina G, Clarke GD, Grugni M, Sbacchi M, Vecchietti V. Central and peripheral analgesic agents: chemical strategies for limiting brain penetration in kappa-opioid agonists belonging to different chemical classes. *Farmaco* 1995; 50:405–418.

Glick EN. Asymmetrical rheumatoid arthritis after poliomyelitis. *BMJ* 1967; 3:26–29.

Gold MS, Levine JD. DAMGO inhibits prostaglandin E_2-induced potentiation of a TTX-resistant Na^+ current in rat sensory neurons in vitro. *Neurosci Lett* 1996; 212:83–86.

Green PG, Levine JD. δ- and κ-opioid agonists inhibit plasma extravasation induced by bradykinin in the knee joint of the rat. *Neuroscience* 1992; 49:129–133.

Gyires K, Budavar I, Fürst S, Molnar I. Morphine inhibits the carrageenan induced edema and the chemoluminescence of leucocytes stimulated by zymosan. *J Pharm Pharmacol* 1985; 37:100–104.

Hassan AHS, Przewlocki R, Herz A, Stein C. Dynorphin, a preferential ligand for kappa-opioid receptors, is present in nerve fibers and immune cells within inflamed tissue of the rat. *Neurosci Lett* 1992; 140:85–88.

Hassan AHS, Ableitner A, Stein C, Herz A. Inflammation of the rat paw enhances axonal transport of opioid receptors in the sciatic nerve and increases their density in the inflamed tissue. *Neuroscience* 1993; 55:185–195.

Heijnen CJ, Kavelaars A, Ballieux RE. Beta-endorphin: cytokine and neuropeptide. *Immunol Rev* 1991; 119:41–63.

Heller PH, Green PG, Tanner KD, et al. Peripheral neural contributions to inflammation. In: Fields HL, Liebeskind JC (Eds). *Pharmacological Approaches to the Treatment of Chronic Pain*. Progress in Pain Research and Management, Vol. 1. Seattle: IASP Press, 1994, pp 31–42.

Hökfelt T, Lundberg JM, Schultzberg M, et al. Cellular localisation of peptides in neural structures. *Proc R Soc Lond B Biol Sci* 1980; 210:63–77.

Hong Y, Abbott FV. Peripheral opioid modulation of pain and inflammation in the formalin test. *Eur J Pharmacol* 1995; 277:1317–1327.

Houghton AK, Valdez JG, Westlund KN. Peripheral morphine administration blocks the development of hyperalgesia and allodynia after bone damage in the rat. *Anesthesiology* 1998; 89:190–201.

Ingram SL, Williams JT. Opioid inhibition of Ih via adenylyl cyclase. *Neuron* 1994; 13:179–186.

Inman RD, Chiu B, Rabinovich S, Marshall W. Neuromodulation of synovitis: capsaicin effect on severity of experimental arthritis. *J Neuroimmunol* 1989; 24:17–22.

Jeanjean AP, Moussaoui SM, Maloteaux J-M, Laduron PM. Interleukin-1β induces long term increase of axonally transported opiate receptors and substance P. *Neuroscience* 1995; 68:151–157.

Jessell TM, Iverson LL. Opiate analgesics inhibit substance P release from rat trigeminal nucleus. *Nature* 1977; 268:549–551.

Ji R-R, Zhang Q, Law P-Y et al. Expression of μ-, δ-, and κ-opioid receptor-like immunoreactivities in rat dorsal root ganglia after carrageenan-induced inflammation. *J Neurosci* 1995; 15:8156–8166.

Kanjhan R. Opioids and pain. *Clin Exp Pharm Physiol* 1995; 22:397–403.

Kayser V, Lee SH, Guilbaud G. Evidence for a peripheral component in the enhanced antinociceptive effect of a low dose of systemic morphine in rats with peripheral mononeuropathy. *Neuroscience* 1995; 64:537–545.

Koltzenburg MK, Reeh PW. The nociceptor sensitization by bradykinin does not depend on sympathetic neurons. *Neuroscience* 1992; 46:465–473.

Kruger L, Halata Z. Structure of nociceptor "endings." In: Belmonte C, Cervero F (Eds). *Neurobiology of Nociceptors*. New York: Oxford University Press, 1996, pp 37–71.

LaMotte C, Pert CB, Snyder SH. Opiate receptor binding in primate spinal cord: distribution and changes after dorsal root section. *Brain Res* 1976; 112:407–412.

Levine JD, Moskowitz MA, Basbaum AI. The contribution of neurogenic inflammation in experimental arthritis. *J Immunol* 1985; 155:843s–847s.

Ley K, Linnemann G, Meinen M, Stoolman LM, Gaehtgens P. Fucoidin, but not polyphosphomannan PPME, inhibits leukocyte rolling in venules of the rat mesentery. *Blood* 1993; 81:177–185.

Machelska H, Cabot PJ, Mousa SA, Zhang Q, Stein C. Pain control in inflammation governed by selectins. *Nature Med* 1998; 4:1425–1428.

Mansour A, Fox CA, Akil H, Watson SJ. Opioid-receptor mRNA expression in the rat CNS: anatomical and functional implications. *Trends Neurosci* 1995; 18:22–29.

Millan MJ, Colpaert FC. Opioid systems in the response to inflammatory pain: sustained blockade suggests role of κ- but not μ-opioid receptors in the modulation of nociception, behaviour and pathology. *Neuroscience* 1991; 42:541–553.

Moises HC, Rusin KI, Macdonald RL. Mu- and kappa-opioid receptors selectively reduce the same transient components of high-threshold calcium current in rat dorsal root ganglion sensory nerves. *J Neurosci* 1994; 14:5903–5916.

Olsson Y. Microenvironment of the peripheral nervous system under normal and pathological conditions. *Crit Rev Neurobiol* 1990; 5:265–311.

Panerai AE, Sacerdote P. β-Endorphin in the immune system: a role at last? *Immunol Today* 1997; 18:317–319.

Parsons CG, Czlonkowski A, Stein C, Herz A. Peripheral opioid receptors mediating antinociception in inflammation. Activation by endogenous opioids and role of the pituitary-adrenal axis. *Pain* 1990; 41:81–93.

Przewlocki R, Hassan AHS, Lason W, et al. Gene expression and localization of opioid peptides in immune cells of inflamed tissue: functional role in antinociception. *Neuroscience* 1992; 48:491–500.

Russell NSW, Jamieson A, Calle A, Rance MJ. Peripheral opioid effects upon neurogenic plasma extravasation and inflammation [Abstract]. *Br J Pharmacol* 1985; 84:788.

Sanderson K, Nyberg F, Khalil Z. Modulation of peripheral inflammation by locally administered hemorphin-7. *Inflamm Res* 1998; 47:49–55.

Sarne Y, Fields A, Gafni M. Stimulatory effects of opioids on transmitter release and possible cellular mechanisms: overview and original results. *Neurochem Res* 1996; 21:1353–1361.

Schäfer MKH, Bette M, Romeo H, Schwaeble W, Weihe E. Localization of kappa-opioid receptor mRNA in neuronal subpopulations of rat sensory ganglia and spinal cord. *Neurosci Lett* 1994; 167:137–140.

Schäfer M, Imai Y, Uhl GR, Stein C. Inflammation enhances peripheral μ-opioid receptor-mediated analgesia, but not μ-opioid receptor transcription in dorsal root ganglia. *Eur J Pharmacol* 1995; 279:165–169.

Schäfer M, Mousa SA, Zhang Q, Carter L, Stein C. Expression of corticotropin-releasing factor in inflamed tissue is required for intrinsic peripheral opioid analgesia. *Proc Nat Acad Sci USA* 1996; 93:6096–6100.

Schäfer M, Mousa SA, Stein C. Corticotropin-releasing factor in antinociception and inflammation. *Eur J Pharmacol* 1997; 323:1–10.

Schäfer M, Zhou L, Stein C. Cholecystokinin inhibits peripheral opioid analgesia in inflamed tissue. *Neuroscience* 1998; 82:603–611.

Schaible HG, Grubb BD. Afferent and spinal mechanisms of joint pain. *Pain* 1993; 55:5–54.

Schaible H-G, Schmidt RF. Neurobiology of articular nociceptors. In: Belmonte C, Cervero F (Eds). *Neurobiology of Nociceptors*. New York: Oxford University Press, 1996, pp 202–219.

Schuligoi R, Donnerer J, Amann R. Bradykinin-induced sensitization of afferent neurons in the rat paw. *Neuroscience* 1994; 59:211–215.

Selley DE, Breivogel CS, Childres SR. Modification of G protein-coupled functions by low pH pretreatment of membranes from NG108-15 cells: increase in opioid agonist efficacy by decreased inactivation of G proteins. *Mol Pharmacol* 1993; 44:731–741.

Sharp BM, Roy S, Bidlack JM. Evidence for opioid receptors on cells involved in host defense and the immune system. *J Neuroimmunol* 1998; 83:45–56.

Smith GD, Seckl JR, Harmar AJ. Distribution of neuropeptides in dorsal root ganglia of the rat; substance P, somatostatin and calcitonin gene related peptide. *Neurosci Lett* 1993; 53:5–8.

Springer TA. Traffic signals for lymphocyte recirculation and leukocyte emigration: the multistep paradigm. *Cell* 1994; 76:301–314.

Stein C. Peripheral mechanisms of opioid analgesia. *Anesth Analg* 1993; 76:182–191.

Stein C. Mechanisms of disease: the control of pain in peripheral tissue by opioids. *N Engl J Med* 1995; 332:1685–1690.

Stein C, Hassan AHS, Przewlocki R, et al. Opioids from immunocytes interact with receptors on sensory nerves to inhibit nociception in inflammation. *Proc Natl Acad Sci USA* 1990; 87:5935–5939.

Stein C, Comisel K, Haimerl E, et al. Analgesic effect of intraarticular morphine after arthroscopic knee surgery. *N Engl J Med* 1991; 325:1123–1126.

Stein C, Hassan AHS, Lehrberger K, Giefing J, Yassouridis A. Local analgesic effect of endogenous opioid peptides. *Lancet* 1993; 342:321–324.

Stein C, Pflüger M, Yassouridis A, et al. No tolerance to peripheral morphine analgesia in presence of opioid expression in inflamed synovia. *J Clin Invest* 1996; 98:793–799.

Stein C, Schäfer M, Cabot PJ, et al. Peripheral opioid analgesia. *Pain Rev* 1997; 4:171–185.

Suarez-Roca H, Maixner W. Activation of kappa opioid receptors by U50488H and morphine enhances the release of substance P from rat trigeminal nucleus slices. *J Pharmacol Exp Ther* 1993; 264:648–653.

Taiwo YO, Levine JD. Kappa- and delta-opioids block sympathetically dependent hyperalgesia. *J Neurosci* 1991; 11:928–932.

Thomas PT, Bhargava HN, House RV. Immunomodulatory effects of in vitro exposure to morphine and its metabolites. *Pharmacology* 1995; 50:51–62.

Walker JS, Chandler AK, Wilson JL, Binder W, Day RO. Effect of μ-opioids morphine and buprenorphine on the development of adjuvant arthritis in rats. *Inflamm Res* 1996; 45:557–563.

Walker JS, Wilson J, Binder W, Scott C, Carmody JJ. The anti-inflammatory effects of opioids: their possible relevance to the pathophysiology and treatment of rheumatoid arthritis. *Res Alerts Rheum Arthritis* 1997; 1:291–299.

Wie ET, Thomas HA, Gjerde EA, et al. Dynorphin A (6–12) analogs suppress thermal edema. *Peptides* 1998; 19:767–775.

Wilson JL, Nayanar V, Walker JS. The site of anti-arthritic action of the kappa agonist, U50488H: importance of local administration. *Br J Pharmacol* 1996; 118:1754–1760.

Wüster M, Schulz R, Herz A. Multiple opiate receptors in peripheral tissue preparations. *Biochem Pharmacol* 1981; 30:1883–1887.

Yaksh TL. Substance P release from knee joint afferent terminals: modulation by opioids. *Brain Res* 1988; 458:319–324.

Yonehara N, Imai Y, Chen J-Q, Takiuchi S, Inoki R. Influence of opioids on substance P release evoked by antidromic stimulation of primary afferent fibers in the hind instep of rats. *Regul Pept* 1992; 38:13–22.

Zhang Q, Schäfer M, Elde R, Stein C. Effects of neurotoxins and hindpaw inflammation on opioid receptor immunoreactivities in dorsal root ganglia. *Neuroscience* 1998; 85:281–291.

Zhou L, Zhang Q, Stein C, Schäfer M. Contribution of opioid receptors on primary afferent versus sympathetic neurons to peripheral opioid analgesia. *J Pharmacol Exp Ther* 1998; 261:1–7.

Correspondence to: Professor Christoph Stein, MD, Klinik für Anaesthesiologie und operative Intensivmedizin, Klinikum Benjamin Franklin, Freie Universität Berlin, Hindenburgdamm 30, D-12200 Berlin, Germany. Tel: 49-30-84452731; Fax: 49-30-84454469; email: cstein@medizin.fu-berlin.de.

Opioid Sensitivity of Chronic Noncancer Pain,
Progress in Pain Research and Management,
Vol. 14, edited by Eija Kalso, Henry J. McQuay,
and Zsuzsanna Wiesenfeld-Hallin, IASP Press,
Seattle, © 1999.

4

Relevance of Proposed Mechanisms of G-Protein-Coupled Receptor Desensitization to Opioid Receptors

Vahri Beaumont and Graeme Henderson

*Department of Pharmacology, University of Bristol,
Bristol, United Kingdom*

Receptor desensitization on prolonged exposure to agonists is a phenomenon common to many G-protein-coupled receptors, including the opioid receptors. Numerous mechanisms have been proposed to explain the desensitization of G-protein-coupled receptors. This chapter describes the main mechanisms of receptor desensitization—phosphorylation by G-protein-coupled receptor kinases (GRKs) with subsequent arrestin binding, phosphorylation by second-messenger kinases, receptor internalization, and receptor downregulation—and reviews the evidence implicating each mechanism in opioid receptor desensitization. Opioid drugs vary in their agonist efficacy at opioid receptors, and the final section addresses the ways in which agonist efficacy can influence both the induction and the expression of receptor desensitization.

RECEPTOR DESENSITIZATION IN OPIOID TOLERANCE

OVERVIEW OF TOLERANCE MECHANISMS

Opioid tolerance is a multimodal phenomenon involving at least four separate mechanisms: (1) desensitization of signal transduction from opioid receptor to cellular effector, (2) compensatory changes in intracellular signaling, (3) compensatory changes in neuronal circuitry, and (4) learning. The purpose of this chapter is to review recent advances in our understanding of the processes involved in the first of these mechanisms, desensitization of the receptor–effector system. Other chapters in this volume discuss the relative importance of the different mechanisms involved in opioid tolerance and address the important question of the extent of opioid tolerance that occurs in clinical situations involving the treatment of pain (see also Mao et al. 1995).

Tolerance, desensitization, tachyphylaxis, and waning are all terms used to describe a decrease in the amplitude of the drug-evoked response on repeated or continuous administration. Desensitization and tachyphylaxis have generally been used to describe rapid events (occurring over seconds or minutes), and tolerance to describe a slower process (occurring over hours or days). However, a slower time scale does not necessarily indicate a different underlying adaptive mechanism. For simplicity, we will use the term desensitization.

Each of the cloned opioid receptors, MOR1 (μ), DOR1 (δ), KOR1 (κ), and ORL1 (opioid-receptor-like 1), is a seven-transmembrane protein that couples through pertussis-toxin-sensitive G proteins of the G_i and G_o families to a variety of cellular effector systems (North 1993). Often these effector systems are shared with other G_i/G_o-coupled receptors (North et al. 1987). Adaptation could thus occur at several potential sites in the receptor–effector pathway following prolonged agonist exposure (Fig. 1).

HOMOLOGOUS VERSUS HETEROLOGOUS DESENSITIZATION

Heterologous desensitization occurs when exposure of cells to an agonist acting at one type of receptor leads to a diminished responsiveness, not only at the receptors activated but also at other types of receptor. A reduction in either effector activity or G-protein expression has been implicated. In dorsal root ganglion (DRG) cultures, heterologous desensitization of opioid receptors has been associated with a decrease in the levels of $G_{i\alpha}$ immunoreactivity (Crain et al. 1982; Attali et al. 1989). A heterologous desensitization of both μ- and δ-opioid receptors following chronic morphine administration has also been described in the periaqueductal gray and thalamus of rats (Noble and Cox 1996), although it did not appear to involve changes in levels of G_i/G_o proteins (Terwilliger et al. 1991). Paradoxically, however, chronic morphine treatment appeared to result in an upregulation of $G_{i\alpha}/G_{o\alpha}$ in other studies (Nestler et al. 1989; Ammer and Schulz 1993), which suggests that adaptive responses occurring during chronic morphine administration are not identical in all opioid-sensitive neuronal populations.

In contrast to heterologous desensitization, homologous desensitization describes a much more circumscribed loss of responsiveness, being specific only to the type of receptor activated, and negating the involvement of altered G-protein expression or effector activity.

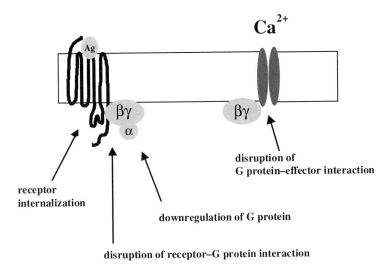

Fig. 1. Potential sites for desensitization of the G-protein-coupled receptor–effector pathway. In this example the effector illustrated is a voltage-operated calcium channel that is inhibited by the βγ dimer of the G protein.

RECEPTOR PHOSPHORYLATION

In common with other G-protein-coupled receptors, each of the cloned opioid receptors possesses multiple consensus sequences for phosphorylation in the third intracellular loop and carboxyl terminal domain. Therefore, phosphorylation on serine and threonine residues by kinases such as G-protein-coupled receptor kinases (GRKs), protein kinase A, and protein kinase C is likely to occur and to modify receptor function.

MECHANISMS OF PHOSPHORYLATION BY GRKs AND ARRESTIN

The processes by which GRKs and subsequent arrestin binding are thought to induce homologous G-protein-coupled desensitization are illustrated in Fig. 2. Agonist binding to the receptor promotes a conformational change in the receptor that results in G-protein activation. Free G-protein βγ subunits facilitate the translocation of some GRKs to the plasma membrane, where they can phosphorylate the receptor at serine/threonine residues on the third intracellular loop and C-terminal tail. The cytoplasmic protein, arrestin, has a high affinity for the phosphorylated receptor and binds to it, resulting in a phosphorylated receptor–arrestin complex that disrupts G-protein binding and renders the receptor nonfunctional, i.e., desensitized. See Krupnick and Benovic (1998) for a detailed review of this process.

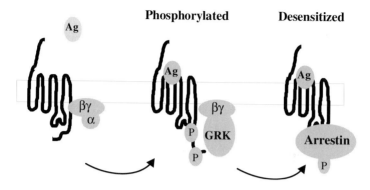

Fig. 2. Mechanism of G-protein-coupled receptor kinase (GRK)-mediated desensitization. The agonist-occupied receptor is phosphorylated by a GRK; arrestin then binds to the phosphorylated receptor, rendering it desensitized.

Phosphorylation by GRKs

Our understanding of the role of GRKs came originally from studies on the β_2 adrenoceptor (β_2AR). Unlike opioid receptors, this receptor couples through G_s proteins to activate adenylyl cyclase. Given that the ability of forskolin or sodium fluoride to activate adenylyl cyclase (via G proteins or the adenylyl cyclase enzyme itself) remained largely unchanged under conditions of marked β_2AR desensitization, it was concluded that the receptor itself, not the subsequent steps in the effector pathway, must be the target of the desensitization mechanism (Hausdorff et al. 1990). In addition, after reconstitution of desensitized β_2ARs, G_s, and adenylyl cyclase in phospholipid vesicles, the desensitized receptors still showed an impaired capacity to mediate agonist stimulation of adenylyl cyclase (Kassis and Fishman 1984; Strulovici et al. 1984). This provided the first evidence that receptors were covalently modified during the desensitization process. Phosphorylation emerged as the prime candidate for this modification when it was demonstrated that stoichiometric phosphorylation of the β_2AR occurred after exposure of intact cells to desensitizing levels of agonist. Furthermore, the kinetics and dose dependence of this phosphorylation paralleled those of desensitization (Sibley et al. 1987). Benovic et al. (1986) demonstrated that agonist-induced phosphorylation of β_2AR also occurred in cell lines that lacked the G-protein αs subunit and that phosphorylation and desensitization occurred in cells lacking protein kinase A (PKA). These findings led to the prediction that a specific receptor kinase existed that would phosphorylate only the agonist-occupied form of the receptor, and thus produce an homologous pattern of desensitization (Lohse et al. 1989; Hausdorff et al. 1990; Palczewski and Benovic 1991). This novel receptor kinase was subsequently isolated and named β-adrenergic receptor kinase or βARK (Benovic et al. 1986); it has since become known as GRK2.

GRK2 is now recognized to be only one of a family of six related serine/ threonine kinases that specifically initiate desensitization of G-protein-coupled receptors. The GRK family includes GRK1 or rhodopsin kinase, GRK2 (βARK1), GRK3 (βARK2), GRK4 (IT11-A), GRK5, and GRK6 (Haga et al. 1994; Palczewski 1997). GRK2, GRK3, and GRK6 are all found in the brain (Inglese et al. 1993; Fehr et al. 1997). They are located in both presynaptic and postsynaptic locations and are thus likely to function in the desensitization of neuronal G-protein-coupled receptors. GRKs must be appropriately localized at the plasma membrane if they are to mediate desensitization of cell-surface receptors. After agonist-mediated receptor activation, some GRK2 and GRK3 molecules can translocate to the plasma membrane by interacting with free G-protein βγ subunits (Inglese et al. 1992). This translocation process creates an extremely precise mechanism for targeting GRKs to activated receptors, as free G-protein βγ subunits are only found in the plasma membrane at sites of receptor activation.

An important question relates to the specificity of action of GRKs. Studies using reconstituted receptors and kinases have shown that GRK2 and GRK3 appear to phosphorylate G_s-, G_q-, and G_i/G_o-coupled receptors (Benovic et al. 1987a, 1991; Kwatra et al. 1989; Kurose and Lefkowitz 1994; Premont et al. 1994, 1996; Debburman et al. 1995; Haga et al. 1996). The use of such reconstituted systems for the analysis of GRK specificity can be problematic, however. In most cases, the GRK levels in reconstituted systems are higher than those found endogenously, which may exaggerate low-level interactions. Furthermore, coupling in transfected cells may utilize a different G-protein with βγ subunits compatible for GRK binding and translocation, whereas the βγ subunits coupled to the receptor in neurons would not support such an effect. GRKs have in fact been shown to exhibit a preference for some βγ-subunit compositions but not others (Daaka et al. 1997).

To elucidate fully the role of GRKs in G-protein-coupled receptor desensitization requires the development of methods for inhibiting the enzyme. GRK activity can be inhibited by the use of relatively nonselective compounds such as Zn^{2+} or heparin (Benovic et al. 1987b; Mundell and Kelly 1998a). These agents are not specific, however, and may also have detrimental effects in intact cells. Studies of the interaction of the GRKs with G-protein βγ subunits have located the βγ-binding domain of the GRKs to a region of the carboxyl terminus (Koch et al. 1994). This finding provides a more specific technique of inhibiting the enzyme, since peptide fragments corresponding to the binding domain should act to inhibit the binding of GRK to the βγ subunits. Intracellular dialysis of a 28-amino-acid fragment of GRK3 corresponding to its βγ-binding domain reduced α_2 adrenoceptor desensitization in chick DRG neurons (Diverse-Pierluissi et al. 1996).

It is also possible to study the role of endogenous GRKs in mediating desensitization using stable expression of dominant negative mutant forms of GRK (Kong et al. 1994). A dominant negative mutant form of GRK2 (DNM GRK2) is able to translocate to, but not phosphorylate target receptors, by virtue of a Lys220Arg mutation in the catalytic domain of wild-type GRK2 that negates its kinase activity. In NG108-15 cells, stable transfection of the mutant resulted in 30- to 60-fold overexpression of the DNM GRK2 protein compared to wild-type GRK2 (Kelly et al. 1996). In intact cells, adenosine A2A- and A2B-receptor-mediated desensitization was significantly reduced, while desensitization at iloprost, secretin, and somatostatin receptors was unaffected (Mundell et al. 1997, 1998; Beaumont et al. 1998). Thus, in intact cells, the selectivity of GRKs for agonist-occupied receptors may be greater than initially suggested by in vitro or reconstituted systems.

Role of arrestins

Phosphorylation of the receptor alone does not significantly reduce its capacity to activate G proteins. It has now been shown that GRK phosphorylation allows the binding of a protein called arrestin to the receptor, which disrupts the interaction between the receptor and G proteins, thereby inducing homologous desensitization (for review see Krupnick and Benovic 1998). Four members of the arrestin family have been cloned, and their receptor recognition and binding domains have been characterized by mutagenesis and generation of chimeric molecules (Dolph et al. 1993; Fuchs et al. 1995). More recently it has been discovered that arrestins are also involved in the targeting of G-protein-coupled receptors to the internalization machinery.

Evidence for GRK- and arrestin-mediated opioid-receptor desensitization

In the human neuroblastoma cell line SK-N-BE, both phosphorylation and desensitization of the δ-opioid receptor was reduced by Zn^{2+} or heparin (Hasbi et al. 1998). Inhibition of δ-receptor desensitization by heparin has also been observed in NG108-15 cells, which contain predominantly GRK2 (Morikawa et al. 1998). Furthermore, in both cell lines the serine/threonine phosphatase-1 and -2A inhibitor, okadaic acid, inhibited the recovery from desensitization. Transfection of COS-7 cells with the DNM GRK2 can inhibit κ-receptor desensitization (Raynor et al. 1994). However, in NG108-15 cells transfected with DNM GRK2, desensitization of δ-opioid-receptor-mediated inhibition of adenylyl cyclase was not reduced (J. Willets and E. Kelly, personal communication), whereas adenosine A2A- and A2B-receptor desensitization was significantly reduced (Mundell et al. 1997). Furthermore, in the same cell line we have observed that the desensitization of the somatostatin sst2 receptor, which is structurally related to the opioid receptors, was not inhibited by either the GRK-βγ-binding inhibitory peptides or by overexpression of DNM GRK2 (Beaumont et al. 1998).

Considerable evidence for the capability of GRKs and arrestins to elicit opioid receptor desensitization has been obtained in studies in which the GRKs and arrestins have been overexpressed in various cell types. GRK2 and GRK5 enhanced the agonist-induced phosphorylation of transfected δ-opioid receptors in HEK293 cells (Pei et al. 1995). Also, in the same cell line, GRK2 enhanced μ-opioid-receptor phosphorylation and desensitization (Zhang et al. 1998), and β-arrestin-1 inhibited κ- and δ- but not μ-opioid-receptor-mediated inhibition of adenylyl cyclase in HEK293 cells, presumably by potentiating receptor desensitization (Cheng et al. 1998).

In the Xenopus oocyte expression system, coexpression of GRK3 and β-arrestin-2 produced a synergistic, rapid ($t_{1/2}$ less than 4 minutes), homologous desensitization of δ-receptor-mediated potassium channel activation. Rapid desensitization was absent in cells expressing δ-receptor mutants that lacked serine and threonine residues at the end of the cytoplasmic C-terminal tail (Kovoor et al. 1997). In the same oocyte expression system, the desensitization of the μ-opioid-receptor-mediated response in the presence of GRK3 and β-arrestin-2 was more than 30-fold slower than that of the δ receptor.

However, none of the above studies have looked at opioid receptor desensitization in neurons. Now that there is sufficient evidence to suggest that GRKs are certainly capable of phosphorylating opioid receptors, it is of primary importance in the near future to establish the role of GRKs and arrestins in opioid receptor desensitization in mature neurons of the central nervous system. It may be significant that in the brainstem nucleus (locus ceruleus), GRK2 and β-arrestin levels are increased after chronic morphine administration (Terwilliger et al. 1994).

PHOSPHORYLATION OF OPIOID RECEPTORS BY SECOND-MESSENGER KINASES

Second-messenger kinases have been shown to phosphorylate various G-protein-coupled receptors, but they do not enhance arrestin binding to the receptor. The amino acid sequences of the opioid receptors reveal consensus sequences in putative intracellular domains for phosphorylation by protein kinase A (PKA), protein kinase C (PKC), and calcium/calmodulin-dependent protein kinase (CaM kinase). The nature of second-messenger kinase desensitization is generally heterologous, in that a kinase activated through one type of receptor may phosphorylate both the agonist-occupied receptors and other types of receptor in their unoccupied state. Second-messenger kinases could also phosphorylate and inactivate components of the receptor–effector pathway other than the receptor itself, such as the ion channel (Kovoor et al. 1995), which would also result in heterologous de-sensitization across receptors that use the same effector pathway.

Protein kinase A

PKA-mediated desensitization is believed to be mainly initiated by G_s-coupled receptors, whereby agonist occupation of the receptor leads to acti-vation of adenylyl cyclase and subsequent PKA activation, which may then phosphorylate other receptor types and render them desensitized (Lohse et al. 1990). However, it has been claimed that PKA plays a role in G_i/G_o-coupled receptor desensitization, and PKA activity has been observed to increase during chronic opioid treatment (Nestler and Tallman 1988; Terwilliger et al. 1994). However, most studies have excluded PKA involve-ment in opioid receptor desensitization. This conclusion has usually been reached by observing that inhibitors of PKA such as adenosine 3´,5´-cyclic phosphorothioate (Rp-cAMPS), as well as the inhibitors KT5720 and H7 had no effect on the rate or extent of opioid receptor desensitization (Narita et al. 1995; Hasbi et al. 1998; Morikawa et al. 1998). Activators of PKA indi-cate that it may in fact exert a negative influence on opioid receptor desen-sitization. In rat locus ceruleus neurons, μ-opioid-receptor desensitization was reduced by forskolin, an activator of adenylyl cyclase (Harris and Will-iams 1991), and in Xenopus oocytes transfected with the μ receptor, PKA activation by 8-chlorophenolthio-cAMP reduced desensitization (Chen and Yu 1994). However, δ-opioid-receptor desensitization in transfected HEK293 cells was unaffected by forskolin (Pei et al. 1995).

Protein kinase C

Upon stimulation, PKC undergoes translocation from the cytosol to dif-ferent sites, including the plasma membrane (Mochly-Rosen 1995), where it can phosphorylate G-protein-coupled receptors. PKC was implicated in opioid receptor tolerance after it was shown that the PKC-αβ isoform was reduced in the brain of heroin addicts and morphine-dependent rats (Busquets et al. 1995). The involvement of PKC in opioid receptor desensitization has been studied using both activators and inhibitors of PKC. Phorbol ester treatment increased the phosphorylation of μ-opioid receptors, but morphine-induced phosphorylation of μ receptors was independent of PKC, suggesting that although a heterologous pathway of PKC-induced desensitization is viable, it is not the mechanism involved in agonist-induced desensitization per se (Zhang et al. 1996). Enhanced desensitization of μ- and δ-opioid receptor-mediated responses has also been observed by others (Chen and Yu 1994; Mestek et al. 1995; Ueda et al. 1995; Zhang et al. 1996). Furthermore, calphostin C, an inhibitor of PKC, has been observed to decrease desensitization (Narita et al. 1995; Ueda et al. 1995; Cai et al. 1996). In contrast, several studies that used long-term phorbol ester treatment to induce downregulation of PKC (Pei et al. 1995; Morikawa et al. 1998) or used H7 to inhibit PKC (Hasbi et al. 1998) have failed to observe any change in δ-opioid-receptor desensitization.

Other kinases

In addition to the above, two other protein kinases have been implicated in opioid receptor desensitization. Desensitization of μ-opioid-receptor-mediated responses was enhanced by injection of activated calcium/calmodulin-dependent protein kinase in transfected oocytes (Mestek et al. 1995) and by expression of a constitutively active form of the enzyme in HEK293 cells (Koch et al. 1997). In addition, a role for mitogen-activated protein kinase (MAPK) was proposed when it was observed that the MAPK inhibitor, PD-98059, reduced μ-opioid receptor desensitization in transfected Chinese hamster ovary (CHO) cells (Polakiewicz et al. 1998).

Other protein kinases have been implicated in G-protein-coupled receptor desensitization, but no studies of their involvement in opioid receptor desensitization have been reported. Desensitization of somatostatin receptors in chick ciliary ganglion neurons was shown to be partially mediated by a calcium guanosine monophosphate (cGMP)-dependent protein kinase (Meriney et al. 1994). Casein kinase may be involved in the phosphorylation of certain G-protein-coupled receptors (Tobin et al. 1997). This kinase is not inhibited by inhibitors of PKA or PKC; it is inhibited by heparin, which inhibits GRK2, but not by zinc chloride, which also inhibits GRK2 .

RECEPTOR INTERNALIZATION

It has been known for some time that agonist stimulation of G-protein-coupled receptors causes a dramatic reorganization of their distribution within the cell (see Koenig and Edwardson 1997 for review). Activation of receptors triggers receptor endocytosis to sites away from the plasma membrane, with a subsequent constitutive recycling of receptors back to the plasma membrane, or degradation in lysosomes (Fig. 3). Agonist-evoked receptor endocytosis has been observed for μ (von Zastrow et al. 1993, 1994; Keith et al. 1996; Whistler and von Zastrow 1998) and δ (Trapaidze et al. 1996; Cvejic and Devi 1997), but not κ (Chu et al. 1997) opioid receptors. Such endocytosis has been observed not only in transfected cell lines, but also in intact neurons (Keith et al. 1996; Sternini et al. 1996). The internalization of μ- and δ-opioid receptors is rapid, with a $t_{1/2}$ of approximately 10 minutes.

Receptor internalization may play a role in desensitization in two very different ways. First, receptor internalization may itself be the mechanism by which desensitization occurs by removing functional receptors from the plasma membrane. Second, receptor internalization may not be a mechanism for desensitization but rather a process by which receptors desensitized by GRK phosphorylation and arrestin binding are resensitized prior to reinsertion in the plasma membrane. One problem is that many investigators have studied internalization in isolation, without relating it to either receptor desensitization or resensitization. Another is that internalization mechanisms may vary in different cell types; the precise details of receptor internaliza-

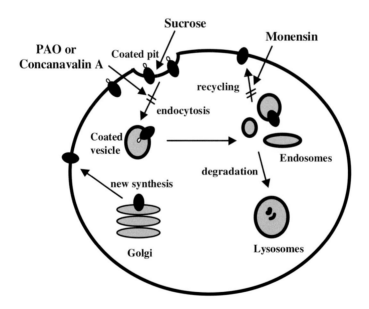

Fig. 3. The endocytosed receptor can either be recycled or degraded (downregulated). Endocytosis by clathrin-coated pits can be inhibited by hyperosmolar sucrose, phenylarsine oxide (PAO), or concanavalin A. Recycling can be inhibited by monensin. Adapted from Koenig and Edwardson (1997), with permission.

tion may be a characteristic of one particular receptor type and should not be generalized to all G-protein-coupled receptors.

THE PROCESS OF RECEPTOR ENDOCYTOSIS

The predominant pathway for agonist-induced internalization of G-protein-coupled receptors is via clathrin-coated pits. Many of the molecules required for clathrin-mediated endocytosis have been identified and characterized, although the endocytic "trigger," that is, the switch to govern the internalization of an agonist–receptor complex is, as yet, ill-defined. Receptor phosphorylation is one candidate for inducing agonist-dependent internalization. Mutation of putative phosphorylation sites in the C-terminus of the δ-opioid receptor or of all phosphorylation sites in the μ-opioid receptor lowered agonist-dependent internalization (Trapaidze et al. 1996; Capeyrou et al. 1997). However, other workers have shown that the δ-opioid receptor can be internalized without phosphorylation (Murray et al. 1998). The δ-opioid receptor converts from a dimer to a monomer prior to internalization (Cvejic and Devi 1997). It is also possible that activation of G proteins and second-messenger generation could be the trigger for endocytosis. An interesting observation was made with the μ-opioid receptor. Truncation of its C-terminus to remove a serine/threonine-rich domain did not result in a reduction of internalization. The mutant receptor did not exhibit elevated basal G-protein coupling but internalized into clathrin-coated vesicles and recycled constitutively (Segredo et al. 1997), which suggests that the C-terminal domain may contain motifs that impair endocytosis. In addition, the two splice variants of the μ-opioid receptor, MOR1 and MOR1B, which differ in the length and composition of their C-terminal domain, undergo different receptor trafficking profiles, with the shorter COOH-terminus MOR1B protein being sequestered and recycled much faster than the longer MOR1 protein (Koch et al. 1998).

The key event in the process of G-protein-coupled receptor internalization is the recruitment of soluble clathrin from the cytoplasm onto the plasma membrane to form clathrin-coated pits. The clathrin assembles into a lattice of hexagons and pentagons, forming a cage-like structure that encloses a membrane vesicle (Kaneseki and Kadota 1969; Robinson 1994; Goodman et al. 1996). Proteins of the dynamin family are thought to assemble in helical collars around the necks of clathrin-coated pits, which allows these pits to pinch off as coated vesicles (Gugliatti et al. 1973). Internalization of G-protein-coupled receptors via uncoated pits has also been described (Dupree et al. 1993; Chun et al. 1994; Roetgger et al. 1995; Rao et al. 1997). The functional implication of these alternative endocytic pathways is not known.

As previously mentioned, recent evidence suggests that the arrestins are also involved in agonist-mediated receptor endocytosis. β-Arrestin-1 and -2 promote internalization and bind with high affinity directly and stoichiometrically to clathrin terminal domain (Goodman et al. 1996, 1997). Moreover, β-arrestin chimeras defective in clathrin binding show a reduced ability to promote receptor endocytosis (Krupnick et al. 1997a,b), whereas overexpression of β-arrestin-1 and -2 rescues agonist-mediated receptor internalization and overexpression of a dominant negative mutant β-arrestin inhibits agonist-induced receptor internalization (Ferguson et al. 1996). In HEK293 cells, overexpression of GRK2 and β-arrestin enhanced μ-opioid receptor internalization (Zhang et al. 1998), and in the same cell type overexpression of these same proteins both enhanced and altered the agonist-specific internalization of the μ-opioid receptor (Whistler and von Zastrow 1998). Thus, arrestins may function as adapter molecules that recruit cellular proteins and thereby facilitate receptor endocytosis, or they may directly mediate endocytosis. Dynamin has been implicated as a protein that interacts with arrestins to enhance endocytosis of some receptors (Zhang et al. 1996).

Little is known about the subsequent stages of endosomal formation and sorting downstream from the initial event. Following internalization from the surface, membrane proteins, lipids, and solutes enter early sorting endosomes. From here, endocytosed receptors are sorted back to the plasma membrane or degraded (downregulated). The process of receptor recycling is constitutive, being unaffected by the presence of the agonist. The recycling pathway can be inhibited by inhibitors of endosomal acidification such as nigericin and monensin; this causes retention of endocytosed receptors within the cell (Grady et al. 1996). From early endosomes, internalized molecules can also proceed to further stages along the endocytic pathway to become late endosomes and lysosomes and then to be degraded.

RECEPTOR INTERNALIZATION AS A MECHANISM OF DESENSITIZATION

Pak et al. (1996) showed that, in transfected CHO cells, μ-opioid-receptor desensitization was associated with a reduction in the number of binding sites present on the plasma membrane, suggesting that endocytosis of the receptors from the surface was responsible for the desensitization. Internalization of receptors also appears to mediate desensitization of m2 muscarinic, sst2 somatostatin, and secretin receptors, since inhibitors of internalization inhibited desensitization (Beaumont et al. 1998; Mundell and Kelly 1998b; Tsuga et al. 1998). Agonist-stimulated phosphorylation of the secretin receptor on serine/threonine residues within the C-terminal tail could be eliminated by truncation of this domain of the receptor (Ozcelebi et al. 1995; Holtmann et al. 1996), but desensitization and internalization still occurred with a similar time course. These results suggest that for the secretin receptor, the main mechanism of agonist-induced desensitization is a rapid phosphorylation-independent receptor internalization. For the CCK receptor, expressed either in CHO cells or in its native pancreatic acinar cells, both phosphorylation of the receptor on agonist binding and internalization of the receptor contributed to receptor desensitization. However, receptor internalization and receptor phosphorylation appeared to be independent of one another (Rao et al. 1997). Furthermore, when PKA and GRK2 are inhibited, internalization contributes to the desensitization of the β_2AR (Lohse et al. 1990). Thus, it remains possible that desensitization of G-protein-coupled receptors may be mediated by more than one mechanism.

RECEPTOR INTERNALIZATION AS A MECHANISM FOR RESENSITIZATION

Once the agonist has bound to the receptor and desensitization has been induced by GRK-mediated phosphorylation and arrestin binding, then sequestration of the receptor from the plasma membrane into an acidified vesicle facilitates subsequent agonist dissociation from the receptor and receptor dephosphorylation by a phosphatase enzyme with consequent dissociation of arrestins (Fig. 4) (see Krupnick and Benovic 1998 for review). A protein phosphatase that dephosphorylates G-protein-coupled receptors has been isolated from bovine brain (Pitcher et al. 1995). The phosphatase inhibitor, okadaic acid, has been shown to prevent resensitization of the NK1-receptor (Garland et al. 1996). Thereafter the receptor, in its nondesensitized form, can be recycled back into the plasma membrane. Resensitization of the β_2AR receptor can be blocked by inhibition of endocytosis with hypertonic media and concanavalin-A pretreatment (Pippig et al. 1995). Inhibitors of endosomal acidification, such as monensin, inhibit neurokinin receptor recycling and resensitization (Bohm et al. 1997). A difference in the internalization, desensitization, and resensitization rates of the two splice variants of the μ-opioid receptor has recently been reported (Koch et al. 1998). MOR1B, which comprises a shorter COOH terminus that differs in its amino acid composition from the longer MOR1 splice variant, desensitized slower than did MOR1 upon agonist activation. Interestingly, the slower desensitization of MOR1B is coupled with a faster resensitization rate, which matches the time course of internalization and rapid recycling back to the membrane. This finding is consistent with internalization as a

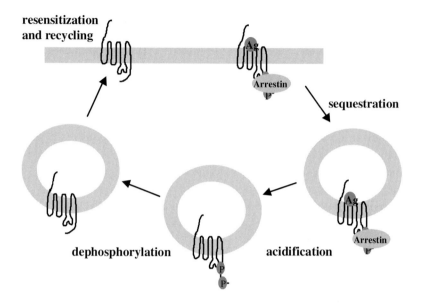

Fig. 4. Resensitization of GRK-phosphorylated receptor by sequestration and dephosphorylation. The agonist-occupied, phosphorylated receptor with bound arrestin is sequestered into a coated vesicle. Following acidification of the vesicle, the agonist unbinds and the receptor is dephosphorylated by a G-protein receptor phosphatase. Thereafter the receptor can be reinserted into the plasma membrane.

mechanism for resensitization and not desensitization, at least for the MOR1B opioid receptor.

RECEPTOR DOWNREGULATION

In addition to internalization, a second mechanism leading to desensitization involves a decrease in the number of receptors at the plasma membrane—receptor downregulation. Downregulation is characterized by a decrease in the total number of receptors in a cell. In some cases the receptors are proteolytically degraded, and new receptor synthesis is required to regenerate them. The process of receptor downregulation takes considerably longer than that of agonist-induced desensitization mediated by second-messenger or specific G-protein-receptor kinases. As the basal turnover of receptors is quite slow, decreases in receptor synthesis can take more than 24 hours to affect the receptor number (Lohse 1993). Downregulation of μ, δ, and κ receptors has been observed (Gucker and Bidlack 1992; Zadina et al. 1992; Baumhaker et al. 1993; Afify et al. 1998; Kato et al. 1998; Zhu et al. 1998).

It is not clear whether receptor internalization is required before downregulation can take place, or whether internalization is even part of the mechanism of downregulation. Mutation of tyrosine residues (which have been proposed to be important in targeting receptors to lysosomal intracellular compartments) in C-terminal tails of the β_2AR and the muscarinic m2 receptor impairs downregulation without affecting internalization, suggesting that endocytosis and downregulation are independent processes that rely on distinct signals (Valiquette et al. 1990; Goldman et al. 1994). Ubiquitination of G-protein-coupled receptors has also been proposed as a mechanism for downregulation, although evidence of this is lacking at present.

At least two signaling pathways contribute to downregulation of β_2AR. First, an agonist-dependent PKA-independent pathway appears to be involved (Hadcock et al. 1989). In support of this is the finding that mutant β_2ARs with defective G-protein coupling show significantly impaired agonist-induced downregulation of receptor number, whereas cells with mutations in signaling proteins downstream of the receptor and G-protein, in which there are defects in cAMP stimulation and PKA activation, nevertheless undergo near-normal agonist-induced downregulation. Second, a PKA-dependent heterologous pathway appears to be involved in receptor downregulation, as cAMP analogues or forskolin can promote receptor downregulation, although at a lower rate compared to full agonists (Collins et al. 1992). GRK-dependent phosphorylation does not appear to contribute to enhanced degradation, as several studies have reported that mutants of the β_2AR that lack GRK phosphorylation sites are downregulated normally (Collins et al. 1992; Hadcock and Malbon 1993).

Downregulation may also result from a reduction in the levels of mRNA. The decline in mRNA levels appears to involve decreases in the stability of mRNA rather than a lowering of the rate of transcription (Lefkowitz et al. 1990). This is strongly dependent on cAMP generation and PKA activation. The involvement of PKA suggests phosphorylation of a factor involved in the selective degradation of receptor mRNA or induction of transcription and translation of such a factor (Tholanikunnel et al. 1995).

ROLE OF AGONIST EFFICACY IN DESENSITIZATION

In the scheme of receptor activation and homologous desensitization shown in Fig. 5, the ability of an agonist to induce a response will be a function of its affinity for the agonist-preferring state of the receptor (Rag) and its ability to induce the subsequent conformational change to the active state (DRag*). Agonist efficacy is dependent on the ability to induce the active state DR*ag**. Although the theory is attractive, there is no need to postulate that agonists of different efficacy induce different active states of the receptor (see Bot et al. 1998); the difference in efficacy is more likely to relate to differing abilities to convert the receptor to the active state (as discussed by Colquhoun 1998). DR´, the desensitized form of the receptor, could represent either the phosphorylated receptor or the internalized receptor (as discussed above), and therefore desensitization is portrayed simply as the conversion of DR*ag** to DR´.

When considering the role of efficacy in receptor desensitization, it is important to distinguish between the *induction* of desensitization (i.e., the conversion of DR*ag** to DR´) and the *expression* of desensitization (the ability of a drug to evoke a response after desensitization has been induced).

INDUCTION OF DESENSITIZATION

With high- and low-efficacy agonists evoking equal, submaximal responses, then at any one time, only a fraction of receptors will be in the active state (DR*ag**). If the efficiency of the desensitization process is low, conversion to DR´ will be small and relatively little tolerance will be induced. However, with saturating concentrations of agonist, high-efficacy agonists will, at any one time, convert a high proportion of receptors to the DR*ag** (from which they can be desensitized) but low-efficacy agonists will

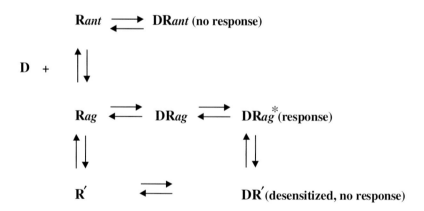

Fig. 5. Multistate model of agonist-induced receptor desensitization. High-efficacy agonists bind to R*ag* to produce DR*ag*, the form of the receptor that evokes the response. Low-efficacy agonists will bind to both R*ag* and R*ant*. DR*ant* does not give rise to a response. DR´ is the desensitized state of the receptor.

convert a smaller proportion of receptors to DR*ag** (because they will also form DR*ant*) and therefore induce less desensitization. This is indeed what is observed experimentally for μ-opioid receptors. Receptor-saturating concentrations of high-efficacy agonists such as DAMGO induced marked homologous desensitization, but the low efficacy agonist, morphine, did not induce desensitization (Yabaluri and Medzihradski 1997; Kovoor et al. 1998; see also the explanation by these authors for the contradictory data obtained by Yu et al. 1997). In HEK293 cells, high-efficacy agonists such as DAMGO and etorphine stimulated receptor endocytosis, whereas morphine failed to do so (Keith et al. 1996; Sternini et al. 1996; Whistler and von Zastrow 1998).

EXPRESSION OF DESENSITIZATION

In the nervous system, endogenous receptors are usually expressed at high enough levels to ensure a receptor reserve. This means that for a high efficacy agonist, the maximal response is evoked when only a proportion of the receptors have been occupied, whereas lower-efficacy agonists must occupy a higher proportion of receptors to evoke the maximal response, and partial agonists cannot evoke the maximal response even when occupying all of the available receptors. When homologous desensitization is induced by prolonged agonist exposure and receptors are functionally removed either by uncoupling or internalization, the concentration-response curve for a high-efficacy agonist will only be shifted to the right in a parallel manner, whereas for lower-efficacy agonists and partial agonists the maximum response will be depressed. In locus ceruleus neurons (Christie et al. 1987) and SH-SY5Y cells (Kennedy and Henderson 1991), chronic opioid exposure shifted the DAMGO concentration-response curve to the right by only three- and sevenfold, respectively, but the concentration-response curves for normorphine and morphine were flattened. This means that with respect to *expression* of desensitization, tolerance was greater for the low-efficacy than for the high efficacy agonist.

COMBINED INDUCTION AND EXPRESSION OF DESENSITIZATION

Some studies compare drugs by analyzing each drug's ability to both induce and express desensitization, i.e., each drug is tested only against the desensitization induced by itself. In such studies conducted in vivo, there is an inverse relationship between opioid agonist efficacy and the degree of tolerance produced, with the relative ability to produce desensitization being morphine > DAMGO > sufentanil (Stevens and Yaksh 1989a,b; Duttaroy and Yoburn 1995). This would indicate that in vivo it is the *expression* of desensitization that is the dominant parameter.

CONCLUSIONS

There is no consensus in the literature on a single mechanism of desensitization for any of the opioid receptors. It is entirely possible that within a cell more than one mechanism may operate to desensitize a single receptor type; this raises the questions of relative importance and redundancy. Furthermore, for the same receptor different mechanisms of desensitization may operate in different cell types. It is now time for the relevance of the processes underlying desensitization, elegantly characterized in expression systems, to be assessed in mature brain neurons where the levels of expression of important components in the different desensitization pathways may vary between cell types.

ACKNOWLEDGMENTS

We thank Dr. Eamonn Kelly for advice and critical reading of the manuscript.

REFERENCES

Afify EA, Law PY, Riedl M, Elde R, Loh HH. Role of the carboxyl terminus of mu and delta opioid receptor in agonist-induced downregulation. *Mol Brain Res* 1998; 54:24–34.

Ammer H, Schulz R. Alterations in the expression of G-proteins and regulation of adenylate cyclase in human neuroblastoma SH-SY5Y cells chronically exposed to low efficacy mu-opioids. *Biochem J* 1993; 95:263–271.

Attali B, Saya D, Vogel Z. Kappa-opiate agonists inhibit adenylate cyclase and produce heterologous desensitization in rat spinal cord. *J Neurochem* 1989; 52:360–369.

Baumhaker Y, Gafni M, Keren O, Sarne Y. Selective and interactive down-regulation of mu-opioid and delta-opioid receptors in human neuroblastoma SK-N-SH Cells. *Mol Pharmacol* 1993; 44:461–467.

Beaumont V, Hepworth MB, Luty JS, Kelly E, Henderson G. Somatostatin receptor desensitization in NG108-15 cells. A consequence of receptor sequestration. *J Biol Chem* 1998; 273:33174–33183.

Benovic J L, Strasser RH, Caron MG, Lefkowitz RJ. Beta-adrenergic receptor kinase: identification of a novel protein kinase that phosphorylates the agonist-occupied form of the receptor. *Proc Natl Acad Sci USA* 1986; 83:2797–2801.

Benovic JL, Regan JW, Matsui H, et al. Agonist-dependent phosphorylation of the alpha 2-adrenergic receptor by the beta-adrenergic receptor kinase. *J Biol Chem* 1987a; 262:17251–17253.

Benovic JL, Mayor F, Staniszewski C, Lefkowitz R, Caron MG. Purification and characterisation of the β-adrenergic receptor kinase. *J Biol Chem* 1987b; 262:9026–9032.

Benovic JL, Onorato JJ, Arriza JL, et al. Cloning, expression, and chromosomal localization of beta-adrenergic receptor kinase 2. A new member of the receptor kinase family. *J Biol Chem* 1991; 266:14939–14946.

Bohm SK, Grady EF, Bunnett NW. Regulatory mechanisms that modulate signalling by G-protein-coupled receptors. *Biochem J* 1997; 322:1–18.

Bot G, Blake, AD, Shuixing L, Reisine T. Fentanyl and its analogs desensitize the cloned mu opioid receptor. *J Pharmacol Exp Ther* 1998; 285:1207–1218.

Busquets X, Escriba PV, Sastre M, Garcia-Sevilla JA. Loss of protein kinase C-alpha beta in brain of heroin addicts and morphine-dependent rats. *J Neurochem* 1995; 64:247–252.

Cai Y, Zhang Y, Wu Y, Pei G. δOpioid receptor in neuronal cells undergoes acute and homologous desensitization. *Biochem Biophys Res Comm* 1996; 21:342–347.

Capeyrou R, Riond J, Corbani M, et al. Agonist-induced signalling and trafficking of the mu-opioid receptor: role of serine and threonine residues in the third cytoplasmic loop and C-terminal domain. *FEBS Letts* 1997; 415:200–205.

Chen Y, Yu L. Differential regulation by cAMP-dependent protein kinase and protein kinase C of the mu opioid receptor coupling to a G protein-activated K+ channel. *J Biol Chem* 1994; 269:7839–7842.

Cheng Z-J, Yu Q-M, Wu Y-L, Ma L, Peng G. Selective interference of βarrestin 1 with κ and δ but not μ opioid receptor/G protein coupling. *J Biol Chem* 1998; 273:24328–24333.

Christie MJ, Williams JT, North RA. Cellular mechanisms of opioid tolerance: studies in single brain neurones. *Mol Pharmacol* 1987; 32:633–638.

Chu P, Murray S, Lissin D, von Zastrow M. δ and κ opioid receptors are differentially regulated by dynamin-dependent endocytosis when activated by the same alkaloid agonist. *J Biol Chem* 1997; 272:27124–27130.

Chun MY, Liyanage UK, Lisanti MP, Lodish HF. Signal-transduction of a G-protein-coupled receptor in caveolae—colocalization of endothelin and its receptor with caveolin. *Proc Natl Acad Sci USA* 1994; 91:11728–11732.

Collins S, Caron Mg, Lefkowitz RJ. From ligand-binding to gene-expression—new insights into the regulation of G-protein-coupled receptors. *Trends Biochem Sci* 1992; 17:37–39.

Colquhoun D. Binding, gating, affinity and efficacy: the interpretation of structure-activity relationships for agonists and of the effects of mutating receptors. *Br J Pharmacol* 1998; 126:924–947.

Crain SM, Crain B, Peterson ER. Development of cross-tolerance to 5-hydroxytryptamine in organotypic cultures of mouse spinal cord-ganglia during chronic exposure to morphine. *Life Sci* 1982; 31:241–247.

Cvejic S, Devi LA. Dimerization of the delta opioid receptor: implication for a role in internalization. *J Biol Chem* 1997; 272:26959–26964.

Daaka Y, Pitcher JA, Richardson M, et al. Receptor and G betagamma isoform—specific interactions with G protein-coupled receptor kinases. *Proc Natl Acad Sci USA* 1997; 94:2180–2185.

Debburman SK, Kanupuli P, Benovic JL, Hosey MM. Agonist-dependent phosphorylation of human muscarinic receptors in *Spodoptera frugiperda* insect cell membranes by G-protein coupled receptor kinases. *Mol Pharmacol* 1995; 47:224–233.

Diverse-Pierluissi M, Inglese J, Stoffel RH, Lefkowitz RJ, Dunlap K. G protein-coupled receptor kinase mediates desensitization of norepinephrine-induced Ca^{2+} channel inhibition. *Neuron* 1996; 16:579–585.

Dolph PJ, Ranganathan R, Colley NJ, et al. Arrestin function in inactivation of G protein-coupled receptor rhodopsin in vivo. *Science* 1993; 260:1910–1916.

Dupree P, Parton RG, Raposo G, Kurzchalia TV, Simons K. Caveolae and sorting in the trans-golgi network of epithelial cells. *EMBO J* 1993; 12:1597–1605.

Duttaroy A, Yoburn BC. The effect of intrinsic efficacy on opioid tolerance. *Anesthesiology* 1995; 82:1226–1236.

Fehr C, Fickova M, Hiemke C, Reuss S, Dahmen N. Molecular cloning of rat G-protein-coupled receptor kinase 6 (GRK6) from brain tissue, and its mRNA expression in different brain regions and peripheral tissues. *Mol Brain Res* 1997; 49:278–282.

Ferguson SSG, Downey WE, Colapietro AM, et al. Role of β-arrestin in mediating agonist-promoted G protein-coupled receptor internalisation. *Science* 1996; 271:363–366.

Fuchs S, Nakazawa M, Maw M, et al. A homozygous1-base pair deletion in the arrestin gene is a frequent cause of Oguchi disease in Japanese. *Nature Genet* 1995; 10:360–362.

Garland AM, Grady EF, Lovett M, et al. Mechanisms of desensitization and resensitization of G-protein-coupled neurokinin(1) and neurokinin(2) receptors. *Mol Pharmacol* 1996; 49:438–446.

Goldman PS, Nathanson NM. Differential role of the carboxyl-terminal tyrosine in down-regulation and sequestration of the m2 muscarinic acetylcholine-receptor. *J Biol Chem* 1994; 269:15640–15645.

Goodman OB, Krupnick JG, Santini F, et al. β-arrestin acts as a clathrin adaptor in endocytosis of the β2-adrenergic receptor. *Nature* 1996; 383:447–450.

Goodman OB Jr, Krupnick JG, Gurevich VV, Benovic JL, Keen JH. Arrestin/clathrin interaction: localization of the arrestin binding locus to the clathrin terminal domain. *J Biol Chem* 1997; 272:15017–15022.

Grady EF, Gamp PD, Jones E, et al. Endocytosis and recycling of neurokinin-1 receptors in enteric neurons. *Neuroscience* 1996; 75:1239–1254.

Gucker S, Bidlack JM. Protein-kinase-C activation increases the rate and magnitude of agonist-induced delta-opioid receptor down-regulation in NG108-15 cells. *Mol Pharmacol* 1992; 42:656–665.

Gugliatti TA, Hall L, Rosenbluth R, Suzuki DT. Temperature sensitive mutants of *Drosophila melanogaster*. XIV. A selection of immobile adults. *Mol Genet* 1973; 120:107–114.

Hadcock JR, Malbon CC. Agonist regulation of gene-expression of adrenergic-receptors and G-proteins. *J Neurochem* 1993; 60:1–9.

Hadcock JR, Ros M, Malbon CC. Activation by G-protein βγ subunits of agonist- or light-dependent phosphorylation of muscarinic acetylcholine receptors and rhodopsin. *J Biol Chem* 1989; 264:13956–13961.

Haga T, Haga K, Kameyama K. G-protein-coupled receptor kinases. *J Neurochem* 1994; 63:400–412.

Haga K, Kameyama K, Haga T, et al. G protein-coupled receptor kinase: phosphorylation of muscarinic receptors and facilitation of receptor sequestration. *J Biol Chem* 1996; 271:2776–2782.

Harris GC, Williams JT. Transient homologous mu-opioid receptor desensitization in rat locus coeruleus neurons. *J Neurosci* 1991; 8:2574–2581.

Hasbi A, Polastron J, Allouche S, et al. Desensitization of the δ-opioid receptor correlates with its phosphorylation in SK-N-BE cells: involvement of a G protein-coupled receptor kinase. *J Neurochem* 1998; 70:2129–2138.

Hausdorff WP, Caron MG, Lefkowitz RJ. Turning off the signal: desensitization of beta-adrenergic receptor function. *FASEB J* 1990; 4:2881–2889.

Holtmann MH, Roetgger BF, Pinon DI, Miller L. Role of receptor phosphorylation in desensitisation and internalisation of the secretin receptor. *J Biol Chem* 1996; 271:23566–23571.

Inglese J, Koch WJ, Caron MG, Lefkowitz RJ. Isoprenylation in regulation of signal transduction by G-protein-coupled receptor kinases. *Nature* 1992; 359:147–150.

Inglese J, Freedman NJ, Koch WJ, Lefkowitz RJ. Structure and mechanism of the G protein-coupled receptor kinases. *J Biol Chem* 1993; 268:23735–23738.

Kaneski T, Kadota K. The 'vesicle in a basket': a morphological study of the coated vesicle isolated from the nerve endings of the guinea pig brain, with special reference to the mechanism of membrane movements. *J Cell Biol* 1969; 42:202–220.

Kassis S, Fishman PH. Functional alteration of the beta-adrenergic receptor during desensitization of mammalian adenylate cyclase by beta-agonists. *Proc Natl Acad Sci USA* 1984; 81:6686–6690.

Kato S, Fukuda K, Morikawa H, et al. Adaptations to chronic agonist exposure of μ-opioid receptor-expressing Chinese hamster ovary cells. *Eur J Pharmacol* 1998; 345:221–228.

Keith DE, Murray SR, Zaki PA, et al. Morphine activates opioid receptors without causing their rapid internalization. *J Biol Chem* 1996; 271:19021–19024.

Kelly E, Benovic JL. Stable expression of G-protein-coupled receptor kinase 2 dominant negative mutant (DNM GRK2) in NG108-15 cells. *Br J Pharmacol* 1996; 118:P142

Kennedy C, Henderson G. μ-Opioid receptor inhibition of calcium current: development of homologous tolerance in single SH-SY5Y cells after chronic exposure to morphine in vitro. *Mol Pharmacol* 1991; 40:1000–1005.

Koch WJ, Hawes BE, Inglese J, Luttrell LM, Lefkowitz RJ. Cellular expression of the carboxyl terminus of a G-protein coupled receptor kinase attenuates $G_{\beta\gamma}$-mediated signalling. *J Biol Chem* 1994; 269: 6193–6197.

Koch T, Wolf R, Raulf E, Mayer P, Holt V. Involvement of phosphorylation in mu opioid receptor desensitization. *Naunyn Schmiedebergs Arch Pharmacol* 1997; 355:SS 118.

Koch T, Schulz S, Schroder H, et al. Carboxyl-terminal splicing of the rat μ opioid receptor modulates agonist-mediated internalization and receptor resensitization. *J Biol Chem* 1998; 273:13652–13657.

Koenig JA, Edwardson JM. Endocytosis and recycling of G protein-coupled receptors. *Trends Pharmacol Sci* 1997; 18:276–287.

Kong G, Penn R, Benovic JL. A β-adrenergic receptor kinase dominant negative mutant attenuates desensitisation of the β₂-adrenergic receptor. *J Biol Chem* 1994; 269:13084–13087.

Kovoor A, Henry DJ, Chavkin C. Agonist-induced desensitization of the mu opioid receptor-coupled potassium channel (GIRK1). *J Biol Chem* 1995; 270:589–595.

Kovoor A, Nappey V, Kieffer BL, Chavkin C. Mu and delta opioid receptors are differentially desensitized by the coexpression of beta-adrenergic receptor kinase 2 and beta-arrestin 2 in Xenopus oocytes. *J Biol Chem* 1997; 272:27605–27611.

Kovoor A, Celver JP, Wu A, Chavkin C. Agonist induced homologous desensitization of mu-opioid receptors mediated by G protein-coupled receptor kinases is dependent on agonist efficacy. *Mol Pharmacol* 1998; 54:704–711.

Krupnick JG, Benovic JL. The role of receptor kinases and arrestins in G protein-coupled receptor regulation. *Ann Rev Pharmacol Toxicol* 1998; 38:289–319.

Krupnick JG, Goodman OB Jr, Keen JH, Benovic JL. Arrestin/clathrin interaction. Localization of the clathrin binding domain of nonvisual arrestins to the carboxy terminus. *J Biol Chem* 1997a; 272:15011–15016.

Krupnick JG, Santini F, Gagnon AW, Keen JH, Benovic JL. Modulation of the arrestin-clathrin interaction in cells. Characterization of beta-arrestin dominant-negative mutants. *J Biol Chem* 1997b; 272:32507–32512.

Kurose H, Lefkowitz RJ. Differential desensitisation and phosphorylation of three cloned and transfected α₂-adrenergic receptor subtypes. *J Biol Chem* 1994; 269:10093–10099.

Kwatra MM, Benovic JL, Caron MG, Lefkowitz RJ, Hosey MM. Phosphorylation of chick heart muscarinic receptors by the β-adrenergic receptor kinase. *Biochemistry* 1989; 28:4543–4547.

Lefkowitz RJ, Hausdorff WP, Caron MG. Role of phosphorylation in desensitisation of the beta-adrenoceptor. *Trends Pharmacol Sci* 1990; 11:190–194.

Lohse MJ. Molecular mechanisms of membrane receptor desensitisation. *Biochim et Biophys Acta* 1993; 1179:171–188.

Lohse MJ, Lefkowitz RJ, Caron MG, Benovic JL. Inhibition of beta-adrenergic receptor kinase prevents rapid homologous desensitization of beta 2-adrenergic receptors. *Proc Natl Acad Sci USA* 1989; 86:3011–3015.

Lohse MJ, Benovic JL, Codina J, Lefkowitz RJ. β-Arrestin: a protein that regulates β-adrenergic receptor function. *Science* 1990; 248:1547–1550.

Mao JR, Price, DD, Mayer DJ. Mechanisms of hyperalgesia and morphine tolerance—a current view of their possible interactions. *Pain* 1995; 62:259–274.

Meriney SD, Gray DB, Pilar GR. Somatostatin-induced inhibition of neuronal calcium current modulated by cGMP-dependent protein kinase. *Nature* 1994; 369:336–339.

Mestek A, Hurley JH, Bye LS, et al. The human mu opioid receptor: modulation of functional desensitization by calcium/calmodulin-dependent protein kinase and protein kinase C. *J Neurosci* 1995; 15:2396–2406.

Mochly-Rosen D. Localization of protein kinases by anchoring proteins: a theme in signal transduction. *Science* 1995; 268:247–251.

Morikawa H, Fukuda K, Mima H, et al. Desensitization and resensitization of δ-opioid receptor-mediated Ca^{2+} channel inhibition in NG108-15 cells. *Br J Pharmacol* 1998; 123:1111–1118.

Mundell SJ, Kelly E. Evidence for co-expression and desensitization of A2a and A2b adenosine receptors in NG108-15 cells. *Biochem Pharmacol* 1998a; 55:595–603.

Mundell SJ, Kelly E. The effect of inhibitors of receptor internalization on the desensitization and resensitization of three G(s)-coupled receptor responses. *Br J Pharmacol* 1998b; 125:1594–1600.

Mundell SJ, Benovic JL, Kelly E. A dominant negative mutant of the G protein-coupled receptor kinase 2 selectively attenuates adenosine A2 receptor desensitization. *Mol Pharmacol* 1997; 51:991–998.

Mundell SJ, Luty JS, Willets J, Benovic JL, Kelly E. Enhanced expression of G protein-coupled receptor kinase 2 selectively increases the sensitivity of A2A adenosine receptors to agonist-induced desensitization. *Br J Pharmacol* 1998; 125:347–356.

Murray SR, Evans CJ, von Zastrow M. Phosphorylation is not required for dynamin-dependent endocytosis of a truncated mutant opioid receptor. *J Biol Chem* 1998; 273:24987–24991.

Narita M, Narita M, Mizoguchi H, Tseng LF. Inhibition of protein kinase C but not protein kinase A blocks the development of acute antinociceptive tolerance to an intrathecally administered μ-opioid receptor agonist in the mouse. *Eur J Pharmacol* 1995; 280:R1–R3.

Nestler EJ, Tallman JF. Chronic morphine treatment increases cyclic AMP-dependent protein kinase activity in the rat locus coeruleus. *Mol Pharmacol* 1988; 33:1127–1132.

Nestler EJ, Erdos JJ, Terwilliger R, Duman RS, Tallman JF. Regulation of G proteins by chronic morphine in the rat locus coeruleus. *Brain Res* 1989; 476:230–239.

Noble F, Cox BM. Differential desensitization of mu- and delta-opioid receptors in selected neural pathways following chronic morphine treatment. *Br J Pharmacol* 1996; 117:161–169.

North RA. Opioid actions on membrane ion channels. In: *Opioids 1. Handb Exp Pharm* 1993; 104/1 Ed Herz:773–792.

North RA, Williams JT, Surprenant A, Christie MJ. Mu-receptor and delta-receptor belong to a family of receptors that are coupled to potassium channels. *Proc Natl Acad Sci USA* 1987; 84:5487–5491.

Ozcelebi F, Holtmann MH, Rentsch RU, Rao R, Miller LJ. Agonist stimulated phosphorylation of the carboxyl terminal tail of the secretin receptor. *Mol Pharmacol* 1995; 48:818–824.

Pak Y, Kouvelas A, Scheideler MA, et al. Agonist-induced functional desensitization of the mu-opioid receptor is mediated by loss of membrane receptors rather than uncoupling from G protein. *Mol Pharmacol* 1996; 50:1214–1222.

Palczewski K. GTP-binding-protein-coupled receptor kinases—two mechanistic models. *Eur J Biochem* 1997; 248:261–269.

Palczewski K, Benovic JL. G-protein-coupled receptor kinases. *Trends Biochem Sci* 1991; 16:387–391.

Pei G, Kieffer BL, Lefkowitz RJ, Freedman NJ. Agonist-dependent phosphorylation of the mouse delta-opioid receptor: involvement of G protein-coupled receptor kinases but not protein kinase C. *Mol Pharmacol* 1995; 48:173–177.

Pippig S, Andexinger S, Lohse MJ. Sequestration and recycling of β_2-adrenergic receptors permit receptor resensitisation. *Mol Pharmacol* 1995; 47:666–676.

Pitcher J, Touhara K, Payne ES, Lefkowitz RJ. Pleckstrin homology domain-mediated membrane association and activation requires co-ordinate interaction with Gβγ and lipid. *J Biol Chem* 1995; 270:11707–11710.

Polakiewicz RD, Schieferl SM, Dorner LF, Kansra V, Comb MJ. A mitogen-activated protein kinase pathway is required for mu-opioid receptor desensitization. *J Biol Chem* 1998; 273:12402–12406.

Premont RT, Koch WJ, Inglese J, Lefkowitz RJ. Identification, purification and characterisation of GRK5, a member of the family of G-protein coupled receptor kinases. *J Biol Chem* 1994; 269:6832–6841.

Premont RT, Macrae AD, Stoffel RH, et al. Characterisation of the G-protein -coupled receptor kinase GRK4. Identification of four splice variants. *J Biol Chem* 1996; 271:6403–6410.

Rao RV, Roetgger BF, Hadac EM, Miller LJ. Roles of cholecystokinin receptor phosphorylation in agonist-stimulated desensitization of pancreatic acinar cells and receptor-bearing Chinese hamster ovary cholecystokinin receptor cells. *Mol Pharmacol* 1997; 51:185–192.

Raynor K, Kong H, Hines J, et al. Molecular mechanisms of agonist-induced desensitization of the cloned mouse kappa opioid receptor. *J Pharmacol Exp Ther* 1994; 270:1381–1386.

Robinson MS. The role of clathrin, adaptors and dynamin in endocytosis. *Curr Opin Cell Biol* 1994; 6:538–544.

Roetgger BF, Rentsch RU, Pinon D, et al. Dual pathways of internalization of the cholecystokinin receptor. *J Cell Biol* 1995; 128:1029–1041.

Segredo V, Burford NT, Lameh J, Sadee W. A constitutively internalizing and recycling mutant of the mu-opioid receptor. *J Neurochem* 1997; 68:2395–2404.

Sibley DR, Daniel K, Strader CD, Lefkowitz RJ. Phosphorylation of the beta-adrenergic receptor in intact cells: relationship to heterologous and homologous mechanisms of adenylate cyclase desensitization. *Arch Biochem Biophys* 1987; 258:24–32.

Sternini C, Spann M, Anton B, et al. Agonist selective endocytosis of mu opioid receptor by neurons in vivo. *Proc Natl Acad Sci USA* 1996; 93:9241–9246.

Stevens CW, Yaksh TL. Potency of infused spinal antinociceptive agents is inversely related to magnitude of tolerance after continuous infusion. *J Pharmacol Exp Ther* 1989a; 250:1–8.

Stevens CW, Yaksh TL. Time course characteristics of tolerance development to continuously infused antinociceptive agents in rat spinal cord. *J Pharmacol Exp Ther* 1989b; 251:216–223.

Strulovici B, Cerione RA, Kilpatrick BF, Caron MG, Lefkowitz RJ. Direct demonstration of impaired functionality of a purified desensitized beta-adrenergic receptor in a reconstituted system. *Science* 1984; 225:837–840.

Terwilliger RZ, Beitner-Johnson D, Sevarino KA, Crain SM, Nestler EJ. A general role for adaptations in G-proteins and the cyclic AMP system in mediating the chronic actions of morphine and cocaine on neuronal function. *Brain Res* 1991; 548:100–110.

Terwilliger RZ, Orti, J, Guitart X, Nestler, EJ. Chronic morphine administration increases β-adrenergic kinase (βARK) levels in rat locus coeruleus. *J Neurochem* 1994; 63:1983–1986.

Tholanikunnel BG, Granneman JG, Malbon CC. The M(R)-35,000 beta-adrenergic-receptor messenger-RNA-binding protein binds transcripts of G-protein-linked receptors which undergo agonist-induced destabilization. *J Biol Chem* 1995; 270:12787–12793.

Tobin AB, Totty NF, Sterlin AE, Nahorski SR. Stimulus-dependent phosphorylation of G-protein coupled receptors by casein kinase 1α. *J Biol Chem* 1997; 269:32522–32527.

Trapaidze N, Keith DE, Cvejic S, Evans CJ, Devi LA. Sequestration of the delta opioid receptor. Role of the C terminus in agonist-mediated internalization. *J Biol Chem* 1996; 271(46):29279–29285.

Tsuga H, Kameyama K, Haga T. Desensitization of human muscarinic acetylcholine receptor m2 subtypes is caused by their sequestration/internalization. *J Biochem* 1998; 124:863–868.

Ueda H, Miyamae T, Hayashi C, et al. Protein kinase C involvement in homologous desensitization of δ-opioid receptor coupled to Gi1-phospholipase C activation in Xenopus oocytes. *J Neurosci* 1995; 15:7485–7499.

Valiquette M, Bonnin H, Hnatowich M. Involvement of tyrosine residues located in the carboxyl tail of the $β_2$-adrenergic receptor in agonist-induced down-regulation of the receptor. *Proc Natl Acad Sci USA* 1990; 87:5089–5093.

von Zastrow M, Kobilka BK. Agonist-dependent and -independent steps in the mechanism of adrenergic receptor internalization. *J Biol Chem* 1994; 269:18448–18452

von Zastrow M, Keith DE Jr, Evans CJ. Agonist-induced state of the delta-opioid receptor that discriminates between opioid peptides and opiate alkaloids. *Mol Pharmacol* 1993; 44:166–172.

Whistler JL, von Zastrow M. Morphine-activated opioid receptors elude desensitization by beta-arrestin. *Proc Natl Acad Sci USA* 1998; 95:9914–9919.

Yabaluri N, Medzihradsky F. Down-regulation of mu-opioid receptor by full but not partial agonists is independent of G protein coupling. *Mol Pharmacol* 1997; 52:896–902.

Yu YK, Zhang L, Yin XX, et al. Mu opioid receptor phosphorylation, desensitization, and ligand efficacy. *J Biol Chem* 1997; 272:28869– 28874.

Zadina JE, Chang SL, Ge LJ, Kastin AJ. Mu opiate receptor downregulation by morphine and upregulation by naloxone in SH-SY5Y human neuroblastoma cells. *J Pharm Exp Ther* 1992; 265:254–262.

Zhang J, Ferguson SSG, Barak LS, Menard L, Caron MG. Dynamin and b-arrestin reveal distinct mechanisms for G protein-coupled receptor internalisation. *J Biol Chem* 1996; 271:18302–18305.

Zhang J, Ferguson SSG, Barak LS, et al. Role for G protein-coupled receptor kinase in agonist-specific regulation of μ-opioid receptor responsiveness. *Proc Natl Acad Sci USA* 1998; 95:7157–7162.

Zhu JM, Luo LY, Mao GF, Ashby B, LiuChen LY. Agonist induced desensitization and downregulation of the human kappa opioid receptor expressed in Chinese hamster ovary cells. *J Pharmacol Exp Ther* 1998; 285:28–36.

Correspondence to: Professor Graeme Henderson, Department of Pharmacology, School of Medical Sciences, University Walk, Bristol BS8 1TD, United Kingdom. Tel: 44-117-928-7630; Fax: 44-117-925-0168; email: graeme.henderson@bris.ac.uk.

Opioid Sensitivity of Chronic Noncancer Pain,
Progress in Pain Research and Management,
Vol. 14, edited by Eija Kalso, Henry J. McQuay,
and Zsuzsanna Wiesenfeld-Hallin, IASP Press,
Seattle, © 1999.

5

Modulation of Opioid Analgesia: Tolerance and Beyond

Gavril W. Pasternak

Cotzias Laboratory of Neuro-Oncology, Memorial Sloan-Kettering Cancer Center, New York, New York, USA

The problem of pain transcends all the boundaries of medical specialties. Although many classes of drugs have been developed to treat pain, the opioids remain the mainstay for managing severe pain (Reisine and Pasternak 1996). Opioids activate pain modulatory systems by mimicking the actions of the endogenous opioid peptides in the central nervous system (Table I). The major peptides are [Met^5]- and [Leu^5]enkephalins, β-endorphin, and dynorphin A, all of which share the same initial pentapeptide sequence as the enkephalins: Tyr-Gly-Gly-Phe-Met or Tyr-Gly-Gly-Phe-Leu. Despite their similar structures, these peptides are generated from three different gene products that are processed to yield numerous active compounds with widely varied binding profiles. Many synthetic peptides have been developed that are far more stable and selective for the various receptor classes.

The opioid peptides work by activating specific receptors (Table II). These opioid receptors comprise a family of related G-protein-coupled receptors, which initiate intracellular cascades through the activation of trimeric G proteins. Three major classes of opioid receptors have been proposed on the basis of detailed pharmacological studies. Morphine and related compounds act through μ receptors. Dynorphin A is the endogenous ligand for the κ receptors, which were initially defined by the pharmacological structure of a series of benzomorphans. Finally, the enkephalins led to the identification of the δ receptors. All three families have well defined and distinct binding profiles. Their regional distributions within the brain also vary. They are distinct members of a complex system designed to modulate the perception of pain.

Pain perception varies widely, both among individuals and according to the circumstances under which the pain occurs. Many factors play a role.

Table I
Opioids and related peptides

[Leu⁵]enkephalin	**Tyr-Gly-Gly-Phe-Leu**
[Met⁵]enkephalin	**Tyr-Gly-Gly-Phe**-Met
Dynorphin A	**Tyr-Gly-Gly-Phe-Leu**-Arg-Arg-Ile-Arg-Pro-Lys-Leu-Lys-Trp-Asp-Asn-Gln
Dynorphin B	**Tyr-Gly-Gly-Phe-Leu**-Arg-Arg-Gln-Phe-Lys-Val-Val-Thr
α-Neoendorphin	**Tyr-Gly-Gly-Phe-Leu**-Arg-Lys-Tyr-Pro-Lys
β-Neoendorphin	**Tyr-Gly-Gly-Phe-Leu**-Arg-Lys-Tyr-Pro
β$_h$-Endorphin	**Tyr-Gly-Gly-Phe-Met**-Thr-Ser-Glu-Lys-Ser-Gln-Thr-Pro-Leu-Val-Thr-Leu-Phe-Lys-Asn-Ala-Ile-Ile-Lys-Asn-Ala-Tyr-Lys-Lys-Gly-Glu
Endomorphin-1	Tyr-Pro-Trp-Phe-NH₂
Endomorphin-2	Tyr-Pro-Phe-Phe-NH₂
Orphanin FQ/nociceptin	**Phe-Gly-Gly-Phe**-Thr-Gly-Ala-Arg-Lys-Ser-Ala-Arg Lys-Leu-Ala-Asp-Glu

The opioid systems, with their profound ability to eliminate pain-related suffering, have been the most intensively studied. However, nonopioid systems also play a major role in shaping pain sensations. Some can enhance the actions of opioids, as demonstrated by the wide use of adjuvant drugs with opioids in the clinical management of pain. Others have actions opposing those of the opioids, leading to increased pain sensitivity. Understanding both of these systems is important for the successful management of pain.

THE ANTI-OPIOID SIGMA SYSTEMS

Anti-opioid systems can act directly on pain perception or by limiting the actions of opioids. These systems include cholecystokinin, neuropeptide FF, σ receptors, and most recently, orphanin FQ/nociceptin. Of these, the σ system is particularly interesting. The σ receptor was originally thought to be a member of the opioid family, but over the years it has become quite clear that it does not belong within this receptor family (Walker et al. 1990; Quirion et al. 1992). In contrast to (–)pentazocine, which is a potent opioid analgesic, (+)pentazocine has little appreciable affinity for any of the opioid receptors. However, (+)pentazocine labels σ receptors very avidly. Despite its inability to bind to opioid receptors, (+)pentazocine dose-dependently reverses opioid analgesia (Chien and Pasternak 1993, 1994). This action is

Table II
Opioid receptor classification and localization of analgesic actions

Receptor	Ligands	Clone	Actions
μ	Morphine	MOR1	Supraspinal/spinal analgesia
$μ_1$			Prolactin release, cetylcholine release, feeding
$μ_2$			Spinal analgesia, respiratory depression, gastrointestinal transit, dopamine release, guinea pig ileum bioassay, feeding
M6G	M6G		Spinal/supraspinal analgesia
κ	Dynorphin A		Psychotomimesis, sedation
$κ_1$	U50,488H	KOR1	Spinal/supraspinal analgesia, diuresis, feeding
$κ_3$	NalBzoH	ORL1/KOR3?	Supraspinal analgesia
δ	Enkephalins		Mouse vas deferens bioassay, dopamine turnover in the striatum, feeding
$δ_1$			Supraspinal analgesia
$δ_2$		DOR1	Spinal/supraspinal analgesia
ORL1	OFQ/ nociceptin	ORL1/KOR3	Supraspinal hyperalgesia (low doses), supraspinal anti-opioid analgesic activity, spinal/ supraspinal analgesia (high doses)

Note: Some of the actions attributed to a general family of receptor have not yet been associated with a specific subtype. All the correlations in this table are based on animal studies, which can show species differences. M6G = morphine-6 β-glucuronide; NalBzoH = naloxone benzoylhydrazone.

antagonized by haloperidol, which blocks σ receptors as potently as it blocks dopamine D2 receptors. The antiopioid actions of the σ system appear to be restricted to analgesia, since (+)pentazocine has no effect upon the inhibition of gastrointestinal transit induced by morphine.

The σ receptor has been cloned from several species, including the mouse (Hanner et al. 1996; Kekuda et al. 1996; Seth et al. 1997, 1998; Pan et al. 1998b). Structurally, it does not resemble any of the known receptor families, and its molecular actions are still unknown. However, cloning of the receptor has enabled researchers to employ antisense methodologies to clearly document its role in anti-opioid actions (Wagner 1994; Wahlestedt 1994; Crooke 1995; Pasternak and Standifer 1995). Short sequences of DNA complimentary to a region of the σ-receptor mRNA bind tightly to the mRNA. This binding destabilizes the mRNA, leading to its degradation and thus to the reduction of receptor levels. The selectivity of this approach far exceeds that of traditional antagonists. Minor changes in the base sequence eliminate the ability of the antisense to modify receptor function. Antisense probes targeting the cloned σ receptor have actions similar to those produced by σ antagonists, confirming at the molecular level the role of the σ receptors in these actions (Pan et al. 1998b).

The σ-receptor system displays tonic activity in animal models, as demonstrated by the ability of a σ antagonist alone to potentiate the analgesic actions of opioids (Chien and Pasternak 1993, 1994). Although morphine analgesia was enhanced by a σ antagonist, the most dramatic effects were observed with κ-opioid drugs. An intriguing aspect of this system is the variability in the levels of σ activity among several strains of mice. Genetically defined differences in analgesic sensitivity among mouse strains has been documented for many years. In some situations, these differences result from variations in the tonic activity of σ systems. For example, BALB-C mice are relatively insensitive to κ analgesics compared to CD-1 mice (Pick et al. 1991). However, these differences in analgesic sensitivity are lost when the two strains are also given a σ antagonist (Chien and Pasternak 1994). Since σ systems can modulate the genetic sensitivity to pain in animal models, it will be interesting to see whether similar situations exist clinically.

ORPHANIN FQ/NOCICEPTIN

The cloning of the opioid receptors quickly uncovered another member of the opioid receptor family, ORL1/KOR3 (Bunzow et al. 1994; Chen et al. 1994; Fukuda et al. 1994; Keith et al. 1994; Mollereau et al. 1994; Pan et al. 1994, 1995). Although structurally homologous to the other cloned opioid receptors, traditional opioids and opioid peptides have very poor affinity for this receptor. The endogenous ligand for the new receptor was identified by two groups and termed orphanin FQ (Reinscheid et al. 1995) or nociceptin (Meunier et al. 1995) (OFQ/N). OFQ/N is a heptadecapeptide that has some structural similarities to dynorphin A (Table II). However, OFQ/N does not label any of the traditional opioid receptors, but acts through a different and unique receptor system.

OFQ/N has a complex pharmacology. Initial reports indicated that it was hyperalgesic (Meunier et al. 1995; Reinscheid et al. 1995). These were soon followed by studies demonstrating the ability of low doses of OFQ/N to reverse the analgesic actions of opioids, despite its inability to label opioid receptors (Grisel et al. 1996; Mogil et al. 1996a,b; Heinricher et al. 1997; King et al. 1998a). However, higher OFQ/N doses are analgesic (Rossi et al. 1996a, 1997; King et al. 1997; Tian et al. 1997; Yamamoto et al. 1997; Hao et al. 1998). The importance of the anti-opioid OFQ/N actions in a clinical setting are unknown, but antagonists would be interesting therapeutic targets.

TOLERANCE

Tolerance is perhaps the most widely recognized modulation of opioid action (Reisine and Pasternak 1996). Repeated opioid administration leads to a gradual decrease in the effectiveness of the drug, requiring increasing doses to maintain an effect. Tolerance almost certainly results from many factors combined. Changes have been observed at the receptor and the cell, but some of the most intriguing observations have been made regarding the role of interacting neuronal circuits.

N-Methyl-D-aspartate (NMDA)/nitric oxide cascade (Fig. 1) has been implicated in the production of morphine tolerance. Initial studies examined the noncompetitive NMDA antagonist MK801 (Trujillo and Akil 1991; Ben-Eliyahu et al. 1992), which prevented morphine tolerance without interfering with the drug's analgesic actions. These observations have now been extended to a series of noncompetitive and competitive NMDA antagonists (Trujillo and Akil 1991; Ben-Eliyahu et al. 1992; Inturrisi 1994; Pasternak et al. 1995; Bilsky et al. 1996; Kest et al. 1997). Even agents acting at the glycine site have been reported to effectively block morphine tolerance (Kolesnikov et al. 1994). Tolerance also develops to enkephalins acting through δ receptors. As in the case of morphine, tolerance to δ analgesics also is blocked by NMDA antagonists, but κ tolerance is not affected (Elliott et al. 1994).

In many systems, activation of NMDA receptors leads to the generation of nitric oxide (NO) through the activity of neuronal nitric oxide synthase (nNOS) (Snyder and Bredt 1991; Bredt and Snyder 1992). As expected, inhibitors of nNOS block morphine tolerance (Kolesnikov et al. 1992, 1993; Babey et al. 1994; Inturrisi 1994; Bhargava and Zhao 1996). There are

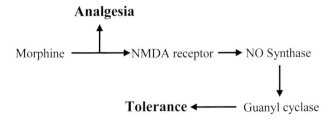

Fig. 1. Schematic of the N-methyl D-aspartate (NMDA)/nitric oxide (NO) cascade.

several NOS isoforms, and the enzymatic inhibitors are not very selective. Antisense approaches have confirmed the importance of nNOS in these actions (Kolesnikov et al. 1997). A number of probes targeting various regions of the nNOS mRNA all prevented morphine tolerance. However, the antisense studies also led to an interesting observation regarding a minor isoform of nNOS that lacks two exons present in the major isoform. Unlike the major isoform of nNOS, which diminishes morphine analgesia through the production of tolerance, the minor isoform enhances morphine analgesia. Selectively downregulating the minor isoform leads to a reduction in morphine analgesia. Thus, NO has opposing roles on opioid analgesia that are mediated through different isoforms of the enzyme by which it is generated.

NMDA receptors and NOS offer two potentially useful therapeutic targets. By minimizing tolerance, it may be possible to maintain clinical pain relief with fewer side effects. However, most NMDA antagonists have a number of side effects that limit their clinical utility, including dysphorias and psychotomimetic effects. NOS inhibitors also have limited clinical potential because NO affects other systems, particularly the vascular system. More selective agents might overcome these difficulties.

Genetic factors also affect tolerance, as illustrated by a recent report that documents lack of morphine tolerance in a strain of mice (Kolesnikov et al. 1998). Aguti 129/SvEv mice display a normal sensitivity to morphine, but with repeated dosing, they do not develop the tolerance seen in other strains. The authors activated the NMDA/NOS cascade at several points to determine where the problem lay. Nitroprusside and L-arginine both lowered morphine analgesia in both 129/SvEv and control CD-1 mice. Nitroprusside is a NO donor, which implies that the target for NO and the remainder of the downstream pathway were intact. L-Arginine is the substrate for NO synthase, and its activity in the 129/SvEv mice indicated that the problem may lie upstream from NO synthase. In contrast to CD-1 mice, NMDA did not affect morphine analgesia in the 129/SvEv mice. This suggests that the defect in the pathway is at either the NMDA receptor itself or at a step in between the NMDA receptor and NOS. This lack of tolerance in 129/SvEv mice is quite unusual, and it is not clear whether it has any clinical significance. However, it further underscores the wide variability of responses that may be genetically determined.

Delta-opioid systems also are important in morphine tolerance, although their relationship to the NMDA/NOS cascade is not clear. Early studies indicated that the δ-selective antagonist naltrindole could block morphine tolerance without interfering with morphine analgesia (Abdelhamid et al. 1991; Fundytus et al. 1994; Hepburn et al. 1997). The importance of δ receptors was further established by the blockade of morphine tolerance by an antisense probe targeting the δ receptor encoded by DOR1 (Kest et al. 1996). The definitive confirmation the role of the δ system came from studies with knockout mice lacking either enkephalins or DOR1 (King et al. 1998b). After repeated daily administration of morphine, neither strain of mouse developed tolerance. Thus, the pathways responsible for morphine tolerance are quite complex, offering many potential therapeutic targets.

INCOMPLETE CROSS-TOLERANCE

Tolerance can develop with chronic opioid use, and although it can be overcome by escalating the drug dosage, side effects often become more troublesome. To avoid this problem, clinicians typically will switch the patient to another opioid analgesics. Over the years, it has become increasingly obvious that various opioids show incomplete cross-tolerance, including drugs thought to be relatively μ selective. Why should drugs that supposedly act through the same receptor show incomplete cross-tolerance? The possibility of more than one subtype of μ receptor might explain these observations. Early studies using several antagonists suggested two pharmacologically distinct μ-receptor subtypes (Pasternak et al. 1980a,b; Wolozin and Pasternak 1981; Pasternak 1993). More recently, a third μ-receptor subtype has been proposed to explain the actions of the potent morphine metabolite morphine-6 β-glucuronide (M6G) (Paul et al. 1989; Pasternak and Standifer 1995; Rossi et al. 1995a,b, 1996b; Chang et al. 1998). The actions of M6G are particularly interesting. Although considered a μ analgesic, M6G does not show cross-tolerance to morphine in some animal paradigms. Furthermore, the drug retains its analgesic actions in CXBK mice, a strain that is not sensitive to morphine. Other μ analgesics also retain analgesic actions in such mice, including fentanyl, methadone, 6-acetylmorphine, and heroin. Clearly, these drugs do not act via the same mechanisms as morphine.

The recent explosion in molecular biology has transformed the opioid field. Cloning studies have isolated cDNAs encoding μ (MOR1), $κ_1$ (KOR1), and δ (DOR1) receptors (Reisine and Bell 1993; Kieffer 1995; Knapp et al. 1995). Expression of these receptors reveals binding selectivities very similar to those previously observed in brain tissues, and antisense approaches have established their pharmacological relevance. The μ receptor has been most extensively examined. Antisense studies have implicated MOR1 in morphine analgesia in both rats and mice (Rossi et al. 1994, 1995). However, antisense mapping studies have revealed some intriguing differences between the two. MOR1 has four exons. Three different antisense probes designed against the first exon effectively lowered morphine analgesia without significantly influencing M6G analgesia (Rossi et al. 1995a,b). Conversely, another three antisense probes based on exon 2 blocked M6G, but not morphine analgesia. Thus, even at the molecular level, there were significant differences between morphine and M6G.

A single gene encoding the μ receptor, MOR1, has been identified (Min et al. 1994; Giros et al. 1995; Mayer et al. 1996). Soon after the initial demonstration of MOR1, two splice variants were reported, which differed at the position of exon 4 (Bare et al. 1994; Zimprich et al. 1995) (Fig. 2); this exon encodes the terminal portion of the intracellular tail of the receptor. More recently, an additional four exons have been described for MOR1, leading to a total of nine exons spanning over 200 kilobases (Pan et al. 1998a, 1999) (Fig. 2). These additional exons encode three more variants, giving a total of six MOR1 splice variants that differ only at the intracellular terminal portion of the receptor. Although all the variants retain μ selectivity as shown by binding assays, there are subtle differences among them. The question remains as to whether these known variants can explain the pharmacologically defined subtypes, or whether additional variants remain to be discovered.

While pharmacological studies suggested the existence of three μ-receptor subtypes, cloning studies have identified six variants of MOR1 that differ only at the terminal portion of the intracellular tail. It seems likely that additional variants with splicing in other regions of the gene will be

MOR 1 Gene Structure

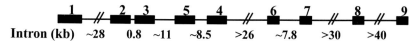

| Intron (kb) | ~28 | 0.8 | ~11 | ~8.5 | >26 | ~7.8 | >30 | >40 |

Alternatively spliced variants

Exon composition

MOR 1 | 1 | 2 | 3 | 4 |
MOR 1A | 1 | 2 | 3 |
MOR 1B | 1 | 2 | 3 | 5 |
MOR 1C | 1 | 2 | 3 | 7 | 8 | 9 |
MOR 1D | 1 | 2 | 3 | 8 | 9 |
MOR 1E | 1 | 2 | 3 | 6 | 7 | 8 | 9 |

Fig. 2. Schematic of the MOR1 gene and splice variants.

uncovered that may help explain the pharmacological differences among the various μ opioids. Although many questions remain, it now seems likely that incomplete cross-tolerance may simply reflect the varying selectivity profile of different μ analgesics for a wide range of μ-receptor splice variants.

CONCLUSION

Opioid systems are quite complex. Although there are only three major families of opioid analgesics, subtypes within these families demonstrate dramatic complexities. Many other systems also modulate opioid actions and analgesia. It remains to be seen whether they represent clinically relevant therapeutic targets in the management of pain.

ACKNOWLEDGMENTS

This work was supported in part by grants from the National Institute on Drug Abuse (DA02615, DA07242, and DA06241) and by a Senior Scientist Award (DA00220).

REFERENCES

Abdelhamid EE, Sultana M, Portoghese PS, Takemori AE. Selective blockage of delta opioid receptors prevents the development of morphine tolerance and dependence in mice. *J Pharmacol Exp Ther* 1991; 258:299–303.

Babey AM, Kolesnikov Y, Cheng J, et al. Nitric oxide and opioid tolerance. *Neuropharmacology* 1994; 33:1463–1470.

Bare LA, Mansson E, Yang D. Expression of two variants of the human μ opioid receptor mRNA in SK-N-SH cells and human brain. *FEBS Lett* 1994; 354:213–216.

Ben-Eliyahu S, Marek P, Vaccarino AL, et al. The NMDA receptor antagonist MK-801 prevents long-lasting non-associative morphine tolerance in the rat. *Brain Res* 1992; 575:304–308.

Bhargava HN, Zhao GM. Effect of nitric oxide synthase inhibition on tolerance to the analgesic action of D-Pen^2, D-Pen^5 enkephalin and morphine in the mouse. *Neuropeptides* 1996; 30:219–223.

Bilsky EJ, Inturrisi CE, Sadée W, Hruby VJ, Porreca F. Competitive and non-competitive NMDA antagonists block the development of antinociceptive tolerance to morphine, but not to selective μ or δ opioid agonists in mice. *Pain* 1996; 68:229–237.

Bredt DS, Snyder SH. Nitric oxide, a novel neuronal messenger. *Neuron* 1992; 8:3–11.

Bunzow JR, Saez C, Mortrud M, et al. Molecular cloning and tissue distribution of a putative member of the rat opioid receptor gene family that is not a μ, δ or kappa opioid receptor type. *FEBS Lett* 1994; 347:284–288.

Chang A, Emmel DW, Rossi GC, Pasternak GW. Methadone analgesia in morphine-insensitive CXBK mice. *Eur J Pharmacol* 1998; 351:189–191.

Chen Y, Fan Y, Liu J, et al. Molecular cloning, tissue distribution and chromosomal localization of a novel member of the opioid receptor gene family. *FEBS Lett* 1994; 347:279–283.

Chien C-C, Pasternak GW. Functional antagonism of morphine analgesia by (+)-pentazocine: Evidence for an anti-opioid σ_1 system. *Eur J Pharmacol* 1993; 250:R7–R8.

Chien C-C, Pasternak GW. Selective antagonism of opioid analgesia by a sigma system. *J Pharmacol Exp Ther* 1994; 271:1583–1590.

Crooke ST. Progress in antisense therapeutics. *Hematol Pathol* 1995; 9:59–72.

Elliott K, Minami N, Kolesnikov YA, Pasternak GW, Inturrisi CE. The NMDA receptor antagonists, LY274614 and MK-801, and the nitric oxide synthase inhibitor, NG-nitro-L-arginine, attenuate analgesic tolerance to the mu-opioid morphine but not to kappa opioids. *Pain* 1994; 56:69–75.

Fukuda K, Kato S, Mori K, et al. cDNA cloning and regional distribution of a novel member of the opioid receptor family. *FEBS Lett* 1994; 343:42–46.

Fundytus ME, Schiller PW, Shapiro M, Weltrowska G, Coderre TJ. The novel and highly selective δ-opioid antagonist TIPP(psi) attenuates morphine tolerance and dependence: comparison with the effects of naltrindole and TIPP. *Regul Pept* 1994; 54:97–98.

Giros B, Pohl M, Rochelle JM, Seldin MF. Chromosomal localization of opioid peptide and receptor genes in the mouse. *Life Sci* 1995; 56:PL369–PL375.

Grisel JE, Mogil JS, Belknap JK, Grandy DK. Orphanin FQ acts as a supraspinal, but not a spinal, anti-opioid peptide. *Neuroreport* 1996; 7:2125–2129.

Hanner M, Moebius FF, Flandorfer A, et al. Purification, molecular cloning, and expression of the mammalian sigma$_1$-binding site. *Proc Natl Acad Sci USA* 1996; 93:8072–8077.

Hao JX, Xu IS, Wiesenfeld-Hallin Z, Xu XJ. Anti-hyperalgesic and anti-allodynic effects of intrathecal nociceptin/orphanin FQ in rats after spinal cord injury, peripheral nerve injury and inflammation. *Pain* 1998; 76:385–393.

Heinricher MM, McGaraughty S, Grandy DK. Circuitry underlying antiopioid actions of orphanin FQ in the rostral ventromedial medulla. *J Neurophysiol* 1997; 78:3351–3358.

Hepburn MJ, Little PJ, Gingras J, Kuhn CM. Differential effects of naltrindole on morphine-induced tolerance and physical dependence in rats. *J Pharmacol Exp Ther* 1997; 281:1350–1356.

Inturrisi CE. NMDA receptors, nitric oxide and opioid tolerance. *Regul Pept* 1994; 54:129–130.

Keith D Jr, Maung T, Anton B, Evans C. Isolation of cDNA clones homologous to opioid receptors. *Regul Pept* 1994; 54:143–144.

Kekuda R, Prasad PD, Fei Y-J, et al. Cloning and functional expression of the human type 1 sigma receptor (hSigmaR1). *Biochem Biophys Res Commun* 1996; 229:553–558.

Kest B, Lee CE, McLemore GL, Inturrisi CE. An antisense oligodeoxynucleotide to the delta opioid receptor (DOR-1) inhibits morphine tolerance and acute dependence in mice. *Brain Res Bull* 1996; 39:185–188.

Kest B, McLemore G, Kao B, Inturrisi CE. The competitive α-amino-3-hydroxy-5-methylisoxazole-4-propionate receptor antagonist LY293558 attenuates and reverses analgesic tolerance to morphine but not to delta or kappa opioids. *J Pharmacol Exp Ther* 1997; 283:1249–1255.

Kieffer BL. Recent advances in molecular recognition and signal transduction of active peptides: receptors for opioid peptides. *Cell Mol Neurobiol* 1995; 15:615–635.

King MA, Rossi GC, Chang AH, Williams L, Pasternak GW. Spinal analgesic activity of orphanin FQ/nociceptin and its fragments. *Neurosci Lett* 1997; 223:113–116.

King M, Chang A, Pasternak GW. Functional blockade of opioid analgesia by orphanin FQ/nociceptin. *Biochem Pharmacol* 1998a; 55:1537–1540.

King MA, Schuller AGP, Zhu J, et al. Requirement of enkephalin/delta receptor systems in morphine tolerance. *Soc Neurosci* 1998b; 24:524.

Knapp RJ, Malatynska E, Collins N, et al. Molecular biology and pharmacology of cloned opioid receptors. *FASEB J* 1995; 9:516–525.

Kolesnikov YA, Pick CG, Pasternak GW. N^G-Nitro-L-arginine prevents morphine tolerance. *Eur J Pharmacol* 1992; 221:339–340.

Kolesnikov YA, Pick CG, Ciszewska G, Pasternak GW. Blockade of tolerance to morphine but not to kappa opioids by a nitric oxide synthase inhibitor. *Proc Natl Acad Sci USA* 1993; 90:5162–5166.

Kolesnikov YA, Maccechini M-L, Pasternak GW. 1-Aminocyclopropane carboxylic acid (ACPC) prevents mu and delta opioid tolerance. *Life Sci* 1994; 55:1393–1398.

Kolesnikov YA, Pan YX, Babey AM, et al. Functionally differentiating two neuronal nitric oxide synthase isoforms through antisense mapping: evidence for opposing NO actions on morphine analgesia and tolerance. *Proc Natl Acad Sci USA* 1997; 94:8220–8225.

Kolesnikov Y, Jain S, Wilson R, Pasternak GW. Lack of morphine and enkephalin tolerance in 129/SvEv mice: evidence for a NMDA receptor defect. *J Pharmacol Exp Ther* 1998; 284:455–459.

Mayer P, Schulzeck S, Kraus J, Zimprich A, Höllt V. Promoter region and alternatively spliced exons of the rat μ-opioid receptor gene. *J Neurochem* 1996; 66:2272–2278.

Meunier JC, Mollereau C, Toll L, et al. Isolation and structure of the endogenous agonist of the opioid receptor like ORL_1 receptor. *Nature* 1995; 377:532–535.

Min BH, Augustin LB, Felsheim RF, Fuchs JA, Loh HH. Genomic structure and analysis of promoter sequence of a mouse μ opioid receptor gene. *Proc Natl Acad Sci USA* 1994; 91:9081–9085.

Mogil JS, Grisel JE, Reinscheid KK, et al. Orphanin FQ is a functional anti-opioid peptide. *Neuroscience* 1996a; 75:333–337.

Mogil JS, Grisel JE, Zhangs G, Belknap JK, Grandy DK. Functional antagonism of μ-, δ- and κ-opioid antinociception by orphanin FQ. *Neurosci Lett* 1996b; 214:1–4.

Mollereau C, Parmentier M, Mailleux P, et al. ORL-1, a novel member of the opioid family: cloning, functional expression and localization. *FEBS Lett* 1994; 341:33–38.

Pan Y-X, Cheng J, Xu J, Pasternak GW. Cloning, expression and classification of a kappa$_3$-related opioid receptor using antisense oligodeoxynucleotides. *Regul Pept* 1994; 54:217–218.

Pan Y-X, Cheng J, Xu J, et al. Cloning and functional characterization through antisense mapping of a kappa$_3$-related opioid receptor. *Mol Pharmacol* 1995; 47:1180–1188.

Pan Y-X, Xu J, Rossi GC, et al. Cloning and expression of a novel splice variant of the mouse mu-opioid receptor (MOR1) gene. *Soc Neurosci* 1998a; 28:524.

Pan Y-X, Mei JF, Xu J, et al. Cloning and characterization of a mouse σ$_1$ receptor. *J Neurochem* 1998b; 70:2279–2285.

Pan Y-X, Xu J, Bolan E, et al. Identification and characterization of three new alternatively spliced mu-opioid receptor isoforms. *Mol Pharmacol* 1999; in press.

Pasternak GW. Pharmacological mechanisms of opioid analgesics. *Clin Neuropharmacol* 1993; 16:1–18.

Pasternak GW, Standifer KM. Mapping of opioid receptors using antisense oligodeoxynucleotides: correlating their molecular biology and pharmacology. *Trends Pharmacol Sci* 1995; 16:344–350.

Pasternak GW, Childers SR, Snyder SH. Naloxazone, long-acting opiate antagonist: effects in intact animals and on opiate receptor binding in vitro. *J Pharmacol Exp Ther* 1980a; 214:455–462.

Pasternak GW, Childers SR, Snyder SH. Opiate analgesia: evidence for mediation by a subpopulation of opiate receptors. *Science* 1980b; 208:514–516.

Pasternak GW, Kolesnikov YA, Babey AM. Perspectives on the N-methyl-D-aspartate nitric oxide cascade and opioid tolerance. *Neuropsychopharmacology* 1995; 13:309–313.

Paul D, Standifer KM, Inturrisi CE, Pasternak GW. Pharmacological characterization of morphine-6β-glucuronide, a very potent morphine metabolite. *J Pharmacol Exp Ther* 1989; 251:477–483.

Pick CG, Cheng J, Paul D, Pasternak GW. Genetic influences in opioid analgesic sensitivity in mice. *Brain Res* 1991; 556:295–298.

Quirion R, Bowen WD, Itzhak Y, et al. A proposal for the classification of sigma binding sites. *Trends Pharmacol Sci* 1992; 13:85–86.

Reinscheid RK, Nothacker HP, Bourson A, et al. Orphanin FQ: a neuropeptide that activates an opioidlike G protein-coupled receptor. *Science* 1995; 270:792–794.

Reisine T, Bell GI. Molecular biology of opioid receptors. *Trends Neurosci* 1993; 16:506–510.

Reisine T, Pasternak GW. Opioid analgesics and antagonists. In: Hardman JG, Limbird LE (Eds). Goodman and Gilman's *The Pharmacological Basis of Therapeutics*. McGraw-Hill, 1996, pp 521–556.

Rossi GC, Pan Y-X, Cheng J, Pasternak GW. Blockade of morphine analgesia by an antisense oligodeoxynucleotide against the mu receptor. *Life Sci* 1994; 54:PL375–379.

Rossi GC, Standifer KM, Pasternak GW. Differential blockade of morphine and morphine-6β-glucuronide analgesia by antisense oligodeoxynucleotides directed against MOR-1 and G-protein α subunits in rats. *Neurosci Lett* 1995a; 198:99–102.

Rossi GC, Pan Y-X, Brown GP, Pasternak GW. Antisense mapping the MOR-1 opioid receptor: Evidence for alternative splicing and a novel morphine-6β-glucuronide receptor. *FEBS Lett* 1995b; 369:192–196.

Rossi GC, Leventhal L, Pasternak GW. Naloxone-sensitive orphanin FQ-induced analgesia in mice. *Eur J Pharmacol* 1996a; 311:R7–R8.

Rossi GC, Brown GP, Leventhal L, Yang K, Pasternak GW. Novel receptor mechanisms for heroin and morphine-6β-glucuronide analgesia. *Neurosci Lett* 1996b; 216:1–4.

Rossi G, Leventhal L, Boland E, Pasternak GW. Pharmacological characterization of orphanin FQ/nociceptin and its fragments. *J Pharmacol Exp Ther* 1997; 282:858–865.

Seth P, Leibach FH, Ganapathy V. Cloning and structural analysis of the cDNA and the gene encoding the murine type 1 sigma receptor. *Biochem Biophys Res Commun* 1997; 241:535–540.

Seth P, Fei YJ, Li HW, et al. Cloning and functional characterization of a σ receptor from rat brain. *J Neurochem* 1998; 70:922–931.

Snyder SH, Bredt DS. Nitric oxide as a neuronal messenger. *Trends Pharmacol Sci* 1991; 12:125–128.

Tian JH, Xu W, Fang Y, et al. Bidirectional modulatory effect of orphanin FQ on morphine-induced analgesia: antagonism in brain and potentiation in spinal cord of the rat. *Br J Pharmacol* 1997; 120:676–680.

Trujillo KA, Akil H. Inhibition of morphine tolerance and dependence by the NMDA receptor antagonist MK-801. *Science* 1991; 251:85–87.

Wagner RW. Gene inhibition using antisense oligodeoxynucleotides. *Nature* 1994; 372:333–335.

Wahlestedt C. Antisense oligonucleotide strategies in neuropharmacology. *Trends Pharmacol Sci* 1994; 15:42–46.

Walker JM, Bowen WD, Walker FO, et al. Sigma receptors: biology and function. *Pharmacol Rev* 1990; 42:355–402.

Wolozin BL, Pasternak GW. Classification of multiple morphine and enkephalin binding sites in the central nervous system. *Proc Natl Acad Sci USA* 1981; 78:6181–6185.

Yamamoto T, Nozaki-Taguchi N, Kimura S. Analgesic effect of intrathecally administered nociceptin, an opioid receptor-like$_1$ receptor agonist, in the rat formalin test. *Neuroscience* 1997; 81:249–254.

Zimprich A, Simon T, Hollt V. Cloning and expression of an isoform of the rat μ opioid receptor (rMOR 1 B) which differs in agonist induced desensitization from rMOR1. *FEBS Lett* 1995; 359:142–146.

Correspondence to: Gavril W. Pasternak, MD, PhD, Department of Neurology, Memorial Sloan-Kettering Cancer Center, 1275 York Avenue, New York, New York 10021, USA. Tel: 212-639-7046; Fax: 212-794-4332; e-mail: pasterng@mskmail.mskcc.org.

Part II

Clinical Pharmacology
of Opioids—
Relevant Aspects

Opioid Sensitivity of Chronic Noncancer Pain,
Progress in Pain Research and Management,
Vol. 14, edited by Eija Kalso, Henry J. McQuay,
and Zsuzsanna Wiesenfeld-Hallin, IASP Press,
Seattle, © 1999.

6

Different Opioids—Same Actions?

Geoffrey K. Gourlay

*Pain Management Unit, Flinders Medical Centre, Bedford Park,
South Australia, Australia*

Epidemiological evidence indicates dramatic increases in the amount of morphine and other opioids being prescribed in many countries since the mid 1980s. A significant proportion (40–90%) of current morphine consumption is for chronic noncancer pain (Richards 1995; Clausen 1997). The use of opioids for this indication is controversial. It is acknowledged that opioids are effective in the treatment of predominantly nociceptive pain, and that some neuropathic pains also respond well to opioid therapy (Jadad et al. 1992; Portenoy 1994). Every effort should be made to optimize nonopioid pharmacological and other locally available treatment options, including behavioral modification programs (if available), before contemplating opioid prescription (Gourlay 1994, 1999). Many national chapters of the International Association for the Study of Pain have taken the pragmatic approach of creating guidelines to aid physicians who elect to prescribe opioids in chronic noncancer pain (Schug et al. 1991; Graziotti and Goucke 1997; Maddox et al. 1997). This chapter will not discuss the arguments for and against the prescription of opioids for chronic noncancer pain, but will consider whether there are any differences between the various opioids and to a lesser extent, differences between various formulations of the same opioid that can be prescribed for chronic noncancer pain.

Almost a decade ago, one of the editors of this volume said: "Overall, there is probably more difference between the effects of the same opiate given by different routes than between the effects of the different opiates given by the same route" (McQuay 1991). While this may well have seemed true at that time, new information prompts a re-evaluation of this statement. Specifically, the binding profiles of opioids to the cloned human receptor, actions at other receptors (e.g., the N-methyl D-aspartate [NMDA] receptor), polymorphic drug metabolism, the role of active metabolites, and the influence of hepatic and renal function must be considered in the selection of the appropriate opioid to treat chronic nonmalignant pain.

OPIOID-RECEPTOR BINDING PROFILES

Morphine occupies a unique place in pharmacological history. As we approach the new millennium, morphine is still considered by many practitioners to be the opioid drug of choice, a place it has essentially occupied throughout recorded history. Nevertheless, morphine falls far short of our concepts of an ideal opioid. It remains in favor because we have a detailed knowledge of its pharmacology, which, when applied appropriately, results in pain relief of a high quality. However, there are still gaps in our knowledge of this and many other opioids. Research promises further improvements in the selection of the appropriate opioid for a particular patient.

While the existence of μ-, κ-, and δ-opioid receptors and various subtypes of these receptors has been proposed for some time, it is only relatively recently that molecular biology techniques have enabled the primary amino acid sequence to be determined. Manipulation and substitution of various amino acids have allowed the identification of critical domains, some of which are different between the various receptor types, which accounts for the selectivity in binding of the various opioids. Other regions are highly conserved, which explains how similar effects (for example, analgesia) can be obtained when agonists and antagonists interact with the various receptors (Befort and Kieffer 1997). This information has allowed the development of more comprehensive models to explain tolerance. Further information on these concepts and on the development of "knock-out" animals that are deficient in a receptor or part of a receptor is provided elsewhere in this volume.

Table I provides the binding affinities of a range of opioids to the μ-, κ-, and δ-opioid receptors in the guinea pig and also to the cloned human μ-opioid receptor. Considering the animal data first, it is apparent that many of the commonly prescribed opioids (morphine, levorphanol, methadone, fentanyl, and buprenorphine) bind to all three receptor types, but generally show a marked preference for the μ receptor. Morphine shows the greatest relative preference for the μ receptor. Normorphine, a minor morphine metabolite (3–5% of the dose is converted to normorphine and normorphine-3-glucuronide), also shows a marked preference for the μ receptor. Alternative data sets characterize the binding of opioids to the three different receptor classes in other animal species (Raynor et al. 1994). While the absolute values usually vary, indicating some species difference, the general trend is reasonably consistent.

Table I
Binding affinities (nmol/L) of various opioids to guinea pig
and cloned human opioid receptors; smaller values
indicate a greater binding affinity

	Guinea Pig Receptors			Cloned Human μ Receptor
	δ	κ	μ	
Morphine	90	317	1.8	2.0
Normorphine	310	149	4.0	—
Levorphanol	5.6	9.6	0.6	1.9
Codeine	>10000	—	2700	65
Methadone	15.1	1628	4.2	5.6
Fentanyl	151	470	7.0	1.9
Pethidine	4345	5140	385	—
Pentazocine	106	22.2	7.0	—
Buprenorphine	1.3	2.0	0.6	0.5
Naloxone	27	17.2	1.8	1.4

Note: Data shown in the table were recompiled from Magnan et al. (1982) and Traynor (1996). Alternative data sets (e.g., Raynor et al. 1994) exist for other animal species.

Codeine is characterized by exceedingly poor binding to at least two receptor types. This raises the possibility that, like heroin (Inturrisi et al. 1983), codeine may be a pro-drug (Sindrup et al. 1991; Mikus et al. 1997). Heroin and codeine generate the pharmacologically active compounds 6-monoacetyl-morphine and morphine, respectively; 6-monoacetyl-morphine is further metabolized to morphine. Codeine also shows low relative efficacy at the μ receptor from cloned human neuroblastoma cells (Traynor 1996). Pethidine is considered to be a μ-receptor agonist, although its binding affinity to all three opioid receptor types is not particularly great. Methadone and buprenorphine show significant binding to δ-opioid receptors at a concentration 2–4 times greater than their μ-receptor-binding affinities. In fact, the binding affinity of buprenorphine to the μ receptor is lower than that of naloxone, which explains why the latter drug only partially reverses buprenorphine toxicity. Ketobemidone has a lower affinity for the μ receptor than does morphine, but shows greater discrimination for this receptor compared to the κ receptor. The binding of both opioids to the δ receptor is similar (Christensen 1993). Recently, it has been suggested that the intrinsic nociceptive effects of oxycodone are mediated via κ receptors (Ross and Smith 1997). Interestingly, κ-opioid agonists produce greater analgesia in women than in men (Gear et al. 1996).

The equivalent data from cloned human μ receptors (Raynor et al. 1995; Traynor 1996) shows excellent congruence with the animal data for morphine,

methadone, buprenorphine, and naloxone. Fentanyl and in particular codeine show greater binding affinity to the cloned human receptor compared
to the analogous animal receptors. Thus, for the commonly administered
opioids, the variability in their affinity for the cloned human μ receptor is
not of sufficient magnitude to account for differences in observed pharmacodynamics. However, more significant variability in their physiochemical
characteristics and pharmacokinetic properties controls the rate and amount
of opioid delivered to the receptor and consequently may account for a
significant proportion of the pharmacodynamic variability.

ACTIONS AT OTHER RECEPTOR TYPES

The NMDA-receptor complex is intimately involved in nociceptive processing and the phenomenon of wind-up, as described in detail elsewhere in
this volume. While experimental competitive and noncompetitive NMDA-
receptor antagonists effectively abolish wind-up (Woolf and Thomson 1991;
Coderre et al. 1993), the combination of an opioid and an NMDA-receptor
antagonist provides profound antinociception (Chapman and Dickenson
1992). The problem is that no potent NMDA antagonists are available for
complementary human studies. Nevertheless, some older drugs do have variable NMDA-antagonist activity (Lodge et al. 1994). For example, the antitussive, dextromethorphan, is one of the more potent drugs and demonstrates noncompetitive NMDA-receptor antagonism (Ebert et al. 1995;
Gorman et al. 1997).

Dextromethorphan and other experimental NMDA-receptor antagonists
appear to delay and even reverse the development of tolerance to morphine,
but not to κ agonists (Elliott et al. 1994a,b). Dextromethorphan is metabolized in the liver to dextrorphan via polymorphically expressed cytochrome
P450 isoform 2D6, and is often used for phenotyping purposes (Chen et al.
1990). Dextrorphan also demonstrates NMDA-receptor antagonist activity,
but its profile of pharmacological effects differs from that of dextromethorphan (Szekely et al. 1991). Dextrorphan has no affinity for the μ-, κ-,
or δ-opioid receptor (Raynor et al. 1994).

Methadone is administered as a racemate in most countries. The L-enantiomer shows between 10 (Kristensen et al. 1995) and 30 times (Horng et al.
1976) greater affinity than the D-enantiomer for opioid receptors and is 50
times more potent as an analgesic in humans (Olsen et al. 1977). Thus, it is
generally accepted that the L-enantiomer is the biologically active component at opioid receptors (see below). There are also pharmacokinetic differences between the enantiomers. Methadone is a noncompetitive NMDA-

receptor antagonist with activity equivalent to that of dextromethorphan, but 30 times greater than that of ketobemidone and 50 times greater than that of pethidine (Ebert et al. 1995). Antagonism at the noncompetitive, but not at the competitive site of the NMDA receptor was confirmed, together with similar affinities of both the L- and D-enantiomers for this site (Gorman et al. 1997). The D-enantiomer was also shown to be antinociceptive in the rat formalin test, demonstrating functional in vivo NMDA-receptor antagonist activity (Shimoyama et al. 1997). Thus, concepts surrounding this opioid have changed in recent times. Not long ago, when renewed interest in the different pharmacological effects of drug enantiomers was applied to methadone, consideration was given to the advantages of administering the active L-enantiomer on a regular basis rather than the racemate. However, the current view supports the administration of the racemate, as the L- and D-enantiomers are active at μ-opioid and NMDA receptors, respectively. The pharmacokinetic profile of methadone makes this drug difficult to use for the novice practitioner.

Ketamine is also an NMDA-receptor blocker and acts at a site different from the NMDA recognition site. However, the D-enantiomer has more potent blocking action at the NMDA receptor than does the L-enantiomer (Lodge et al. 1994). Dextropropoxyphene has also recently been shown to be a noncompetitive NMDA-receptor antagonist (Ebert et al. 1998).

Morphine, hydromorphone, codeine, fentanyl, and naltrexone have no NMDA-receptor antagonist activity (Gorman et al. 1997; Ebert et al. 1998), while levorphanol has a very weak blocking action compared to dextromethorphan.

Tramadol is administered as a racemate and has a dual mechanism of action; the D-enantiomer exhibits preferential but weak binding activity at μ receptors and is a more potent inhibitor of serotonin reuptake, while the L-enantiomer is more efficient in blocking noradrenaline uptake (Kovelowski et al. 1998).

PHARMACOKINETIC CONSIDERATIONS AND THE ROLE OF ACTIVE METABOLITES

ABSORPTION

Table II shows selected pharmacokinetic parameters for commonly administered opioids. The oral bioavailability ranges from almost zero for fentanyl to quite high values for methadone and codeine; most opioids fall somewhere between these extremes. It is significant that this pharmacokinetic parameter is the most variable of all parameters for some opioids; for example, for morphine the range varies from 10% to 50% (Gourlay et al. 1986). However, while interpatient variability in morphine bioavailability is high, bioavailability in individual patients is nevertheless reproducible over time (Gourlay et al. 1991). The variability in oral bioavailability for opioid drugs is not a major clinical problem, as pain clinicians have adopted a careful dose titration procedure to achieve an optimal balance between analgesia and side effects. This procedure is essentially a bioassay to determine the effective opioid dose according to the oral bioavailability and analgesia requirements specific to each patient.

The influence of food on oral morphine absorption depends on the type of formulation administered. For example, ingesting food results in an increased area under the curve (AUC) following immediate-release formulations (Gourlay et al. 1989), but has more variable effects with modified-release preparations (Gourlay 1998). We have little information on the influence of food on the absorption of many opioid drugs. Studies in this area are often generated by mandatory testing of new sustained- or modified-release formulations, and often prompt complementary studies with immediate-release formulations. Sustained- and modified-release morphine formulations are now extensively prescribed in chronic noncancer pain and vary in the mechanisms by which they delay the absorption of morphine. These formulations are not necessarily bioequivalent (Gourlay 1998), and practitioners should closely monitor and possibly retitrate patients if they elect to change sustained-release formulations.

Morphine displays chronopharmacokinetic variability; that is, the resultant blood-concentration time profile for the same dose varies depending on the time of day the dose is administered (Barberi-Heyob et al. 1991; Gourlay et al. 1995; Gourlay 1998). Following the administration of immediate-release formulations at steady state, the maximum morphine concentration following the 1400-hour dose was significantly less than that observed following both the 1000- and 1800-hour doses, and essentially similar changes were seen in AUC. Chronopharmacokinetic variability has also been reported with sustained-release formulations in cancer pain patients where the day/night AUC ratio was 1.7 (Barberi-Heyob et al. 1991, Gourlay 1998). The precise mechanism of this effect has not been established but may be related to variability in absorption, because (1) there were no changes in the half-life for morphine for the three doses of immediate-release morphine (according to our best estimate), and (2) there was an apparent congruence (albeit with a lag phase) between the blood-concentration time profiles of morphine and morphine-6-glucuronide (M6G) (Gourlay et al. 1995). This could be important, as chronopharmacokinetic variability for morphine may not match the reported diurnal variation in pain scores (Glynn and Lloyd

1976; Sandrini et al. 1986; Strian et al. 1989). Such chronopharmacokinetic variability has not been reported for other opioids.

Some studies of factors that influence absorption of opioid drugs have obtained interesting results with other means of administration, such as transdermal and rectal routes. The rectal route is frequently used in patients who have difficulty swallowing or have significant vomiting despite optimized anti-emetic therapy. For morphine, various modified-release oral formulations have been administered rectally (Gourlay 1998). Several studies have shown a significantly greater AUC following rectal administration compared to equivalent oral doses (Wilkinson et al. 1992; Darke et al. 1995), probably as a result of partial avoidance of the hepatic first-pass effect. However, the precise anatomical location of the solid dosage form in the rectum is a crucial factor governing the extent of avoidance of hepatic first-pass metabolism. The venous drainage of the upper part of the rectum is directed to the portal system, whereas that of the lower portion is directed to the systemic circulation. Theoretically, the closer the suppository is to the anal sphincter, the greater will be the avoidance of first-pass metabolism (Gourlay 1998). Specific rectal formulations of immediate-release morphine and methadone have been studied (Bruera et al. 1995; Morley and Makin 1998).

Codeine and oxycodone show good oral bioavailability from both immediate- and modified-release formulations. The rectal (Leow et al. 1995) and nasal (Takala et al. 1997) bioavailability of oxycodone was quite variable and averaged approximately 60% and 45%, respectively.

Fentanyl has negligible oral bioavailability, as the drug undergoes N-dealkylation catalyzed by cytochrome P450 isoform 3A4 to form norfentantyl in both the liver and intestines (Mather and Gourlay 1984; Labroo et al. 1997). However, this drug has been successfully administered via the buccal mucosa as a lollipop in pediatric patients (Schechter et al. 1995), and the same technique could be used for the rapid treatment of incident pain in adults. Thus, fentanyl dissolved in saliva that is swallowed can be ignored as the drug has almost zero oral bioavailability. Similarly, heroin has zero oral bioavailability. In addition, fentanyl has desirable physiochemical properties that enable analgesic blood concentrations to be achieved following transdermal administration (Mather and Gourlay 1991; Gourlay 1999). The fentanyl pharmacokinetics from the transdermal formulation (transdermal therapeutic systems fentanyl [TTS-fentanyl]; Duragesic [Janssen]) are characterized by a slow onset, but a long duration of effect of up to 3 days (Gourlay and Mather 1991). A reservoir in the stratum corneum immediately below the patch is established over 12–16 hours once a system is applied, and constant blood fentanyl concentrations are then maintained for up to 3 days. This depot becomes desaturated after system removal, which maintains pain relief while analgesic blood concentrations are being established from a new system. Studies in cancer pain suggest that TTS-fentanyl has similar pain control to MS Contin (controlled-release morphine sulfate [Purdue Frederick]), but a lower incidence of constipation (Ahmedzai et al. 1997).

METABOLISM

There are substantial differences among the various opioids regarding their fate following absorption. The free aliphatic and aromatic hydroxyl groups of opiates undergo conjugation with glucuronic acid, while both N- and O-dealkylations (usually demethylations) are catalyzed by various isoforms of the predominantly hepatic cytochrome P450 (notably 3A4 and 2D6), some of which are polymorphically expressed. Furthermore, there are differences among the opioids in the pharmacological status of the resultant metabolites with respect to pain relief and toxicity.

The terminal half-life for most opioids varies between 2 and 7 hours, the notable exception being methadone, where the extremes are as short as 6 hours and as long as 150 hours (Table II), although most patients will be in a range of 12–60 hours (Plummer et al. 1988). Correspondingly, the clearance of most opioids is high, and hepatic blood flow has a major impact on their rate of elimination. These opioids are frequently grouped together as *flow-limited* opioids. They generally require significant hepatic compromise before their pharmacokinetics are influenced, with the exception of pethidine, where clearance is reduced in patients with cirrhosis (Pond et al. 1981). The clearance of methadone is much lower (Table II) and depends on the amount of functional cytochrome P450 isoform 3A4 in the liver, which means that methadone metabolism can be either stimulated or inhibited by the concurrent administration of other drugs. Methadone is termed a *capacity-limited* opioid.

Table II
Opioid pharmacokinetics and the role of metabolites

Opioid	Terminal Half-life (h)	Clearance (L/min)	Oral Bioavail-ability (%)	Active Metabolites
Morphine	2–4	0.8–1.2	10–50	M6G
Pethidine	3–4	0.6–0.8	30–60	Norpethidine
Methadone	6–150	0.1–0.3	60–90	No
Fentanyl	3–7	0.7–1.5	<2	No
Codeine	3–4	0.6–0.9	60–90	Morphine
Oxycodone	2–6	0.4–1.1	40–130	Oxymorphone
Hydromorphone	2–4	0.4	35–80	No

The metabolic fate of morphine is well known, with the formation of 3- and 6-glucuronides by conjugation as well as normorphine by N-demethylation. Morphine-6-glucuronide (M6G) and to a lesser extent normorphine have intrinsic analgesic activity. The status of morphine-3-glucuronide (M3G) is still controversial, ranging from claims that it is inactive (Hewett et al. 1993) to suggestions that it is a functional antagonist at other receptors (Gong et at. 1992) because it does not bind to opioid receptors (Pasternak et al. 1987). Animal studies have implicated M3G (or more particularly the M3G:morphine molar ratio) in delaying the development of tolerance to morphine (Smith and Smith 1995). The problem is that the ratio of M3G:morphine and M6G:morphine do not vary substantially among various formulations, between single or multiple doses, in most routes of administration (except for intravenous and rectal routes, where the molar ratios are lower, or in the presence of renal disease, where the ratios are higher) (Faura et al. 1998). Thus, we must evoke a combination of unusual partition of the metabolites and quite specialized dose-response relationships for morphine and M3G if the antagonist role of M3G is to have any clinical relevance. Clinical evidence for this role is lacking at the present time.

Heroin (3,6-diacetlymorphine or diamorphine) does not bind to opioid receptors (Inturrisi et al. 1983) and undergoes metabolic activation by successive deacetylations to form 6-monoacetyl-morphine and then morphine. The initial deacetylation is catalyzed by plasma esterase and has a half-life of approximately 2 minutes. While high-quality pain relief is observed after heroin administration, it offers no advantages over other opioids in patients with chronic noncancer pain, where there is always a concern of possible drug-seeking behavior. It does have two advantages in other situations, both related to its physiochemical characteristics: (1) high aqueous solubility, which is a benefit in terminal care patients with high opioid dose requirements (as these can be administered in a small volume of fluid), and (2) rapid dural permeation (because of the greater heroin lipophilicity) but a prolonged analgesic action (as a consequence of deacetylation) following epidural administration. Epidural heroin is mainly used for controlling postoperative pain. The heroin metabolite 6-monoacetyl-morphine appears to behave in a similar manner to morphine in the cerebrospinal fluid.

Codeine is considered to be a pro-drug and undergoes metabolic activation to morphine via hepatic metabolism catalyzed by cytochrome P450 isoform 2D6 (Chen et al. 1988; Desmeules et al. 1991; Poulsen et al. 1996; Eckhardt et al. 1998). One problem is that there is a polymorphic distribution of this isoform in Caucasians; 8–10% of the population lack the capacity to perform this transformation and consequently will not experience analgesia following codeine administration. Furthermore, codeine metabolism could be inhibited in fast metabolizers by the concurrent administration of other drugs metabolized by this isoform (Desmeules et al. 1991). It has been suggested that codeine itself and not the derived morphine is predominantly responsible for the side effects observed following codeine administration (Desmeules et al. 1991; Poulsen et al. 1996; Eckhardt et al. 1998). Thus, poor codeine metabolizers could experience side effects without the benefit of analgesia (Eckhardt et al. 1998). However, even relatively high doses of codeine (60 mg) do not provide particularly impressive analgesia, as this drug shows low relative efficacy at the human μ-opioid receptor (Traynor 1996). For example, an acute-pain study indicated that only 1 in 18 patients reported >50% pain relief compared to the response with placebo (Moore et al. 1997). Codeine is sometimes administered with NSAIDs, where the response is greater. Thus, while high-dose codeine does provide analgesia, uncertainty surrounds the therapeutic response due to variable bioactivation (a consequence of polymorphic metabolism), possible drug interactions, and significant side effects at higher doses. It makes more sense to use opioids with a more predictable outcome. While one possible advantage of poor metabolizers over extensive metabolizers is a lower risk of oral opiate dependency (Tyndale et al. 1997), this is of little benefit if the patient experiences minimal pain relief. The major metabolite is codeine-6-glucuronide, which unlike M6G, would not be expected to have significant analgesic activity, as the 3-phenolic group is methylated and thus would have low affinity for the phenolic binding site on the μ-opioid receptor.

Essentially similar metabolic considerations apply to oxycodone (Otton et al. 1993a), hydrocodone (Otton et al. 1993b), and dihydrocodeine (Fromm et al. 1995), as each undergoes an O-demethylation catalyzed by cytochrome P450 2D6.

Methadone is metabolized by hepatic cytochrome P450 3A4 (Iribarne et al. 1997). The pharmacokinetics of the L- and D-enantiomer show some differences: for example, the terminal half-life is longer, the volume of distribution greater, and the clearance higher for the analgesically active L-enantiomer than for the D-enantiomer (Kristensen et al. 1996). However, there are no differences in oral bioavailability between the enantiomers. There is also stereoselective plasma protein binding to α_1-acid glycoprotein (Eap et al. 1990). As methadone elimination depends on the amount of functional cytochrome P450 3A4 in the hepatocyte, the clearance can be significantly influenced by both environmental factors and concomitantly administered drugs. The anticonvulsants (notably phenytoin) and rifampicin markedly stimulate methadone metabolism (Plummer et al. 1988), while fluconazole (Cobb et al. 1998), human immunodeficiency virus type 1 protease inhibitors (Iribarne et al. 1998), and the new selective serotonin reuptake inhibitors

(SSRIs) such as fluvoxamine (Alderman and Frith 1999) competitively inhibit methadone clearance. Methadone clearance was lower in malignant disease (perhaps due to increased amounts of plasma α_1-acid glycoprotein), but somewhat surprisingly, it was not influenced by tumor activity in the liver. While there is an age-related increase in methadone half-life, there is no sex difference, nor did a history of smoking or alcohol consumption influence the resultant pharmacokinetics (Plummer et al. 1988). The metabolites of methadone are not considered to be pharmacologically active.

Pethidine (meperidine) undergoes significant metabolism and is also excreted unchanged in the urine (Mather and Gourlay 1984). The pKa for pethidine is such that the rate of urinary elimination can be manipulated by consciously altering urinary pH. Norpethidine (normeperidine) is a significant metabolite formed in appreciable quantities by N-demethylation in the liver. Norpethidine accumulates on repeated doses or prolonged infusions as a consequence of a slower clearance (relative to pethidine), especially in patients with renal disease. It is thought that norpethidine produces a gradation of effects in the central nervous system, depending on its concentration in the blood. These effects range from unpleasant feelings to myoclonic jerks and even grand mal seizures. As the blood norpethidine concentration increases, more patients display signs of pethidine-associated neurotoxicity (PAN), and the severity of PAN is greater in sensitive patients. However, there is not a direct relationship between blood norpethidine concentration and PAN in all patients; clearly other, as yet unknown factors influence this relationship. Acute-pain studies indicate that pethidine provides inferior analgesia to morphine (Plummer et al. 1997a). Moreover, pethidine appears to be disproportionately represented in terms of abuse in chronic noncancer patients with pronounced drug-seeking behavior. Staff at the Pain Management Unit at Flinders Medical Centre use the acronym ROPI (Responds Only to Pethidine Injections) to describe patients who indicate that pethidine administered by injection is the only option to relieve their pain. Extreme caution should be exercised in sanctioning the continued administration of any opioid in general and pethidine in particular in such patients. It is commonly believed that pethidine causes less spasm of the sphincter of Oddi and that other biliary effects are more benign with this drug compared to other opioids (Ruskis 1982). However, differences between pethidine and other opioids are only observed at subanalgesic, not at analgesic doses. Thus, pethidine use should be consciously minimized based on its propensity to deliver less analgesia (in some pain models) and its high abuse liability, while it possesses no overt advantages over other opioids. Animal studies indicate that dextromethorphan (but not dextrorphan) potentiates the neurotoxic effects of norpethidine (Plummer et al. 1997b).

Fentanyl is metabolized in the liver by N-dealkylation catalyzed by the 3A4 isoform of cytochrome P450 to form norfentanyl. Other minor routes of metabolism include amide hydrolysis and hydroxylation (Mather and Gourlay 1984; Labroo et al. 1997). The metabolites are believed to be inactive. The 3A4 isoform is also the major determinant of both alfentanil and sufentanil metabolism (Yun et al. 1992; Labroo et al. 1995; Tateishi et al. 1996).

RENAL ELIMINATION

The majority of the metabolites of most opioids are excreted renally following hepatic biotransformation. Consequently, there is a potential for enhanced pharmacological effects following the administration of opioids that have active metabolites (Table II) to patients with compromised renal function. Any analgesic and toxic effects following morphine administration to patients with poor renal function are probably due to M6G rather than morphine, as the former accumulates (Portenoy et al. 1991), while the latter often cannot be detected in the bloodstream within a few hours of administration. The contribution of M6G to the analgesia observed after morphine administration to patients with normal renal function is more controversial. Norpethidine accumulates at a greater rate in patients with renal insufficiency, with a corresponding greater potential for PAN (discussed in the previous section). Thus, it is appropriate to consider the use of fentanyl, methadone, or possibly hydromorphone in chronic noncancer pain patients with significantly reduced renal function.

OPIOID RESPONSIVENESS OF NOCICEPTIVE AND NEUROPATHIC PAIN

Nociceptive pain is generally regarded as being opioid sensitive, while opinion regarding the opioid sensitivity of neuropathic pain is divided. One view places neuropathic pain toward the upper regions of a continuous dose-response relationship such that suboptimal pain responses are observed with standard opioid doses and effective pain control can only be achieved following higher opioid doses (Portenoy et al. 1990; Portenoy 1994). The main consideration is the balance between degree of pain relief and the incidence and severity of side effects. The opposing view is that neuropathic pain is essentially insensitive to opioid therapy and that clinical characteristics of the pain predict this insensitivity (Arner and Meyerson 1988). More recently, Bennett (Chapter 19 of this volume) suggested that it is more appropriate to consider that patients suffer neuropathic *pains* (rather than the more general neuropathic *pain*), and that these various pains may show differential responses to opioids and other pharmacological therapies. While experimental evidence in the form of randomized controlled trials is available to support both views, most of these studies have limitations. Often, we do not know whether the dose used was sufficiently large to have the possibility of detecting an opioid sensitive pain, particularly in patients with neuropathic pain. Side effects may have been inadequately assessed, and appropriate inclusion criteria for neuropathic pain may be lacking. A study that allowed patients to titrate their morphine dose via a patient-controlled analgesia pump indicated that some neuropathic pains were indeed opioid sensitive, while all nociceptive pains showed significant opioid responsiveness (Jadad et al. 1992). Thus, the generally accepted view is that nociceptive pains are opioid sensitive, while neuropathic pains may be opioid sensitive, but at higher opioid doses. In some patients, unacceptable side effects may be observed in the absence of adequate analgesia.

PHARMACODYNAMIC EFFECTS

I see little benefit in subdividing opioids into the so-called *weak* or *strong* classes, as the weak opioids have little of the benefits and essentially all of the disadvantages of the strong opioids. Once the decision has been made to administer opioids to chronic noncancer pain patients, opioids that provide the most predictable outcome (i.e., opioids normally included at Step 3 of the World Health Organization analgesic ladder) should be prescribed. However, no randomized, appropriately blinded, controlled studies exist comparing the analgesic efficacy of these opioids at steady state in chronic noncancer pain. A view held by many is that an equivalent extent of analgesia could be obtained for opioid-sensitive pain by prescribing and optimizing different opioids (e.g., heroin, morphine, methadone, fentanyl, and hydromorphone). But is this really true, and at what comparative doses? Even if we accept that an equivalent degree of analgesia can be achieved, what about other effects? In the cancer pain area, fentanyl administered transdermally had a lower incidence of constipation than that observed with MS Contin (Ahmedzai et al. 1997), while oxycodone had a lesser extent of delirium (Maddocks et al. 1996) and of nausea and hallucinations (Kalso and Vainio 1990) than was observed following morphine administration. However, frequently there is no overwhelming patient preference for a particular opioid. Thus, pharmacodynamic differences between various opioids may have as much or more to do with effects at nonopioid as opioid receptors. Of all the available opioids, morphine is considered by many to have the best balance between providing pain relief and the incidence and sever-ity of side effects in treating both chronic cancer and noncancer pain. This position is reflected by data from the International Narcotic Control Board, which documents morphine consumption in many countries of the world. However, the consumption rates of both TTS-fentanyl and oxycodone are increasing in the treatment of chronic noncancer pain. There is an urgent need for appropriately blinded, randomized, controlled trials of morphine, fentanyl, oxycodone, and perhaps methadone to provide objective data that will allow clinicians to make the best choices for their patients. Such studies would require large numbers of patients because of the variability in analge-sic outcomes and the size of the placebo response in analgesic studies (McQuay et al. 1995).

CONCLUSIONS

Let us return to the quotation mentioned at the beginning of this chap-ter, indicating that there are "probably greater differences between the same opioid given by different routes than between different opioids given by the same route" (McQuay 1991). For chronic noncancer pain, the oral route is overwhelmingly preferred. For most patients with nociceptive pain, then, the above statement is true, and it is of no consequence which opioid the practi-tioner selects, despite the different profiles of affinity of the various opioids for the μ-, κ-, and δ-opioid receptors as well as a range of nonopioid recep-tors. The NMDA receptor is perhaps the most significant of the "other" receptors, with its documented role in nociceptive processing and the phe-nomenon of wind-up.

However, for other patients, this statement is not true. Some patients lack specific isoforms of critical enzymes, which means they cannot under-take the necessary transformations to convert some opioids, which are pro-drugs, to an active form. Concomitant drug therapy may have one of two effects, causing a significant reduction in the rate of these bioactivations either by competitive inhibition or by changing (stimulating or inhibiting) the rate of elimination of methadone. Some opioids have altered pharmaco-kinetics in the presence of hepatic or renal disease. In these patients, there can be differences between the opioids, sometimes of a significant magni-tude; perhaps fentanyl (Jeal and Benfield 1997), methadone, or possible hydromorphone would be better choices.

The type of pain can also be significant; is it better described as nocice-ptive or as neuropathic pain(s)? This raises the issue of the opioid respon-siveness of neuropathic pain. Methadone may be superior in cases where there are neuropathic elements because of the NMDA-receptor activity of the D-enantiomer in addition to the μ-receptor activation by the L-enantiomer. Using the clinically available NMDA-receptor antagonists (dextromethorphan or ketamine) is difficult on a long-term basis because of the lack of suitable formulations with appropriate dose strengths for this indication (Cherry et al. 1995). Particularly in the case of dextromethorphan, antitussive formulations can be used, but they suffer from the disadvantages of low concentration and the presence of additional unwanted compounds. Cost can also be a consideration.

In summary, the magnitude of the differences between opioids for chronic noncancer pain is variable. The differences are relatively minor for the majority of patients, but for others they can be very significant.

REFERENCES

Ahmedzai S, Brooks D. Transdermal fentanyl versus sustained-release oral morphine in cancer pain: efficacy, and quality of life. *J Pain Symptom Manage* 1997; 13:254–261.

Alderman CP, Frith PA. Fluvoxamine-methadone interaction. *Aust N Z J Psychiatry* 1999; 33:99–101.

Arner S, Meyerson BA. Lack of analgesic effects of opioids on neuropathic and idiopathic forms of pain. *Pain* 1988; 33:11–23.

Barberi-Heyob M, Merlin JL, Poulain P, et al. Circadian variations in morphine and morphine-6-glucuronide pharmacokinetics after oral and subcutaneous administration: first results. *Eur J Cancer* 1991; 27(Suppl 2):286.

Befort K, Kieffer BL. Structure-activity relationships in the δ-opioid receptor. *Pain Reviews* 1997; 4:100–121.

Bruera E, Watanabe S, Fainsinger RL, et al. Custom made capsules and suppositories of methadone for patients on high dose opioids for cancer pain. *Pain* 1995; 62:141–146.

Chapman V, Dickenson AH. The combination of NMDA antagonism and morphine produces profound antinociception in the rat dorsal horn. *Brain Res* 1992; 573:321–323.

Chen ZR, Somogyi AA, Bochner F. Polymorphic-O-demethylation of codeine. *Lancet* 1988; 2:914–915.

Chen J Somogyi A, Bochner F. Simultaneous determination of dextromethorphan and three metabolites in plasma and urine using high performance liquid chromatography with application to their disposition in man. *Ther Drug Monit* 1990; 12:97–104.

Cherry DA, Plummer JL, Gourlay GK, et al. Ketamine as an adjunct to morphine in the treatment of pain. *Pain* 1995; 62:119–121.

Christensen CB. The opioid receptor binding profiles of ketobemidone and morphine. *Pharmacol Toxicol* 1993; 73:344–345.

Clausen TG. International opioid consumption. *Acta Anaesthesiol Scand* 1997; 41:162–165.

Cobb MN, Desai J, Brown LS, Zannikos PN, Rainey PM. The effect of fluconazole on the clinical pharmacokinetics of methadone. *Clin Pharmacol Ther* 1998; 63:655–662.

Coderre TJ, Katz J, Vaccarino AL, Melzack R. Contribution of central neuroplasticity to pathological pain: review of clinical and experimental evidence. *Pain* 1993; 52:259–285.

Darke A, Moulin D, Provencher L, et al. Efficacy, safety and pharmacokinetics of controlled release morphine suppositories and tablets in cancer pain. *Clin Pharmacol Ther* 1995; 57:165.

Desmeules J, Gascon MP, Dayer P, Magistris M. Impact of environmental and genetic factors on codeine analgesia. *Eur J Clin Pharmacol* 1991; 41:23–26.

Eap CB, Cuendet C, Baumann P. Binding of *d*-methadone, *l*-methadone and *dl*-methadone to protein in plasma of healthy volunteers: role of variants of α_1-acid glycoprotein. *Clin Pharmacol Ther* 1990; 47:338–346.

Ebert B, Andersen S, Krogsgaard-Larsen P. Ketobemidone, methadone and pethidine are non-competitive N-methyl-D-aspartate (NMDA) antagonists in the rat cortex and spinal cord. *Neurosci Lett* 1995; 187:165–168.

Ebert B, Andersen S, Hjeds H, et al. Dextropropoxyphene acts as a non-competitive N-methyl-D-aspartate antagonist. *J Pain Symptom Manage* 1998; 15:269–274.

Eckhardt K, Li S, Ammon S, et al. Same incidence of adverse drug events after codeine administration irrespective of the genetically determined differences in morphine formation. *Pain* 1998; 76:27–33.

Elliott K, Minami K, Kolesnikov YA, et al. The NMDA receptor antagonists LY274614 and MK-801, and the nitric oxide synthase inhibitor N_G-nitro-L-arginine, attenuate analgesic tolerance to the mu-opioid morphine but not to kappa opioids. *Pain* 1994a; 56:69–74.

Elliott KJ, Hynansky A, Inturrisi CE. Dextromethorphan attenuates and reverses analgesic tolerance to morphine. *Pain* 1994b; 59:361–368.

Faura CC, Collins C, Moore RA, McQuay HJ. Systematic review of factors affecting the ratios of morphine and its major metabolites. *Pain* 1998; 74:43–53.

Fromm MF, Hofmann U, Griese EU, Mikus G. Dihydrocodeine: a new opioid substrate for the polymorphic CYP2D6 in humans. *Clin Pharmacol Ther* 1995; 58:374–382.

Gear RW, Maiskowski C, Gordon NC, et al. Kappa-opioids produce significantly greater analgesia in women than in men. *Nature Med* 1996; 2:1248–1250.

Glynn CJ, Lloyd JW. The diurnal variation in the perception of pain. *Proc Roy Soc Med* 1976; 69:369–372.

Gong QL, Hedner J, Bjorkman R, Hedner T. Morphine-3-glucuronide may functionally antagonize morphine-6-glucuronide induced antinociception and ventilatory depression in the rat. *Pain* 1992; 48:249–255.

Gorman AL, Elliott KJ, Inturrisi CE. The *d*- and *l*-isomers of methadone bind to the non-competitive site on the N-methyl-D-aspartate (NMDA) receptor in rat forebrain and spinal cord. *Neurosci Lett* 1997; 223:5–8.

Gourlay GK. Long-term use of opioids in chronic pain patients with nonterminal disease states. *Pain Reviews* 1994; 1:45–59.

Gourlay GK. Sustained relief of chronic pain: pharmacokinetics of SR morphine. *Clin Pharmacokin* 1998; 35:173–190.

Gourlay GK. Clinical pharmacology of the treatment of chronic non-cancer pain. In: Max MB (Ed). *Pain 1999—An Updated Review*. Seattle: IASP Press, 1999, in press.

Gourlay GK, Mather LE. Postoperative pain management with TTS-fentanyl: pharmacokinetics and pharmacodynamics. In: Lehmann KA, Zech D (Eds). *Transdermal Fentanyl*. Berlin: Springer-Verlag, 1991, pp 119–140.

Gourlay GK, Cherry DA, Cousins MJ. A comparative study of the efficacy and pharmacokinetics of oral methadone and morphine in the treatment of severe pain in patients with cancer. *Pain* 1986; 25:297–312.

Gourlay GK, Plummer JL, Cherry DA, et al. Influence of a high fat meal on the absorption of morphine from oral solutions. *Clin Pharmacol Ther* 1989; 46:463–468.

Gourlay GK, Plummer JL, Cherry DA, et al. The reproducibility of bioavailability of oral morphine from solution under fed and fasted conditions. *J Pain Symptom Manage* 1991; 6:431–436.

Gourlay GK, Plummer JL, Cherry DA. Chronopharmacokinetic variability in plasma morphine concentrations following oral doses of morphine solution. *Pain* 1995; 61:375–381.

Graziotti PJ, Goucke CR. The use of oral opioids in patients with chronic non-cancer pain: management strategies. *Med J Aust* 1997; 167:30–34.

Horng JS, Smits SE, Wong DT. The binding of the optical isomers of methadone, α-acetylmethadol and their N-demethylated derivatives to the opiate receptors of rat brain. *Res Commun Chem Pathol Pharmacol* 1976; 14:621–629.

Hewett K, Dickenson AH, McQuay HJ. Lack of effect of morphine-3-glucuronide on the spinal antinociceptive actions of morphine in the rat: an electrophysiological study. *Pain* 1993; 53:59–63.

Inturrisi CE, Schultz M, Shin S, et al. Evidence from opiate binding studies that heroin acts through its metabolites. *Life Sci* 1983; 33:773–776.

Iribarne C, Dreano Y, Bardou LG, et al. Interaction of methadone with substrates of human hepatic cytochrome P450 3A4. *Toxicology* 1997; 117:13–23.

Iribarne C, Berthou F, Carlhant D, et al. Inhibition of methadone and buprenorphine-N-demethylations by three HIV-1 protease inhibitors. *Drug Metab Dispos* 1998; 26:257–260.

Jadad AR, Carroll D, Glynn CJ, Moore RA. Morphine responsiveness of chronic pain: double-blind randomised crossover study with patient-controlled analgesia. *Lancet* 1992; 339:1367–1371.

Jeal W, Benfield P. Transdermal fentanyl: a review of its pharmacological properties and therapeutic efficacy in pain control. *Drugs* 1997; 53:109–138.

Kalso E, Vainio A. Morphine and oxycodone hydrochloride in the management of cancer pain. *Clin Pharmacol Ther* 1990; 47:639–646.

Kovelowski CJ, Raffa RB, Porreca F. Tramadol and its enantiomers differentially suppress c-fos-like immunoreactivity in rat brain and spinal cord following acute noxious stimulus. *Eur J Pain* 1998; 2:211–219.

Kristensen K, Christensen CB, Christrup LL. The mu₁, mu₂, delta, kappa opioid receptor binding profiles of methadone stereoisomers and morphine. *Life Sci* 1995; 56:45–50.

Kristensen K, Blemmer T, Angelo HR, et al. Stereoselective pharmacokinetics of methadone in chronic pain patients. *Ther Drug Monit* 1996; 18:221–227.

Labroo RB, Thummel KE, Kynze KL, et al. Catalytic role of cytochrome P4503A4 in multiple pathways of alfentanil metabolism. *Drug Metab Dispos* 1995; 23:490–496.

Labroo RB, Paine MF, Thummel KE, et al. Fentanyl metabolism by human hepatic and intestinal cytochrome P450 3A4: implications for inter-individual variability in disposition, efficacy, and drug interactions. *Drug Metab Dispos* 1997; 25:1072–1080.

Leow KP, Cramond T, Smith M. Pharmacokinetics and pharmacodynamics of oxycodone when given intravenously and rectally to adult patients with cancer pain. *Anesth Analg* 1995; 80:296–302.

Lodge D, Jones M, Fletcher E. Non-competitive antagonists of N-methyl-D-aspartate. In: Collingridge GL, Watkins JC (Eds). *The NMDA Receptor*, 2nd ed. Oxford: Oxford University Press, 1994, pp 105–131.

Maddocks I, Somogyi A, Abbott F, et al. Attenuation of morphine-induced delirium in palliative care by substitution with infusion of oxycodone. *J Pain Symptom Manage* 1996; 12:182–189.

Maddox JD, Joranson D, Angarola RT, et al. The use of opioids for the treatment of chronic pain [position statement]. *Clin J Pain* 1997; 13:6–8.

Magnan J, Paterson SJ, Tavani A, Kosterlitz HW. The binding spectrum of narcotic analgesic drugs with different agonist and antagonist properties. *Naunyn Schmiedebergs Arch Pharmacol* 1982; 319:197–205.

Mather LE, Gourlay GK. The biotransformation of opioids: significance for pain therapy. In: Nimmo WS, Smith G (Eds). *Opioid Agonist/Antagonist Drugs in Clinical Practice*. Amsterdam: Excerpta Medica, 1984, pp 31–47.

Mather LE, Gourlay GK. Pharmacokinetics of fentanyl. In: Lehmann KA, Zech D (Eds). *Transdermal Fentanyl*. Berlin: Springer-Verlag, 1991, pp 73–79.

McQuay HJ. Opioid clinical pharmacology and routes of administration. *Br Med Bull* 1991; 47:703–717.

McQuay H, Carroll D, Moore A. Variation in the placebo effect in randomised controlled trials of analgesics: all is as blind as it seems. *Pain* 1995; 64:331–335.

Mikus G, Trausch B, Rodewald C, et al. Effect of codeine on gastrointestinal motility in relation to CYP2D6 phenotype. *Clin Pharmacol Ther* 1997; 61:459–466.

Moore A, Collins S Carroll D, McQuay H. Paracetamol with and without codeine in acute pain: a quantitative systematic review. *Pain* 1997; 70:193–201.

Morley JS, Makin MK. The use of methadone in cancer pain poorly responsive to other opioids. *Pain Reviews* 1998; 5:51–58.

Olsen GD, Wendel HA, Livermore JD, et al. Clinical effects and pharmacokinetics of racemic methadone and its optical isomers. *Clin Pharmacol Ther* 1977; 21:147–157.

Otton SV, Wu D, Joffe RT, Cheung SW, Sellers EM. Inhibition of fluoxetine by cytochrome P450 2D6 activity. *Clin Pharmacol Ther* 1993a; 53:401–409.

Otton SV, Schadel M, Cheung SW, et al. CYP2D6 phenotype determines the metabolic conversion of hydrocodone to hydromorphone. *Clin Pharmacol Ther* 1993b; 54:463–472.

Pasternak GW, Bodnar RJ, Clark JA, Inturrisi CE. Morphine-6-glucuronide, a potent mu agonist. *Life Sci* 1987; 41:2845–2849.

Plummer JL, Gourlay GK, Cherry DA, Cousins MJ. Estimation of methadone clearance: application in the management of cancer pain. *Pain* 1988; 33:313–322.

Plummer JL, Owen H, Ilsley AH, et al. Morphine patient-controlled analgesia is superior to meperidine patient-controlled analgesia for postoperative pain. *Anesth Analg* 1997a; 84:794–799.

Plummer JL, Tran KD, Gourlay GK. Interaction between dextromethorphan and nor-pethidine in rats. *Eur J Pain* 1997b; 1:191–196.

Pond SM, Tong T, Benowitz N, et al. Presystemic metabolism of meperidine to normeperidine in normal and cirrhotic subjects. *Clin Pharmacol Ther* 1981; 30:183–188.

Portenoy RK. Opioid therapy for chronic non-malignant pain: current status. In: Fields HL, Liebeskind JC (Eds). *Pharmacological Approaches to the Treatment of Chronic Pain: New Concepts and Critical Issues.* Progress in Pain Research and Management, Vol. 1. Seattle: IASP Press, 1994, pp 247–287.

Portenoy RK, Foley KM, Inturrisi CE. The nature of opioid responsiveness and its implications for neuropathic pain: new hypotheses derived from studies of opioid infusions. *Pain* 1990; 43:273–286.

Portenoy RK, Foley KM, Stulman J, et al. Plasma morphine and morphine-6-glucuronide during chronic morphine therapy for cancer pain: plasma profiles, steady state concentrations and the consequences of renal failure. *Pain* 1991; 47:13–19.

Poulsen L, Brosen K, Arendt-Nielson L, et al. Codeine and morphine in extensive and poor metabolisers of sparteine: pharmacokinetics, analgesic effect and side effects. *Eur J Clin Pharmacol* 1996; 51:289–295.

Raynor K, Kong H, Chen Y, et al. Pharmacological characterization of the cloned κ-, δ- and μ-opioid receptors. *Molec Pharmacol* 1994; 45:330–334.

Raynor K, Kong H, Mestek A, et al. Characterization of the cloned human mu opioid receptor. *J Pharmacol Exp Ther* 1995; 272:423–428.

Richards AH. The use of controlled release morphine sulfate (MS Contin) in Queensland 1990–1993. *Med J Aust* 1995; 163:181–182.

Ross FB, Smith MT. The intrinsic antinociceptive effects of oxycodone appear to be κ-opioid receptor mediated. *Pain* 1997; 73:151–157.

Ruskis AF. Effects of narcotics on gastrointestinal tract, liver and kidneys. In: Kitahata LM, Collins JG (Eds). *Narcotic Analgesics in Anesthesiology.* Baltimore: Williams and Wilkins, 1982, pp 143–156.

Sandrini G, Alfonsi E, Bono G, et al. Circadian variations of human flexion reflex. *Pain* 1986; 25:403–410.

Schechter NL, Weisman SJ, Rosenblum M, et al. The use of oral transmucosal fentanyl citrate for painful procedures in children. *Pediatrics* 1995; 95:335–339.

Schug SA, Merry AF, Acland RH. Treatment principles for the use of opioids in pain of non-malignant origin. *Drugs* 1991; 42:228–232.

Shimoyama N, Shimoyama M, Elliott KJ, Inturrisi CE. *d*-Methadone is antinociceptive in the rat formalin test. *J Pharmacol Exp Ther* 1997; 283:648–652.

Sindrup SH, Brosen K, Bjerring P, et al. Codeine increases pain thresholds to copper vapour laser stimuli in extensive but not poor metabolisers of sparteine. *Clin Pharmacol Ther* 1991; 49:686–693.

Smith GD, Smith MT. Morphine-3-glucuronide: evidence to support its putative role in the development of tolerance to the antinociceptive effects of morphine in the rat. *Pain* 1995; 62:51–60.

Strian F, Lautenbacher S, Golfe G, Holzl R. Diurnal variations in pain perception and thermal sensitivity. *Pain* 1989; 36:123–131.

Szekely JL, Sharpe LG, Jaffe JH. Induction of phencyclidine-like behaviour in rats by dextrorphan but not dextromethorphan. *Pharmacol Biochem Behav* 1991; 40:381–386.

Takala A, Kaasalainen V, Seppala T, et al. Pharmacokinetic comparison of intravenous and intranasal administration of oxycodone. *Acta Anaesthesiol Scand* 1997; 41:309–312.

Tateishi T, Krivoruk Y, Ueng YF, et al. Identification of human cytochrome P450 3A4 as the enzyme responsible for fentanyl and sufentanil N-dealkylation. *Anesth Analg* 1996; 82:167–172.

Traynor JR. The μ-opioid receptor. *Pain Reviews* 1996; 3: 221–248.

Tyndale RF, Droll KP, Sellers EM. Genetically deficient CYP2D6 metabolism provides protection against oral opiate dependence. *Pharmacogenetics* 1997; 7:375–379.

Wilkinson TJ, Robinson BA, Begg EJ, et al. Pharmacokinetics and efficacy of rectal versus oral sustained-release morphine in cancer patients. *Cancer Chemother Pharmacol* 1992; 31:251–254.

Woolf CJ, Thomson SWN. The induction and maintenance of central sensitization is dependent on N-methyl-D-aspartic acid receptor activation: implications for the treatment of post-injury pain hypersensitivity states. *Pain* 1991; 44:293–299.

Yun CH, Wood M, Wood AJ, et al. Identification of the pharmacogenetic determinants of alfentanil metabolism: cytochrome P450 3A4. An explanation of the variable elimination clearance. *Anesthesiology* 1992; 77:467–474.

Correspondence to: Geoffrey K Gourlay, BPharm, PhD, Chief Medical Scientist, Pain Management Unit, Flinders Medical Centre, Bedford Park, South Australia 5042, Australia. Fax: 61-8-8374-1758; email: geoff.gourlay @flinders.edu.au.

Opioid Sensitivity of Chronic Noncancer Pain,
Progress in Pain Research and Management,
Vol. 14, edited by Eija Kalso, Henry J. McQuay,
and Zsuzsanna Wiesenfeld-Hallin, IASP Press,
Seattle, © 1999.

7

Route of Opioid Administration: Does It Make a Difference?

Eija Kalso

Pain Relief Unit, Department of Anesthesia, Helsinki University Central Hospital, Helsinki, Finland

The effects of opioids on the brain have been known for millennia, but it was only in the 1970s that the spinal cord was shown to play a crucial role in opioid analgesia. The assumption that opioid analgesia is restricted to the central nervous system (CNS) was not seriously challenged until the 1990s. Today the existence of peripheral opioid receptors is generally accepted.

While the mechanisms of the actions of opioids, particularly in the spinal cord but also in the periphery, have been studied extensively and are fairly well understood, the supraspinal effects of opioids remain elusive. The three main mechanisms of supraspinal action of opioids are activation of descending inhibititory controls, diffuse noxious inhibitory controls (DNIC), and disinhibition of GABAergic interneurons. All these mechanisms involve the spinal cord. Coactivation of supraspinal and spinal opioid receptors can yield up to a 30-fold increase in the effect of morphine (Yeung and Rudy 1980; Miyamoto et al. 1991). As Ossipov and colleagues suggest in Chapter 10 of this volume, the loss of this synergy between the supraspinal and spinal sites may significantly reduce the effectiveness of opioids in neuropathic pain. We lack data on the possible enhancing effects of the simultaneous activation of spinal or supraspinal opioid receptors on peripheral opioid analgesia.

Opioids have important effects on various neural circuits in the CNS. In some persons opioids may have euphoric, antidepressive, and anxiolytic effects, whereas others may experience dysphoria and depression. Opioids also activate various neurohumoral systems. These effects cannot be ignored when assessing the total effect of opioids in a chronic pain patient.

Adverse effects are a significant factor in the effectiveness of opioids. Spinal administration was originally expected to result in segmental analgesia.

However, it was soon recognized that epidural administration of opioids had both a spinal and a systemic effect due to rapid uptake of the opioid into circulation. It was also obvious that particularly hydrophilic opioids show significant cephalad spread in the cerebrospinal fluid (CSF), with the potential for severe respiratory depression.

To separate the supraspinal, spinal, and peripheral effects of opioids it would be necessary to achieve and maintain the desired concentrations only at the target organs, which cannot be done in clinical practice. Oral administration is the preferred route because it is easy and cheap and does not require sophisticated technology. The role of first-pass metabolism and the problems of active and harmful metabolites complicate comparisons of the effectiveness of the oral and other routes of administration.

Answers to some interesting questions would help us to define the role of more advanced routes for administering opioids: What systemic doses of opioids result in sufficient concentrations in the spinal cord and periphery? How important is the proposed synergy between different sites of opioid actions? Do any pain conditions respond differently to different routes of opioid administration? Can the cost/benefit ratio of opioid therapy be improved by changing the route of administration? Does development of tolerance vary with different routes of administration?

SOME ANSWERS FROM BASIC RESEARCH

ROUTE AND EFFICACY

Animal models provide some information about the effects of route of administration of different drugs in the same model of nociception, and also about the effect of route of opioid administration in different pain models. Several examples will elucidate both aspects.

Antinociceptive effects of morphine and oxycodone were studied in the tail-flick and hot-plate tests after intraperitoneal (i.p.), intrathecal (i.t.), and subcutaneous (s.c.) administration (Pöyhiä and Kalso 1992). Subcutaneous injections represent systemic administration, whereas i.p. administration resembles oral administration as it will show differences in first-pass metabolism. Oxycodone and morphine were administered i.p. and s.c. in doses of 2.5–10 and 5–20 mg/kg, respectively, and i.t. in doses of 12.5 µg and 100 µg of oxycodone and 6.25 µg and 50 µg of morphine. In both nociceptive tests, oxycodone administered s.c. and i.p. was 2–4 times more potent than morphine, while i.t. morphine was over 14 times more potent than oxycodone. These results indicate that the route of administration significantly alters the respective potencies of these two drugs. The difference may be due to several factors, but the two most obvious explanations are that oxycodone needs active metabolites for full effect or that the two drugs differ in receptor-binding profile. Lipid solubility has been advocated as an important factor for the i.t. potency of opioids (McQuay et al. 1989), but oxycodone and morphine do not differ significantly in this respect (Pöyhiä and Seppälä 1994).

ADVERSE EFFECTS

Few studies on rats have looked at clinically relevant adverse effects. Rats neither vomit nor sweat, nor complain of dry mouth and nightmares. Studies have suggested that opioids with higher lipid-solubility would enable easier passage through the blood–brain barrier and thus cause less constipation (Megens et al. 1998), but no cross-route comparisons have been made. Sedation is an important adverse effect, as it may interfere with the assessment of nociception (Yu et al. 1997). The study by Pöyhiä and Kalso (1992) indicated that CNS depression was more profound with oxycodone than with morphine after i.p. and s.c. administration, but was not observed after i.t. administration of either drug.

EFFECT OF ROUTE OF ADMINISTRATION
IN TWO MODELS OF NEUROPATHIC PAIN

Many chapters of this book have highlighted the central role of the spinal cord in the modulation of nociception. It might be assumed that i.t. injection would be the most effective way to administer opioids. However, this is not always the case, and the spinal nerve ligation (SNL) model of neuropathic pain (Kim and Chung 1992) and the spinal cord injury model of central pain serve as good examples to show how some pain states can show differential efficacy to various routes of opioid administration.

As can be seen in Table I, even very high doses of up to 100 µg of intrathecal morphine were ineffective against mechanical allodynia in the SNL model of neuropathic pain. High doses of i.p. and intracerebroventricular (i.c.v.) morphine showed efficacy. These results could indicate an important differential effect. However, another likely explanation is that high doses of systemic or i.c.v. morphine caused significant sedation that interfered with the testing of the animals, as will be discussed below.

Yu et al. (1997) studied the effects of different routes of morphine administration on both thermal nociceptive pain (tail-flick reflex) and neuropathic pain (spinal cord injury). Morphine administered by all three routes (s.c., i.t., and i.c.v.) produced powerful antinociception in the tail-flick test in normal animals. However, only i.t. morphine relieved the mechanical

Table I

Efficacy of various routes and doses of morphine
administration in the spinal nerve ligation
model of neuropathic pain

Route of Administration	Dose	Effect (+/–)*
Intraperitoneal	3 mg/kg	–
	>6 mg/kg	+ +
Intrathecal	10–100 μg	– – – – – ±
Intracerebroventricular	1–3 μg	+
	10 μg	+

Source: Based on data from Bian et al. (1995); Lee et al.
(1995); Nichols et al. (1995, 1997); Wegert et al. (1997);
Yaksh et al. (1995).
* All studies tested mechanical allodynia with von Frey hairs.
Each + indicates a study with a significant antiallodynic effect,
whereas – indicates a study with a negative outcome.

allodynia-like responses measured with von Frey hairs in spinally injured
rats in doses (1–10 μg) that were not sedative.

EVIDENCE FROM THE CLINIC

TESTING DIFFERENT ROUTES OF ADMINISTRATION

Most of the first controlled clinical trials on opioid sensitivity of different pain states were performed using intravenous (i.v.) opioid administration, and subsequent trials have investigated long-term administration of
oral and transdermal (t.d.) opioids. It would be interesting to examine how
the different routes of administration compare in their clinical effects and
required dosages.

Dellemijn and colleagues have conducted two studies on the same group
of neuropathic pain patients. In the first randomized and controlled study by
Dellemijn and Vanneste (1997), the patients received an i.v. fentanyl infusion of 5 $\mu g \cdot kg^{-1} \cdot h^{-1}$ for up to 5 hours and either a saline or a diazepam
infusion as a control. The second study was an open follow-up protocol
using t.d. fentanyl with 48 of the 50 patients in the first study participating.
Table II shows that the daily t.d. dose was one-fourth of the i.v. titration
dose and that only 29% of the patients were good responders (i.e., they had
50% pain relief), compared with 58% of patients after the i.v. infusion. The
important message of these two studies was the significant positive correlation ($r = 0.59$, $P < 0.0001$) between pain relief obtained with i.v. fentanyl
and prolonged t.d. fentanyl. In brief, 58% of the patients were good re-

Table II
Effectiveness of intravenous and transdermal
fentanyl in patients with neuropathic pain

	Intravenous	Transdermal
Mean dose/24 h	4.190 mg	1.077 mg
Duration of dosing	5 h	12 wk
Patients with ≥50% pain relief	58%	29%
Withdrawals (adverse effects or inadequate pain relief)	90%	38%

Source: Dellemijn and Vanneste (1997); Dellemijn et al. (1998).

sponders after a 5-hour i.v. infusion and 29% after 12 weeks on t.d. fentanyl; 19% continued with the treatment for more than 2 years.

Table III shows information about studies that tested opioid sensitivity with i.v. or i.t. morphine titration and with chronic administration of i.t. or oral morphine. All studies on i.v. morphine titration and chronic oral morphine were randomized, controlled, and double blind, but it is difficult to draw conclusions as the pain populations differed. It is obvious, however, that the doses used in the i.v. titration represent daily oral doses 16–25 times higher than those that the patients were able to take in the oral study. The i.t. study indicates that a 16-fold dose escalation occurred during long-term treatment.

The clinically relevant routes of administration in long-term management of chronic noncancer pain would include oral, sublingual/buccal, subcutaneous/transdermal, and spinal (epidural and intrathecal) administration of opioids. The advantage of administering opioids sublingually, subcutaneously, or transdermally is that first-pass metabolism is avoided, as are possibly harmful metabolites (e.g., morphine-3-glucuronides). The superiority of

Table III
Mean intravenous, intrathecal, and oral doses of morphine in
studies of opioid effectiveness of chronic noncancer pain

Route of Administration	Neuropathic Pain	Mixed Types of Pain	Nociceptive Pain
Intrathecal	Initial: 0.46 mg/24 h[d] Long-term: 7.6 mg/24 h[d]	—	—
Intravenous	19 mg/1 h (target)[a]	230 mg/8 h (on demand)[b]	—
Oral	1368 mg/24 h*[a]	2070 mg/24 h*[b]	83.5 mg/24 h[c]

Source: Rowbotham et al. (1991)[a]; Jadad et al. (1992)[b]; Moulin et al. (1996)[c]; Angel et al. (1998)[d].
*These doses were calculated from the intravenous doses, assuming a 33% oral bioavailability.

spinal administration would imply that pain relief could be improved significantly by increasing the opioid concentrations in the CSF. To make any
sensible comparisons, the same opioid should be compared using different
routes of administration. Conclusions about adverse effects should be drawn
only if equianalgesia was achieved.

LESSONS FROM CHRONIC CANCER PAIN

Only a few controlled clinical trials have performed cross-route comparisons of the same opioid. The only opioid that has been studied in this
respect is morphine. As there are no controlled studies of cross-route comparisons in chronic noncancer pain, I will present examples from chronic
cancer pain.

Vainio and Tigerstedt (1988) studied the effectiveness of oral and epidural morphine in a randomized open parallel group of 30 cancer patients
suffering from severe pain caused by tumor involvement of the brachial or
lumbar nerve plexus. Ten patients were treated with oral morphine and 20
with an epidural catheter with or without port. The doses were adjusted daily
during the first week and once a week thereafter. The patients were followed
for at least 90 days.

Satisfactory pain relief was achieved with both oral and epidural administration. Mean doses were 151 mg (range 24–480 mg) with oral administration and 45 mg (range 2–800 mg) with epidural administration. Pain intensi-
ties measured with a visual analogue scale (VAS) did not differ significantly
between the groups. However, adverse effects were more prevalent in the
oral (16 reports of adverse effects in 10 patients) compared with the epidural group (10 reports in 20 patients). The most common adverse effects for
the oral group were drowsiness, hallucinations, and constipation. Dose escalation occurred in both groups. Technical or infectious complications occurred in 12 patients in the epidural group.

Kalso et al. (1996) compared the effectiveness of epidural and subcutaneous morphine in a crossover study in cancer patients with mainly nerve
infiltration pain. The study was randomized and double blind, and was pre-
ceded by a open titration to the optimum dose with oral morphine. During
the randomized part of the study, the patients were able to titrate themselves
to a pain-free state using a patient-controlled analgesia (PCA) technique for
48 hours. The median daily dose of subcutaneous morphine, as calculated
from the "steady state," was three times (range 1–10 times) the median
epidural dose. The two modes of administration provided equal pain relief
both at rest and during movement, and there were no significant differences

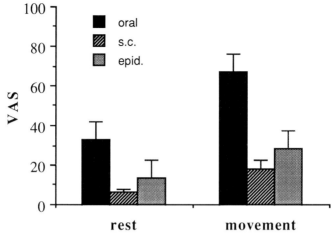

Fig. 1. Pain at bedrest and when moving in a study of morphine in cancer pain (from Kalso et al. 1996; reprinted with permission). Pain was estimated on a horizontal 100-mm visual analogue scale (VAS) at bedrest (rest) and when moving (movement) before the study (oral morphine) and at the end of each titration phase (s.c. = subcutaneous morphine, epid. = epidural morphine). Mean values with SEM are given. The number of patients was 10, except during the epidural treatment when it was nine. The mean VAS was significantly lower during s.c. administration compared with oral administration both at rest ($P < 0.05$) and during movement ($P < 0.01$). During epidural administration the mean VAS was lower than during oral administration ($P < 0.05$) during movement only. There were no statistically significant differences between the mean VAS values during epidural compared with s.c. administration.

in adverse effects (Figs. 1 and 2). However, s.c. morphine provided significantly better analgesia than did oral morphine. When the VAS values of all adverse effects were summed, the total amount of adverse effects was significantly higher during oral compared with s.c. morphine.

This study was limited by the small number of patients (10) and the short duration of 48 hours per stage of treatment. Also, the oral morphine was titrated in the open phase. However, with the lower daily dose of oral morphine (median 225 mg), the patients had significantly more adverse effects (and more pain) than with a higher dose of s.c. morphine (median 372 mg/24 hours). It could be concluded that there is a greater difference in the analgesic effect/adverse effect ratio between oral and s.c. administration of morphine than between s.c. and epidural administration. The difference in doses was only threefold and for plasma concentrations only 1.5-fold between s.c. and epidural administration. Therefore, a comparison between systemic and i.t. administration of morphine would be relevant.

124   E. KALSO

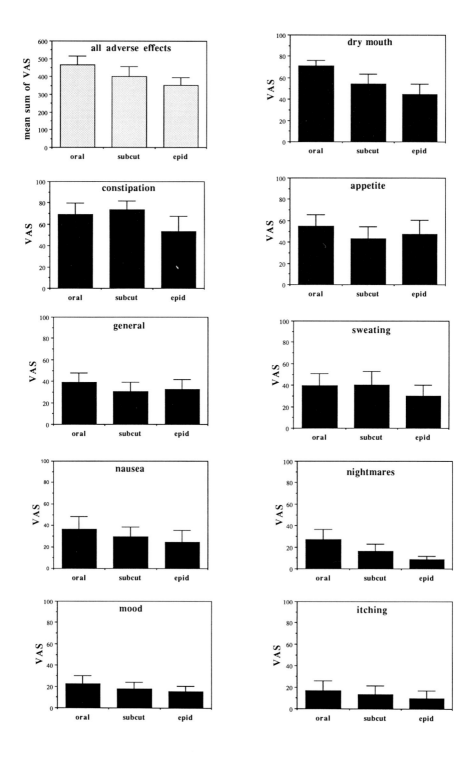

SYSTEMIC AND SPINAL MORPHINE
IN CHRONIC NONCANCER PAIN

As oral or subcutaneous administration of morphine has not been compared with intrathecal administration in any randomized study, answers must be sought by considering separate studies where morphine was administered orally (Moulin et al. 1996) over 9 weeks or i.t. (Winkelmüller and Winkelmüller 1996) over a period of 0.5–5.7 years (Table IV). The studies are of course very different; the former is a randomized, controlled crossover study, whereas the latter is a long-term retrospective analysis. However, certain interesting observations can be made. Constipation, nausea, and vomiting were equally frequent in the two groups, whereas dizziness, fatigue, and dry mouth were more common after oral administration. In accordance with studies on acute administration of segmental morphine, urinary retention was common after i.t. administration. Interestingly, patients' activity and mood improved significantly during i.t. treatment, whereas no significant

Table IV
Incidence of adverse effects after long-term treatment
with oral and intrathecal morphine

	Oral Morphine (60–120 mg/24 h)	Intrathecal Morphine (3–5 mg/24 h)
Number of patients	46	82
Type of pain	Musculoskeletal	Mixed
Follow-up	9 wk	0.5–5.7 y
Adverse Effects		
Nausea	39%	39%
Vomiting	39%	27%
Dizziness	37%	2%
Constipation	41%	50%
Fatigue	22%	5%
Itching/pruritis	15%	15%
Dry mouth	17%	4%
Urinary retention	Not reported	43%
Sexual dysfunction	Not reported	27%

Source: Moulin et al. (1996); Winkelmüller and Winkelmüller (1996).

⟵   **Fig. 2.** Adverse effects of morphine treatment (Kalso et al. 1996), measured on a horizontal 100-mm VAS before treatment (oral) and at the end of both titration periods (subcut = subcutaneous, epid = epidural). Mean values and SEM are given for each adverse effect. The number of nightmares was significantly lower during s.c. compared with oral administration of morphine ($P < 0.05$). No other statistically significant differences were detected.

psychological or functional improvement was achieved with oral morphine. This difference, however, could also be due to different pain patient populations.

CSF CONCENTRATIONS OF MORPHINE AFTER SYSTEMIC AND SPINAL ADMINISTRATION

The few studies that have measured the CSF concentrations of morphine and its metabolites after oral administration suggest a significant passage of both morphine and its glucuronides through the blood–brain barrier. The difficulty in drawing any conclusions from the CSF and plasma concentrations of morphine (or its metabolites) lies in the significant interindividual variation in the concentrations resulting from standard dosing. The median steady-state CSF/plasma concentration ratio after slow-release oral morphine varied from a mean of 0.8 (±0.1) (Wolff et al. 1995) to a median of 1.3 (range 0.6–1.5) (Goucke et al. 1994). The concentration ratio after epidural administration of morphine varied from 2.5 to 806, with a median of 66 (Samuelsson et al. 1993).

PERIPHERAL ADMINISTRATION OF OPIOIDS

The therapeutic potential of peripherally acting opioids has been discussed in detail by Machelska et al. in Chapter 3 of this book and by Schäfer in Chapter 20. This mode of administration, if it proves as effective as we hope, has the advantage of no adverse central effects. At present, opioids can be administered peripherally only to a restricted number of sites via intra-articular injection, for example, into the knee joint. Opioids that do not penetrate the blood–brain barrier would be a natural solution, and such compounds (Barber et al. 1994) are now being tested in the clinic.

CONCLUSIONS

All conclusions should be drawn cautiously as controlled clinical trials have produced little evidence to support them. Cross-route comparisons require the use of double-dummy techniques that make these studies more difficult to run. However, the more invasive the techniques we want to use, the more we should be able to show that they provide significant benefit. Intrathecal opioid administration with implantable pumps is an invasive therapy, and so randomized, if not double-blind, controlled prospective studies should be performed to show that the time and money that is invested in these therapies is worthwhile.

Eliminating the first-pass metabolism of morphine may improve the effect/adverse effect profile of morphine analgesia. Intrathecal administration of morphine seems to cause a somewhat different adverse effect profile from that of oral morphine. Tolerance develops to all modes of opioid administration.

The available clinical studies do not indicate that spinal administration of opioids would cause a more sensory-discriminative type of analgesia compared with systemic opioid administration. We can hope that the possibilities offered by modern imaging techniques will shed more light on the supraspinal effects of opioids.

Finally, if future pharmacological studies can provide us with drugs that can be targeted to specific sites in the nervous system, we may eventually know whether the route of administration truly makes a difference.

REFERENCES

Angel IF, Gould HJ, Carey ME. Intrathecal morphine pump as a treatment option in chronic pain of nonmalignant origin. *Surg Neurol* 1998; 49:92–99.

Barber A, Bartoszyk GD, Bender HM, et al. A pharmacological profile of the novel, peripherally-selective κ-opioid receptor agonist, EMD 61753. *Br J Pharmacol* 1994; 113:1317–1327.

Bian D, Nichols ML, Ossipov MH, Lai J, Porreca F. Characterization of the antiallodynic efficacy of morphine in a model of neuropathic pain in rats. *Neuroreport* 1995; 6:1981–1984.

Dellemijn PLI, Vanneste JAL. Randomised double-blind active-placebo-controlled crossover trial of intravenous fentanyl in neuropathic pain. *Lancet* 1997; 349:753–758.

Dellemijn PLI, van Duijn H, Vanneste JAL. Prolonged treatment with transdermal fentanyl in neuropathic pain. *J Pain Symptom Manage* 1998; 16:220–229.

Goucke CR, Hackett LP, Ilett KF. Concentrations of morphine, morphine-6-glucuronide and morphine-3-glucuronide in serum and cerebrospinal fluid following morphine administration to patients with morphine-resistant pain. *Pain* 1994; 56:145–149.

Jadad AR, Carroll D, Glynn CJ, Moore RA, McQuay HJ. Morphine responsiveness of chronic pain: double-blind randomised crossover study with patient-controlled analgesia. *Lancet* 1992; 339:1367–1371.

Kalso E, Heiskanen T, Rantio M, Rosenberg PH, Vainio A. Epidural and subcutaneous morphine in the management of cancer pain: a double-blind cross-over study. *Pain* 1996; 67:443–449.

Kim SH, Chung JM. An experimental model for peripheral neuropathy produced by segmental spinal nerve ligation in the rat. *Pain* 1992; 50:355–363.

Lee Y-W, Chaplan SR, Yaksh TL. Systemic and supraspinal, but not spinal opiates suppress allodynia in a rat neuropathic pain model. *Neurosci Lett* 1995; 186:111–114.

McQuay HJ, Sullian AF, Smallman K, Dickenson AH. Intrathecal opioids, potency and lipophilicity. *Pain* 1989; 36:111–115.

Megens A, Artois K, Vermeire J, Meert T, Awouters FHL. Comparison of the analgesic and intestinal effects of fentanyl and morphine in rats: relevance for side-effect liability of TTS fentanyl. *J Pain Symptom Manage* 1998; 15:253–257.

Miyamoto Y, Morita N, Kitabata Y, et al. Antinociceptive synergism between supraspinal and spinal sites after subcutaneous morphine evidenced by CNS morphine content. *Brain Res* 1991; 552:136–140.

Moulin DE, Iezzi A, Amireh R, Sharpe WKJ, Merskey H. Randomised trial of morphine for chronic non-cancer pain. *Lancet* 1996; 347:143–147.

Nichols ML, Bian D, Ossipov MH, Lai J, Porreca F. Regulation of morphine antiallodynic efficacy by cholecystokinin in a model of neuropathic pain in rats. *J Pharmacol Exp Ther* 1995; 275:1339–1345.

Nichols ML, Lopez Y, Ossipov MH, Bian D, Porreca F. Enhancement of the antiallodynic and antinociceptive efficacy of spinal morphine by antisera to dynorphin A (1–13) or MK-801 in a nerve-ligation model of peripheral neuropathy. *Pain* 1997; 69:317–322.

Pöyhiä R, Kalso EA. Antinociceptive effects and central nervous system depression caused by oxycodone and morphine in rats. *Pharmacol Toxicol* 1992; 70:125–130.

Pöyhiä R, Seppälä T. Liposolubility and protein binding of oxycodone in vitro. *Pharmacol Toxicol* 1994; 74:23–27.

Rowbotham MC, Reisner-Keller LA, Fields HL. Both intravenous lidocaine and morphine reduce the pain of postherpetic neuralgia. *Neurology* 1991; 41:1024–1028.

Samuelsson H, Hedner T, Venn R, Michalkiewicz A. CSF and plasma concentrations of morphine and morphine glucuronides in cancer patients receiving epidural morphine. *Pain* 1993; 52:179–185.

Vainio A, Tigerstedt I. Opioid treatment for radiating cancer pain: oral administration vs. epidural techniques. *Acta Anaesth Scand* 1988; 32:179–185.

Wegert S, Ossipov MH, Nichols ML, et al. Differential activities of intrathecal MK-801 or morphine to alter responses to thermal and mechanical stimuli in normal or nerve-injured animals. *Pain* 1997; 71:57–64.

Winkelmüller M, Winkelmüller W. Long-term effects of continuous intrathecal opioid treatment in chronic pain of nonmalignant etiology. *J Neurosurg* 1996; 85:458–467.

Wolff T, Samuelsson H, Hedner T. Morphine and morphine metabolite concentrations in cerebrospinal fluid and plasma in cancer pain patients after slow-release oral morphine administration. *Pain* 1995; 62:147–154.

Yaksh TL, Pogrel JW, Lee YW, Chaplan SR. Reversal of nerve ligation-induced allodynia by spinal alpha-2 adrenoceptor agonists. *J Pharmacol Exp Ther* 1995; 272:207–214.

Yeung JC, Rudy TA. Multiplicative interaction between narcotic agonisms expressed at spinal and supraspinal sites of antinociceptive action as revealed by concurrent intrathecal and intracerebroventricular injections of morphine. *J Pharmacol Exp Ther* 1980; 215:633–642.

Yu W, Hao J-X, Xu X-J, Wiesenfeld-Hallin Z. Comparison of the anti-allodynic and antinociceptive effects of systemic, intrathecal and intracerebroventricular morphine in a rat model of central neuropathic pain. *Eur J Pain* 1997; 1:17–29.

Correspondence to: Eija Kalso, MD, DMedSci, Karolinska Institute, Department of Anesthesia and Intensive Care, Huddinge University Hospital, S-14186 Huddinge, Sweden. Fax: 46-8-7795424; email: eija.kalso@helsinki.fi.

Opioid Sensitivity of Chronic Noncancer Pain,
Progress in Pain Research and Management,
Vol. 14, edited by Eija Kalso, Henry J. McQuay,
and Zsuzsanna Wiesenfeld-Hallin, IASP Press,
Seattle, © 1999.

8

Clinical Status of Opioid Tolerance in Long-Term Therapy of Chronic Noncancer Pain

Roman Dertwinkel, Michael Zenz, Michael Strumpf, and Barbara Donner

Department of Anesthesiology, Intensive Care, and Pain Therapy, Bergmannsheil University Hospital, Ruhr University of Bochum, Bochum, Germany

LONG-TERM OPIOID THERAPY IN CHRONIC PAIN

Most patients diagnosed with cancer will require opioid analgesics at some time during their disease, and many will eventually require strong opioids (Grond et al. 1990). In industrialized countries, 30–80% of cancer patients receive insufficient pain therapy (Ventafridda et al. 1987a, 1997), although physicians could ensure at least moderate pain relief for most patients by following the World Health Organization (WHO) guidelines for treatment of cancer pain (Zech et al. 1995; Ventafridda et al. 1997).

Patients with chronic noncancer pain can also be treated safely and effectively with opioids when other therapeutic approaches fail (Dertwinkel et al. 1996). Many studies have demonstrated excellent results for opioid therapy in chronic noncancer pain (Grond et al. 1990; Schug et al. 1992; Zenz et al. 1992; Haythornthwaite et al. 1998). A study that followed chronic noncancer pain patients for over a decade found opioid therapy to be effective in 85% of subjects (Taub 1982). Three placebo-controlled studies have also demonstrated the effectiveness of opioid therapy for noncancer pain (Moran 1991; Arkinstall et al. 1995; Moulin et al. 1996).

Nonetheless, the required dose of opioids is often underestimated. Physicians are concerned about serious side effects such as respiratory depression, addiction (Schofferman 1993), and opioid abuse. One survey showed that patients and their relatives not only share their physicians' concerns about addiction, but also are anxious about opioid efficacy during long-term treatment (Hodes 1989); such concerns may lead to reduced patient compliance.

In the treatment of chronic noncancer pain, a progression to strong opioid analgesics may involve long-term or even life-long therapy, so the possibility that patients may develop tolerance is of great concern to physicians. Diminution of opioid efficacy in the course of long-term treatment has been noted as a frequent problem (Halpern 1997; Osipova et al. 1991; Crews et al. 1993), and development of clinically relevant opioid tolerance could impede the use of opioids in chronic noncancer pain. However, opioid tolerance often is not clinically relevant and may not require limitation of opioid therapy (Drexel et al. 1989; Cherny et al. 1995). In fact, most problems with opioid therapy are the result of therapeutic mistakes, such as failing to follow WHO guidelines or to include adjuvant therapy (Grond et al. 1991); if defined standards are followed, opioid therapy can be a very effective long-term therapy for chronic noncancer pain.

A fixed dosage must be regarded as unethical in cancer pain therapy, as the pain level fluctuates and the nature of the pain can change. For patients with chronic noncancer pain, however, once the initial titration phase has been completed, the opioid dosage should stay at about the same level as long as the underlying cause of pain does not change.

CLINICAL RELEVANCE OF OPIOID TOLERANCE

Opioid tolerance is pharmacologically defined as a reduced analgesic effect following repeated application or the need for increasing dosages to maintain the same therapeutic effect. This results in a shift to the right on the dose-effect curve (Mercadante 1998).

The development of opioid tolerance has been described mainly in animal studies. In most of these studies opioids were applied to pain-free animals, and their reaction to induced pain was registered secondarily (Detweiler et al. 1995; Thornton and Smith 1997). Other experiments employed a chronic pain stimulus, but the opioids were not applied continuously, nor did the researchers measure pharmacological properties such as duration of action (Yu et al. 1997). Regardless of the kind of pain induced, the opioid was used in a mostly discontinuous monotherapeutic approach, and so the application of these experimental results to the clinical setting is questionable.

Clinical investigations show that even years of pain therapy with strong opioids do not necessarily lead to an escalation of dosage or to decreased pain relief. On the contrary, patients can be treated effectively with stable dosages for a long time (Walker et al. 1988; Zenz et al. 1992).

The effectiveness of opioid therapy for patients with chronic noncancer pain was documented in an excellent prospective study over about 6 months (Haythornthwaite et al. 1998). After opioid titration, patients reported significantly lower pain scores and significantly better performance at work and greater participation in leisure activities.

An investigation of patients with chronic noncancer pain under opioid therapy revealed that 32 of 40 patients received stable pain relief on a constant opioid dose. The duration of opioid therapy ranged from 3 to 10 years (mean 4.9 years). After the initial titration of the required dose, only three patients needed a moderate increase in dosage, which could be explained by a progression of their disease. After surgery, two patients intermittently required higher doses of the opioid, whereas a reduction was possible for another two patients (Strumpf et al. 1998). In other investigations a higher dosage was prescribed for patients with cancer pain, but an increase in dosage could be explained by a progression of their disease (Follett et al. 1992; Collin et al. 1993; Donner et al. 1998).

The literature that describes the development of opioid tolerance mostly consists of case reports (Greenberg et al. 1982; Coombs et al. 1985; Clark and Kalan 1995), and their clinical relevance is difficult to assess. Most controlled studies on the development of tolerance in cancer and noncancer pain (Table I) should also be regarded critically because of certain methodological problems: (1) Opioids were not applied according to a fixed schedule (Crawford et al. 1983; Pfeifer et al. 1989; Bouckoms et al. 1992; Ebel et al. 1993; Santillan et al. 1994). (2) Immediate-release opioids were used with inadequate time intervals between doses (Bouckoms et al. 1992). (3) An adjuvant medical therapy was not applied or was insufficient (Crawford et al. 1983; Dennis et al. 1987; Pfeifer et al. 1989; Swanson et al. 1989). Dennis et al. (1987) noted that patients with bone metastases or infiltration of the plexus by the tumor required rapidly increasing amounts of opioids; however, neither NSAIDs, antidepressant drugs, nor anticonvulsants were prescribed concomitantly. Some authors postulated a development of tolerance but did not mention whether a progression of the disease had taken place. The progression of cancer can lead to the development of new, opioid-resistant pain that can be clinically more relevant than any opioid tolerance (Ventafridda et al. 1987b).

Table I
Controlled studies reporting opioid tolerance in cancer and noncancer pain

Reference	Design	n	Opioid	Route	Mistakes in Therapy	Missing Data	Comments
Santillan et al. 1994	PR	23 3	Morphine Morphine	p.o. spinal	No adjuvant medication; no time schedule	Progression of disease	
Santillan et al. 1998	PR	54	Morphine	p.o.			
Pfeifer et al. 1989	PR	3 18 3	Morphine Morphine Morphine	p.o. s.c. i.m.	Insufficient adjuvant medication (only diazepam or NSAID); no time schedule; different routes of administration	Etiology of pain	Tolerance described despite low opioid dosages during long-term therapy
Drexel et al. 1989	PR	36	Morphine	s.c.			Patients included only when oral opioid therapy had failed; tolerance in two patients
Crawford et al. 1983	RT	105	Morphine	epidural	No adjuvant medication; no time schedule	Progression of disease	
Dennis et al. 1987	PR	10	Morphine	spinal	No adjuvant medication	Progression of disease	Marked tolerance only in patient with bone metastasis/plexopathy
Ebel et al. 1993	RT	25	Morphine	spinal	No time schedule	Adjuvant medication	
Swanson et al. 1989	PR	117	Morphine	s.c.	No adjuvant medication	Progression of disease	
Osipova et al. 1991	PR	26	Morphine	p.o.		Etiology of pain; progression of disease	
Bouckoms et al. 1992	PR	28 11 7 5 7	Oxycodone Codeine Methadone Meperidine Variable	?	No time schedule; immediate-release opioids	Opioid dosages; routes of administration	

Abbreviations: i.m. = intramuscular; p.o. = per os; PR = prospective; RT = retrospective; s.c. = subcutaneous.

OPIOID RESISTANCE

Pain that responds only slightly or not at all to opioid analgesics is termed opioid resistant. Clinically, opioid resistance seems to be more frequent than opioid tolerance. The pathophysiology of opioid resistance has important clinical implications (Table II).

Reduced opioid sensitivity may be due to a loss of opioid receptors at the spinal level. Up to 70% of presynaptic μ-opioid receptors may be lost due to mechanical, thermal, chemical, or metabolic injuries to afferent C-fibers (Besse et al. 1990). Opioid resistance, however, cannot be explained by this mechanism alone, as postsynaptic and supraspinal receptors cannot be harmed by injuries to the afferent nerve. In one investigation, animals in chronic pain maintained a significantly higher number of nociceptive postsynaptic receptors (α_2-adrenergic, δ-, and μ-opioid receptors) compared with healthy animals; the receptors' susceptibility to opioids remained unchanged (Brandt and Livingston 1990). The clinical role of this mechanism may be of secondary importance, however.

Changes involving the anti-opioid peptides, represented predominantly by cholecystokinin (CCK), seem more relevant. CCK receptors are found close to opioid receptors at the spinal (pre- and postsynaptic) and supraspinal level. CCK itself does not bind to opioid receptors, but by binding to its own receptor it may induce allosteric changes at the μ receptor, thereby reducing the body's response to μ-opioid agonists.

Animal experiments have shown that higher CCK levels were followed by a reduction in opioid effectiveness, whereas the application of CCK antagonists led to improved opioid sensitivity (Dickenson 1994). The pathophysiological mechanisms behind the increased release of CCK remain unclear. One study found that persistent nociceptive stimuli might induce an

Table II
Possible mechanisms of poor opioid response

Resistance
  Loss of opioid receptors
  Activation of nonopioid peptids
  Activation of NMDA antagonists

Tolerance
  Changed metabolism
  Psychological processes
    Increasing psychological distress
    Conditioned behavior

Pseudotolerance
  Treatment of opioid-resistant pain

increased release of CCK (Xu et al. 1993), while another investigation concluded that opioids themselves may lead to an enhanced release of CCK (Zhou et al. 1993). Xu's study most likely addresses opioid resistance, as the pathological mechanism began before opioid therapy was initiated, whereas Zhou's findings apply to opioid tolerance.

Regardless which pathophysiological theory is correct, CCK antagonists most likely will play an important role as adjuvant substances in opioid therapy for chronic pain. In a preliminary double-blind cross-over study, Bernstein et al. (1998) showed that opioid requirements of patients with cancer pain could be reduced to half the dose after the CCK antagonist proglumide was added. The pain intensity, however, remained stable, and all patients had constant drug requirements without any indication of developing opioid tolerance.

The activation of N-methyl-D-aspartate (NMDA) receptors in the area of the substantia gelatinosa probably is the most important mechanism of reduced opioid sensitivity. Repetitive stimulation of nociceptive C-fibers leads to a changed depolarization pattern of central nociceptive neurons, mediated by activation of NMDA receptors. This pattern consists of prolonged and enhanced depolarizations, even though the C-fiber stimulation continues unchanged or ceases. This phenomenon, known as wind-up, seems to be mainly responsible for the initiation of what is termed the central hypersensitive state. Opioids applied during experimentally induced wind-up-phenomena had a reduced efficacy, whereas opioids given before the NMDA mechanisms were activated showed the expected effect, according to preliminary clinical reports that indicate that opioid-resistant pain can be treated successfully with NMDA antagonists (Mercadante et al. 1995; Persson et al. 1995).

In chronic noncancer pain, we can assume that pathological mechanisms such as wind-up have already been well established when opioid therapy is initiated. It may thus be possible to diagnose opioid resistance before therapy begins (Dertwinkel et al. 1998). In contrast, cancer is a dynamic process whereby growth of the tumor, metastases, and inflammatory processes can lead to an increased activation of peripheral nociceptive receptors and neuropathic pathways (Portenoy 1994). This may result in secondary development of opioid-refractory pain even after effective long-term opioid therapy. A careful clinical history and extended diagnostic procedures may help to distinguish between opioid tolerance and developed opioid resistance.

OPIOID TOLERANCE

Opioid tolerance may develop in certain patients during the course of pain therapy. One possible reason is a change in the distribution or metabolism of the drug when repetitively applied, which results in a lower concentration of opioids at the receptor site. However, one study found that in cancer patients, over 5–8 months the plasma concentration of morphine and its metabolites morphine-3-glucuronide and morphine-6-glucuronide still showed a linear increase with increased doses of morphine. The relation between morphine and its metabolites was constant and independent of the dosage or length of therapy (Säwe et al. 1983). We can therefore assume that a pharmacokinetic tolerance does not play a clinically relevant role in long-term opioid treatment.

Conditioned tolerance seems to have much greater clinical importance (Collett 1998). In the course of pain therapy, patients learn to use expressions of pain, often involving pleading for help, to articulate physical and psychological problems. Statements of pain are often used to express reactive depression or anxiety. Patients may receive more attention from their physicians and others by describing persistent pain. Increasingly higher doses of opioids might be prescribed if physicians misinterpret conditioned tolerance as opioid tolerance.

Patient noncompliance (failure to take drugs as prescribed) is another aspect that might lead to false conclusions about opioid-sensitive pain. Several investigations have demonstrated that about one-third of patients showed questionable drug compliance (Lewis et al. 1983; Basch et al. 1985). Patients also may take drugs but deny having taken them. In a controlled study, 17% of patients with noncancer pain showed positive urinalysis results for benzodiazepine metabolites, although none of them admitted having received prescriptions for such drugs from other physicians. In these patients the side effects of opioid therapy were significantly higher and more severe than in other patients (Schulzeck et al. 1993).

PSEUDOTOLERANCE

If a patient with opioid-refractory pain is treated with opioid analgesics, effects on the central nervous system such as sedation and euphoria can lead to mental dissociation from the pain, which patients and physicians can easily misinterpret as an analgesic effect. As these effects often decline rapidly, higher doses of opioids are needed to keep up the dissociative effect. These higher opioid requirements can be mistaken for opioid toler-

Table III
Standards for opioid treatment of noncancer pain

Interdisciplinary Approach
Correct diagnosis
Compliance
Test of Opioid Sensitivity
Adjuvant Therapy
Psychological therapy
Physiotherapy
Co-medication
Control of Therapy
Close follow up
Documentation

ance. Thus chronic noncancer pain should be managed according to a standardized schedule (Table III). The indication for opioid therapy should be confirmed by an interdisciplinary team consisting of pain clinicians and psychologists, and sometimes including neurologists, orthopedic surgeons. internists, or physical therapists, depending on the nature of the case. Pain disorders of psychosomatic origin should be excluded. Physicians must determine whether the patient is willing and able to tolerate long-term opioid therapy. In almost all patients an adjuvant medical or nonmedical therapy is necessary.

ADJUVANT PAIN THERAPY

PSYCHOLOGICAL THERAPY

Chronic pain is a complex biopsychosocial phenomenon, which is maintained by physical, behavioral, cognitive, and affective components. Therefore a behaviorally oriented psychological therapeutic intervention can be an indispensable part of most pain treatments (Pappagallo and Heinberg 1997; Willweber-Strumpf and Aschke 1998).

PHYSIOTHERAPY

Often initial pharmaceutical intervention is needed to break the vicious cycle of pain–tension–more pain–more tension before intensive physiotherapy can be used to address the actual cause of pain, not only in patients with primary musculoskeletal pain, but also for those with pain of neuropathic origin who have secondary tension or muscle pain.

ADJUVANT MEDICATION

Numerous clinical studies have demonstrated that adjuvant therapy with coanalgesics and suitable nonanalgesic drugs was able to reduce the intensity of pain significantly (Ferrer-Brechner and Ganz 1984; Frank et al. 1988; Ernst et al. 1992; Dellemijn et al. 1994; Rodriguez et al. 1994). The prescription must be adjusted according to the character of pain and the etiology and symptoms of the disease (Grond et al. 1991). A study of 550 patients with cancer pain over 22,000 days of therapy showed that an appropriate adjuvant medication was able to reduce the necessary dosage of morphine; even with long-term treatment no development of opioid tolerance could be observed (Schug et al. 1992).

TESTING OPIOID SENSITIVITY

Patients with noncancer pain should be tested for opioid sensitivity (by intravenous opioid infusion) to avoid treating opioid-refractory pain with

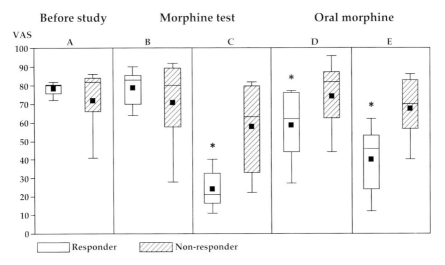

Fig. 1. Pain intensity as measured on a visual analogue scale (mean, median, and standard error) in a test of opioid sensitivity using morphine infusion (adapted from Dertwinkel et al. 1998). (A) Prestudy period (7 days); (B) immediately before morphine infusion; (C) immediately after morphine infusion; (D) before the first oral opioid medication; and (E) at the end of the 30-day observation period. Open bars show responders (*n* = 5); hatched bars show nonresponders (*n* = 15). Asterisks (*) denote statistical significance (*P* < 0.05). Doses for morphine test (at 20 mg/h) were 35–100 mg (mean 51.3 mg) for responders and 22–75 mg (mean 53.4 mg) for nonresponders. Doses for oral morphine were 10–100 mg (mean 40 mg) for responders and 10–80 mg (mean 42 mg) for nonresponders.

opioids. A placebo-controlled double-blind study demonstrated that patients with a good opioid response could be differentiated by this means from those for whom morphine would be ineffective. All patients were then given an oral sustained-release preparation of morphine on a fixed schedule; the results of the morphine testing were mirrored exactly (Dertwinkel et al. 1998) (Fig. 1). Haythornthwaite et al. (1998) demonstrated that patients who were regarded as responders at the end of a period of observation needed significantly lower opioid dosages than those categorized as nonresponders. Alternative predictors for opioid sensitivity have not yet been identified.

CONTROL OF THERAPY

Patients with long-term opioid treatment should visit their physician regularly. Visits should be more frequent during the titration phase and less frequent during the stable phase of opioid therapy to ensure the safety and efficiency of the therapy. Documentation of the therapeutic course should not only focus on the patient's pain intensity, but also take into account aspects such as pain quality, frequency of pain attacks, emotional content, habits (including interference with sleep), physiological effects, and quality of life (Nilges 1998). Clinicians can adapt therapy to such ongoing changes and thereby prevent the development of opioid tolerance.

CONCLUSIONS

Opioid tolerance may develop in the course of therapy (Drexel et al. 1989; Santillan et al. 1998), although the incidence is low when pain responds to opioids adequately (Schug et al. 1991). In most cases of opioid tolerance the primary problem is not pharmacodynamic or pharmacokinetic but rather iatrogenic in origin. Use of opioid therapy for opioid-refractory pain, failure to prescribe adjuvant treatment, or provision of opioids on demand are examples of improper prescription of opioids and should not detract from the effectiveness of opioid therapy in general. Opioid therapy that follows a standardized approach can offer a safe and effective long-term therapy, which can successfully be applied for patients with chronic noncancer pain.

REFERENCES

Arkinstall W, Sandler A, Goughnour B, et al. Efficacy of controlled-release codeine in chronic non-malignant pain: a randomized, placebo-controlled clinical trial. *Pain* 1995; 62:169–178.

Basch EC, Gold RS, McDermott RJ, Richardson CE. Confounding variables in the measurement of cancer patient compliance. *Cancer Nurs* 1985; 285–293.

Bernstein ZP, Yucht S, Battista E, Lema M, Spaulding MB. Proglumide as a morphine adjunct in cancer pain management. *J Pain Symptom Manage* 1998; 15:314–320.

Besse D, Lombard MC, Zajac JM, et al. Pre and postsynaptic distribution of mu, delta and kappa opioid receptors in the superficial layers of the cervical dorsal horn of the rat spinal cord: a quantitative autoradiographic study. *Brain Res* 1990; 521:15–22.

Bouckoms AJ, Masand P, Murray GB, et al. Chronic nonmalignant pain treated with long-term oral narcotic analgesics. *Ann Clin Psych* 1992; 4:185–192.

Brandt SA, Livingston A. Receptor changes in the spinal cord of sheep associated with exposure to chronic pain. *Pain* 1990; 42:323–329.

Cherny NI, Portenoy RK, Raber M, Zenz M. Medikamentöse Therapie von Tumorschmerzen. *Schmerz* 1995; 9:3–19.

Clark JL, Kalan GE. Effective treatment of severe cancer pain of the head using low-dose ketamine in an opioid-tolerant patient. *J Pain Symptom Manage* 1995; 10:310–314.

Collett B-J. Opioid tolerance: the clinical perspective. *Br J Anaesth* 1998; 81:58–68.

Collin E, Poulain P, Gauvain-Piquard A, Petit G, Pichard-Leandri E. Is disease progression the major factor in morphine 'tolerance' in cancer pain treatment? *Pain* 1993; 55:319–326.

Coombs DW, Saunders RL, Lachance D, et al. Intrathecal morphine tolerance: use of intrathecal clonidine, DADLE, and intraventricular morphine. *Anesthesiology* 1985; 62:358–363.

Crawford ME, Andersen HB, Augustenborg G, et al. Pain treatment on outpatient basis utilizing extradural opiates. A Danish multicentre study comprising 105 patients. *Pain* 1983; 16:41–47.

Crews JC, Sweeney NJ, Denson DD. Clinical efficacy of methadone in patients refractory to other mu-opioid receptor agonist analgesics for management of terminal cancer pain. Case presentations and discussion of incomplete cross-tolerance among opioid agonist analgesics. *Cancer* 1993; 72:2266–2272.

Dellemijn PLI, Verbiest HBC, Van Vliet JJ, et al. Medical therapy of malignant nerve pain. A randomised double-blind explanatory trial with naproxen versus slow-release morphine. *Eur J Cancer* 1994; 30A:1244–1250.

Dennis GC, DeWitty R. Management of intractable pain in cancer patients by implantable infusion systems. *J Nat Med Assoc* 1987; 79:939–944.

Dertwinkel R, Wiebalck A, Zenz M, Strumpf M. Orale Opioide zur Langzeittherapie chronischer Nicht-Tumorschmerzen. *Anaesthesist* 1996; 45:495–505.

Dertwinkel R, Strumpf M, Willweber-Strumpf A, et al. Intravenous testing of opioid sensibility in patients with chronic non-cancer pain and consecutive oral adjustment of pain medication. *Br J Anaesth* 1998; 80(Suppl 1):170.

Detweiler DJ, Rohde DS, Basbaum AI. The development of opioid tolerance in the formalin test in the rat. *Pain* 1995; 63:251–254.

Dickenson AH. Neurophysiology of opioid poorly responsive pain. *Cancer Surv* 1994; 21:5–16.

Donner B, Zenz M, Strumpf M, Raber M. Long-term treatment of cancer pain with transdermal fentanyl. *J Pain Symptom Manage* 1998; 15:168–175.

Drexel H, Dzien A, Spiegel RW, et al. Treatment of severe cancer pain by low-dose continuous subcutaneous morphine. *Pain* 1989; 36:169–176.

Ebel H, Buschmann D, Conzen M, Oppel F. Erste Erfahrungen mit implantierbaren Pumpensystemen zur intrathekalen Therapie chronischer Schmerzen. *Nervenarzt* 1993; 64:468–473.

Ernst DS, MacDonald RN, Paterson AH, et al. A double-blind, crossover trial of intravenous clodronate in metastatic bone pain. *J Pain Symptom Manage* 1992; 7:4–11.

Ferrer-Brechner T, Ganz P. Combination therapy with ibuprofen and methadone for chronic cancer pain. *Am J Med* 1984: 78–83.

Follett KA, Hitchon PW, Piper J, et al. Response of intractable pain to continuous intrathecal morphine: a retrospective study. *Pain* 1992; 49:21–25.

Frank RG, Kashani JH, Parker JC, et al. Antidepressant analgesia in rheumatoid arthritis. *J Rheumatol* 1988; 15:1632–1638.

Greenberg HS, Taren J, Ensminger WD, Doan K. Benefit from and tolerance to continuous intrathecal infusion of morphine for intractable cancer pain. *J Neurosurg* 1982; 57:360–364.

Grond S, Zech D, Horrichs-Haermeyer G, Lehmann KA. Schmerztherapie in der Finalphase maligner Erkrankungen. *Schmerz* 1990; 4:22–28.

Grond S, Zech D, Schug SA, Lynch J, Lehmann KA. The importance of non-opioid analgesics for cancer pain relief according to the guidelines of the World Health Organization. *Int J Pharm Res* 1991; XI:253–260.

Halpern LM. Analgesic drugs in the management of pain. *Arch Surg* 1977; 112:661–669.

Haythornthwaite JA, Menefee LA, Quatrano-Piacentini AL, Pappagallo M. Outcome of chronic opioid therapy for non-cancer pain. *J Pain Symptom Manage* 1998; 15:185–194.

Hodes RL. Cancer patients' needs and concerns when using narcotic analgesics. In: Hill CS Jr, Fields WS (Eds). *Advances in Pain Research and Therapy*, Vol. 11. New York: Raven Press, 1989, pp 91–99.

Lewis C, Linet MS, Abeloff MD. Compliance with cancer therapy by patients and physicians. *Am J Med* 1983; 74:673–678.

Mercadante S. Opioid rotation in cancer pain. *Curr Rev Pain* 1998; 3:131–142.

Mercadante S, Lodi F, Sapio M. Long-term ketamine subcutaneous continuous infusion in neuropathic cancer pain. *J Pain Symptom Manage* 1995; 10:564–568.

Moran C. MST continus tablets and pain control in severe rheumatoid arthritis. *Br J Clin Res* 1991; 2:1–12.

Moulin DE, Iezzi A, Amireh R, et al. Randomised trial of oral morphine for chronic non-cancer pain. *Lancet* 1996; 347:143–147.

Nilges P. Outcome measures in pain therapy. *Baillieres Clin Anaesth* 1998; 12:1–1.

Osipova NA, Novikov GA, Beresnev VA, Loseva NA. Analgesic effect of tramadol in cancer patients with chronic pain: a comparison with prolonged-action morphine sulfate. *Curr Ther Res* 1991; 50:812–821.

Pappagallo M, Heinberg LJ. Ethical issues in the management of chronic nonmalignant pain. *Semin Neurol* 1997; 17:203–211.

Persson J, Axelsson G, Hallin RG, Gustafsson LL. Beneficial effects of ketamine in a chronic pain state with allodynia, possibly due to central sensitization. *Pain* 1995; 60:217–222.

Pfeifer BL, Sernaker HL, Ter Horst UM, Porges SW. Cross-tolerance between systemic and epidural morphine in cancer patients. *Pain* 1989; 39:181–187.

Portenoy RK. Tolerance to opioid analgesics: clinical aspects. *Canc Surv* 1994; 21:49–65.

Rodriguez M, Barutell C, Rull M, et al. Efficacy and tolerance of oral dipyrone versus oral morphine for cancer pain. *Eur J Cancer* 1994; 30A:584–587.

Santillan R, Maestre JM, Hurle MA, Florez J. Enhancement of opiate analgesia by nimodipine in cancer patients chronically treated with morphine: a preliminary report. *Pain* 1994; 58:129–132.

Santillan R, Hurle MA, Armijo JA, de los Mozos R, Florez J. Nimodipine-enhanced opiate analgesia in cancer patients requiring morphine dose escalation: a double-blind, placebo-controlled study. *Pain* 1998; 76:17–26.

Säwe J, Svensson JO, Rane A. Morphine metabolism in cancer patients on increasing oral doses—no evidence for autoinduction or dose-dependence. *Br J Clin Pharmacol* 1983; 16:85–93.

Schofferman J. Long-term use of opioid analgesics for the treatment of chronic pain of nonmalignant origin. *J Pain Symptom Manage* 1993; 8:279–288.

Schug SA, Merry AF, Acland RH. Treatment principles for the use of opioids in pain of nonmalignant origin. *Drugs* 1991; 42:228–239.

Schug SA, Zech D, Grond S, et al. A long-term survey of morphine in cancer pain patients. *J Pain Symptom Manage* 1992; 7:259–266.

Schulzeck S, Gleim M, Maier C. Morphintabletten bei chronischen nicht-tumorbedingten Schmerzen. *Anaesthesist* 1993; 42:545–556.

Strumpf M, Zenz M, Dertwinkel R, Rothstein D. Long-term oral opioid therapy in patients with non-cancer pain. *Br J Anaesth* 1998; 80 (Suppl 1):170.

Swanson G, Smith J, Bulich R, New P, Shiffman R. Patient-controlled analgesia for chronic cancer pain in the ambulatory setting: a report of 117 patients. *J Clin Oncol* 1989; 7:1903–1908.

Taub A. Opioid analgesics in the treatment of chronic intractable pain of non-neoplastic origin. In: Kitahata LM, Collins D (Eds). *Narcotic Analgesics in Anesthesiology*. Baltimore: Williams and Wilkins, 1982, pp 199–208.

Thornton SR, Smith FL. Characterization of neonatal rat fentanyl tolerance and dependence. *J Pharmacol Exp Ther* 1997; 281:514–521.

Ventafridda V, Tamburini M, Caraceni A, et al. A validation study of the WHO method for cancer pain relief. *Cancer* 1987a; 59:850–856.

Ventafridda V, Spoldi E, Caraceni A, De Conno F. Intraspinal morphine for cancer pain. *Acta Anaesthesiol Scand* 1987b; 85(Suppl):47–53.

Ventafridda V, Sbanotto A, Burnhill R. Ten years of World Health Organization guidelines—do they really work? *Curr Opin Anaesth* 1997; 10:386–390.

Walker VA, Hoskin PJ, Hanks GW, White ID. Evaluation of WHO analgesic guidelines for cancer pain in a hospital-based palliative care unit. *J Pain Symptom Manage* 1988; 3:145–149.

Willweber-Strumpf A, Aschke M. Psychologische Schmerztherapie. *Z Arztl Fortbild Qualitatssich* 1998; 92:57–63.

Xu XJ, Puke MJ, Verge VM, et al. Up-regulation of cholecystokinin in primary sensory neurons is associated with morphine insensitivity in experimental neuropathic pain in the rat. *Neurosci Lett* 1993; 152:129–132.

Yu W, Hao JX, Xu XJ, Wiesenfeld-Hallin Z. The development of morphine tolerance and dependence in rats with chronic pain. *Brain Res* 1997; 756:141–146.

Zech DF, Grond S, Lynch J, Hertel D, Lehmann KA. Validation of World Health Organisation guidelines for cancer pain relief: a 10-year prospective study. *Pain* 1995; 63:65–76.

Zenz M, Strumpf M, Tryba M. Long-term opioid therapy in patients with chronic nonmalignant pain. *J Pain Symptom Manage* 1992; 7:69–77.

Zhou Y, Sun YH, Shen JM, Han JS. Increased release of immunoreactive CCK-8 by electroacupuncture and enhancement of electroacupuncture analgesia by CCK-B antagonist in rat spinal cord. *Neuropeptides* 1993; 24:139–144

Correspondence to: Professor Dr. med. Michael Zenz, Department of Anesthesiology, Intensive Care, and Pain Therapy, Bergmannsheil University Hospital, Ruhr University of Bochum, Bürkle-de-la-Camp-Platz 1, D-44789 Bochum, Germany. Tel: 49-234-3026825; Fax: 49-234-3026834; email: michael.zenz@ruhr-uni-bochum-de.

Part III

Understanding and Improving Opioid Sensitivity—New Perspectives

Opioid Sensitivity of Chronic Noncancer Pain,
Progress in Pain Research and Management,
Vol. 14, edited by Eija Kalso, Henry J. McQuay,
and Zsuzsanna Wiesenfeld-Hallin, IASP Press,
Seattle, © 1999.

9

Phenotypic Changes Induced in Dorsal Root Ganglion Neurons by Nerve Injury

Tomas Hökfelt,[a] Tie-Jun Sten Shi,[a] J.-G. Cui,[b] Björn
Meyerson,[b] Bengt Linderoth,[b] Yong-Guang Tong,[c]
Hui Fredrik Wang,[a] Zhi-Qing David Xu,[a] Gong Ju,[c]
Gunnar Grant,[a] and Xu Zhang[c]

*[a]Department of Neuroscience, Karolinska Institute, Stockholm, Sweden;
[b]Department of Clinical Neuroscience, Section of Neurosurgery, Karolinska
Hospital/Institute, Stockholm, Sweden; and [c]Department of Neurobiology,
Institute of Neurosciences, The Fourth Military Medical University,
Xi'an, P.R. China*

Transection of a peripheral nerve causes major changes in the expression of various molecules in the neurons of the dorsal root ganglia (DRG), including peptides, peptide receptors, and enzymes (Shehab and Atkinson 1986; see Hökfelt et al. 1987, 1994; Zigmond et al. 1996). This chapter describes the results of two studies, both dealing with the effect of peripheral nerve injury on DRG neurons (Shi et al. 1999; Tong et al. 1999). The results emphasize the dramatic changes induced by peripheral nerve lesion.

REGULATION OF PEPTIDES AND PEPTIDE RECEPTORS IN DRG NEURONS

Nielsch et al. (1987) demonstrated that peripheral nerve injury leads to a reduction in substance P (SP) synthesis in DRG neurons, and similar findings have been reported for calcitonin gene-related peptide (CGRP) (Noguchi et al. 1990; Dumoulin et al. 1991). The first evidence for peptide upregulation in DRG neurons was presented for vasoactive intestinal polypeptide (VIP) (Shehab and Atkinson 1986), followed by galanin (Hökfelt et al. 1987), neuropeptide tyrosine (NPY) (Wakisaka et al. 1991), and pituitary adenylate cyclase-activating peptide (PACAP) (Q. Zhang et al. 1995; Y.-Z. Zhang et al. 1996). Peptide upregulation occurs, at least partly, in different neuron populations: for VIP it occurs mostly in small DRG neurons, for galanin mostly in small but also in some large neurons, for NPY mostly in large and a few small neurons, and for PACAP in both small and large neurons. (Small DRG neurons are mostly associated with nociception and large ones with mechanoreception.)

At least one receptor exists for virtually every known peptide, and some neuropeptides may have half a dozen or more receptor subtypes (see Meyerhof et al. 1993; Schwartz et al. 1995; Betancur et al. 1997). Peptide receptors exist in DRG neurons and are regulated by nerve injury. Under normal circumstances the cholecystokinin-B (CCK_B) receptor (Kopin et al. 1992) is expressed at very low levels in rat DRG neurons, but it is strongly upregulated after peripheral nerve injury, when approximately 60% of all neuron profiles express CCK_B-receptor mRNA (Zhang et al. 1993a). (A neuron profile is a slice of a neuron within our 14-µm thick sections of DRG. Only profiles containing the nucleus are counted.) A neurotensin receptor (Tanaka et al. 1990) has been detected in about one-third of all small DRG neuron profiles, and its synthesis is downregulated after axotomy (complete nerve transection) (X. Zhang et al. 1995). The first cloned galanin receptor, the GAL-R1 receptor (Habert-Ortoli et al. 1994; Burgevin et al. 1995; Parker et al. 1995), is expressed mostly in large neuron profiles and exists in about 20% of DRG neurons; virtually all of these neurons also contain CGRP mRNA (Xu et al. 1996b) (Fig. 1). Axotomy induces a marked downregulation of expression of GAL-R1 receptor mRNA, and inflammation causes a transient decrease in the mRNA levels (Xu et al. 1996b). The GAL-R2 receptor (Ahmad et al. 1996; Fathi et al. 1997; Howard et al. 1997; Smith et al. 1997; Wang et al. 1997) is present in around 25% of all neuron profiles, mainly small and often CGRP mRNA positive (Shi et al. 1997), and is weakly downregulated by axotomy.

The µ-, δ-, and κ-opioid receptors have also been cloned (see Minami and Satoh 1995) and identified in DRG neurons and in the dorsal horn of the spinal cord by using in situ hybridization and immunohistochemistry techniques (Dado et al. 1993; Maekawa et al. 1994, 1995; Mansour et al. 1994, 1995, 1996; Minami et al. 1994, 1995; Arvidsson et al. 1995a,b,c; Cheng et al. 1995; Honda and Arvidsson 1995; Ji et al. 1995; Minami and Satoh 1995; Zhang et al. 1998). Mu-opioid-receptor (MOR) mRNA was found in more than half of all DRG neurons (Minami et al. 1995); 40% of these neurons expressed preprotachykinin (ppTK) mRNA. Almost all neurons that were ppTK mRNA positive also expressed MOR mRNA (Minami et al. 1995). The levels of MOR mRNA and MOR-like immunoreactivity were downregulated

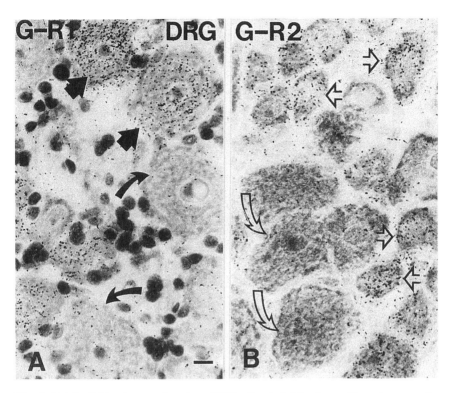

Fig. 1. Bright-field micrographs of rat DRG after hybridization with probes complementary to mRNA for (A) GAL-R1 and (B) GAL-R2 receptor. (A) GAL-R1 mRNA is
mainly localized in many large neurons (*arrows*) and some medium-sized neurons.
Curved arrows point to large unlabeled neurons. (B) GAL-R2 mRNA is seen in many
small neurons (*arrows*). Curved arrows point to large unlabeled neurons. Bar indicates
10 μm.

after peripheral nerve injury, particularly in a study using monkeys (Zhang
et al. 1998). This finding is analogous to the downregulation of opioid receptors, as revealed with ligand-binding techniques (Jessell et al. 1979; Fields
et al. 1980; Besse et al. 1992), and may account for the decreased sensitivity
to morphine in neuropathic pain. Table I summarizes the effects of axotomy
on messengers and receptors in DRG neurons.

CHOLERATOXIN-B SUBUNIT UPTAKE IN MONKEY
AND RAT DRG NEURONS

Several studies provide strong evidence that peripheral nerve injury in
the rat induces sprouting of myelinated primary afferent fibers from deeper
laminae into laminae I and II of the spinal cord. Such changes may be

Table 1
Effect of axotomy on neuropeptides and reptors in
dorsal root ganglion neurons

	Regulation*
Neuropeptides	
Substance P	↓↓↓(↑)
CGRP	↓↓↓(↑)
Somatostatin	↓↓
VIP/PHI	↑↑↑
Galanin	↑↑↑
CCK	(↑)
NPY	↑↑↑
PACAP	↑↑↑
NOS (enzyme)	↑↑
Receptors	
δ-opioid receptor	↓
μ-opioid-receptor	↓
α_2A-adrenoceptor	↑
α_2C-adrenoceptor	↓
NPY-Y1 receptor	↓(↑)
NPY-Y2 receptor	↑
CCK_B receptor	↑↑↑
GAL-R1 receptor	↓
GAL-R2 receptor	(↑)
Neurotensin receptor	↓

Abbreviations: CCK = cholecystokinin; CGRP = calcitonin gene-related peptide; GAL = galanin; NOS = nitric oxide synthase; NPY = neuropeptide tyrosine; PACAP = pituitary adenylate cyclase-activating peptide; PHI = peptide histidine, isoleucine; VIP = vasoactive intestinal polypeptide. *Arrows indicate up- or downregulation following axotomy. Parentheses indicate weak regulation or opposite regulation in subpopulations of neurons.

related to the development of chronic pain (see Woolf 1997), so it would be useful to analyze to what extent they may occur in other species, including primates. To our knowledge, only one study has observed this phenomenon in the monkey spinal cord after peripheral nerve injury (Florence et al. 1993). We therefore used choleratoxin-B subunit (CTB) as a tracer to investigate the possibility of neural sprouting in the monkey (Tong et al. 1999; method originally introduced by Stoeckel et al. 1977). CTB is known to bind to cell membrane glucoconjugates, in particular monoganglioside GM1 (Cuatrecacas 1973; Holmgren et al. 1973; King and van Heyningen 1973).

We also used the lectin B4 of the plant lectin *Griffonia simplicifolia I* as a marker for a subtype of small DRG neurons (Streit et al. 1985, 1986).

We deeply anesthetized adult male *Macaca mulatta* monkeys and resected part of the left sciatic nerve at mid-thigh level. Two weeks later we exposed the sciatic nerves bilaterally and slowly injected 1% CTB 7 mm proximal to the nerve stump on the transected side and into the contralateral, intact nerve at the same level. Six days later the animals were deeply anesthetized and perfused with formalin and picric acid to preserve the tissue. The ganglia and spinal cord were then cut in a cryostat and the sections processed for immunohistochemistry using goat antiserum raised against CTB and secondary donkey antibodies conjugated with fluorescein isothiocyanate (FITC). We examined the DRG and spinal cord at the L5 level and observed a marked difference in the percentage of CTB-labeled neuron profiles between the ipsi- and contralateral sides. More than 70% of the counted neuron profiles were stained (i.e., positive) ipsilaterally (Fig. 2A), but only 11.5% were stained on the unlesioned side (Fig. 2B). Moreover, on the ipsilateral side most of the CTB-labeled neuron profiles were small, whereas those on the contralateral side were larger. In the contralateral dorsal horn we observed only a moderately dense CTB-positive fiber plexus in laminae I and II, with a few fibers in deeper laminae. Ipsilaterally we noted a marked increase in positive fibers in laminae I and II and detected distinct patches of densely packed fibers in lamina II. B4 binding sites were found in about 60% of the small neuron profiles in the contralateral DRG, compared to less than 1% in the ipsilateral DRG.

We performed a similar experiment on rats (Tong et al. 1999) to find out whether the results would be similar to our results with monkeys or to the results of previous studies with rats (see Woolf 1997). On examining the DRG 18 days after unilateral axotomy, we found that 43% of neuron profiles, mainly large ones, were CTB positive in the contralateral DRG. On the axotomized side more than 80% of all neuron profiles were CTB positive. The results are summarized in Figs. 3 and 4. In the contralateral dorsal horn many CTB-positive fibers were localized in laminae III–V, with only scattered positive fibers in the superficial laminae (Fig. 2D). On the lesioned side, however, we observed a dense CTB-positive fiber plexus in laminae I and II, with more intense CTB labeling in the deeper lamina (Fig. 2C). In the contralateral DRG about 50% of small neuron profiles were B4 positive, compared to around 15% ipsilaterally.

These results show, unexpectedly, that axotomy dramatically changes the uptake properties for CTB into axons and alters B4 binding properties to DRG neurons, both in the monkey and in the rat (Tong et al. 1999). These changes are particularly evident in the monkey, where 70% of all DRG neuron profiles were CTB positive after axotomy versus only 10% in the intact sciatic nerve. We found a similar, although less pronounced difference in rats, where the corresponding figures for CTB were around 80% versus 40%, and also observed a marked change for B4 binding. The percentage of labeling of DRG neuron profiles in the rat after injection of tracer into the intact sciatic nerve is similar to that previously reported by Woolf et al. (1995), whose study did not observe the same dramatic increase we saw on the axotomized side. Importantly, the increase in CTB labeling was mainly confined to small DRG neuron profiles, both in rats and monkeys.

The changes in cell body labeling were paralleled by the CTB labeling patterns in the dorsal horn. Thus, there was a strong increase in the number and intensity of CTB labeling in laminae I and II in the monkey dorsal horn, whereas the main features in the rat dorsal horn were the new appearance of labeled fibers in laminae I and II and an intensity increase in the deeper layers. These findings in the rat dorsal horn confirm the results of many earlier studies (see Woolf 1997). Several conclusions can be drawn from our results:

1) Transection of DRG neurons dramatically changes the uptake and binding properties for certain lectins in both rats and monkeys. Nerve injury induces uptake of CTB into small DRG neurons, which apparently do not have this capacity under normal circumstances. This finding indicates modification of carbohydrate-rich sphingolipids on the membrane surface, especially monoganglioside GM1, the receptor for CTB (Cuatrecacas 1973; Holmgren et al. 1973). The binding of B4 lectin is also dramatically attenuated by axotomy.

2) The projection sites for small and large neurons are different in monkeys compared to rats, at least in *M. mulatta*, where hardly any CTB-positive fibers were seen in the deeper lamina, in sharp contrast to the rat. Moreover, part of the strong ipsilateral increase in CTB labeling was observed in

Fig. 2. Immunofluorescence micrographs of ipsilateral (Ipsi) (A, C) and contralateral (Con) (B, D) monkey L5 DRGs (A, B) and rat dorsal horn (C, D) 20 days (in monkeys) or 18 days (in rats) after unilateral sciatic nerve cut, labeled for CTB. (A, B) The number of CTB-labeled neurons is markedly increased in the ipsilateral (A) as compared to the contralateral (B) DRG. (C) Intense CTB labeling is observed in laminae I (*arrowhead*), II (*curved arrow*), III (*arrow*), and deeper laminae of the ipsilateral dorsal horn. (D) Weak CTB labeling is seen in only a few nerve fibers in the contralateral laminae I and II. Strongly labeled fibers are seen in laminae III–V. Bar indicates 50 μm in A and B, and 100 μm in C and D. Adapted from Tong et al. (1999) with permission from Wiley-Liss, Incorporated, a subsidiary of John Wiley and Sons, Incorporated. ⟶

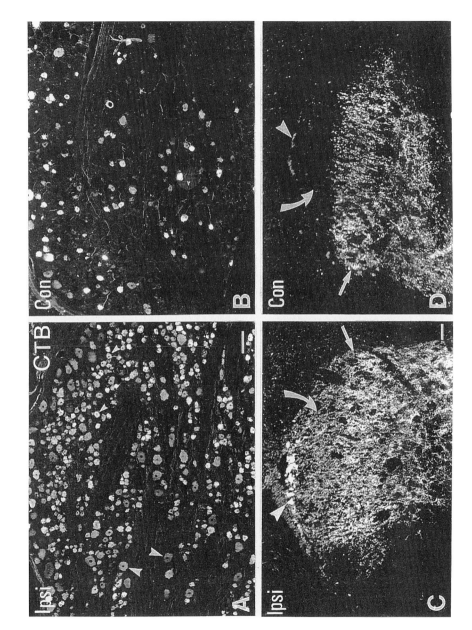

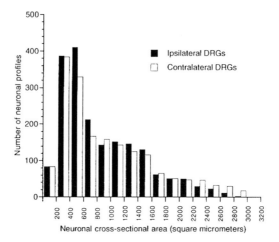

Fig. 3. Cross-sectional area of neuronal profiles in rat L5 DRG 18 days after unilateral axotomy. The size distributions of neuron profiles are similar in the DRG on both sides. One peak representing small neuron profiles is located at 200–800 μm², and another for larger profiles at 800–1600 μm². Adapted from Tong et al. (1999) with permission from Wiley-Liss, Incorporated, a subsidiary of John Wiley and Sons, Incorporated.

"patches" in lamina II. Such patches contain somatostatin and galanin in the monkey dorsal horn after axotomy (Zhang et al. 1993b) and are similar to primary afferent fiber patterns in lamina II of rats (Ygge and Grant 1983; Molander and Grant 1985) and cats (Réthelyi 1977).

3) The increase in CTB labeling in the superficial laminae in the dorsal horn in rats after peripheral nerve injury has generally been interpreted to indicate neural sprouting (see Woolf 1997), a view also supported by the results seen after injecting single large-diameter fibers with horseradish peroxide (Woolf et al. 1992; Koerber et al. 1994). Moreover, neural sprouting could represent an important anatomical basis for neuropathic pain encountered after peripheral nerve injury (see Woolf 1997). Our findings suggest, however, that mechanisms other than sprouting may also be involved in the increase in CTB labeling in the superficial laminae after nerve injury. Thus, nerve injury seems to change the capacity to take up CTB, which after nerve injury is conferred to small DRG neurons. Further studies are necessary to validate this hypothesis, including demonstration that CTB can be found in axons and terminals of small DRG neurons in the dorsal roots and dorsal horn. The concept of neural sprouting as an anatomical basis for neuropathic pain should be viewed with some caution until further studies can test our hypothesis.

4) Our findings help clarify the changes in phenotype that occur after nerve injury. Messenger molecules, such as peptides, are either downregulated

(SP, CGRP) or upregulated (VIP, galanin, NPY). Peptide receptors are also distinctly regulated; for example, CCK_B receptors are upregulated, and NPY-Y1 and GAL-R1 receptors are downregulated after axotomy. We have shown that availability of gangliosides is strongly upregulated after axotomy (Tong et al. 1999). Trophic factors and neuroimmune molecules of various types, often localized to non-neuronal cells, are also regulated in response to axotomy (Kreutzberg 1996; Raivich et al. 1996; Zigmond et al. 1996; Jonakait 1997).

5) An important question is whether the changes in phenotype of peptides and receptors are specific to DRG neurons. Are they a particular feature of pseudounipolar neurons, which have one peripheral and one central branch, and do they occur only when the lesion is confined to the peripheral branch? We now know that lesion of motoneuron axons causes dramatic changes in the expression of several types of molecules in the somata (Arvidsson et al. 1993; Raivich et al. 1996) and also in certain central systems, such as the hypothalamic magnocellular neurons (e.g., Villar et al. 1994). It is therefore possible that such changes may occur in many parts of the nervous system when neurons are injured, and that similar events may play a role in several neurodegenerative diseases.

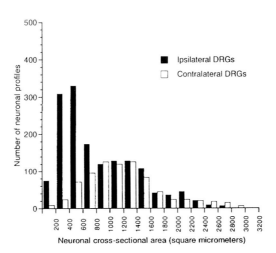

Fig. 4. Cross-sectional area of CTB-labeled neuron profiles in rat L5 DRG 18 days after unilateral axotomy; the peak is shifted toward small profiles. In the contralateral DRG the peak is in the range of medium-sized and large neuron profiles. Adapted from Tong et al. (1999) with permission from Wiley-Liss, Incorporated, a subsidiary of John Wiley and Sons, Incorporated.

REGULATION OF GALANIN IN RAT
MONONEUROPATHIC MODELS

Several studies have demonstrated that transection of the sciatic nerve causes a dramatic increase in levels of galanin and galanin mRNA in neurons of the L4 and L5 DRG (see Hökfelt et al. 1994 for review). Until recently, little information has been available to document similar changes in other models of mononeuropathy. However, Nahin et al. (1994) and Ma and Bisby (1997) demonstrated that galanin, NPY, and VIP are strongly upregulated after chronic nerve constriction. They used the model of Bennett and Xie (1988), as did Wakisaka and collaborators (1992), who also showed upregulation of NPY. Ma and Bisby (1997) also studied partial nerve transection and showed increases in galanin expression. Recently Gazelius et al. (1996) introduced a new model of rat neuropathy based on photochemically induced lesion of the rat sciatic nerve (see also Kupers et al. 1998; Hao et al. 1999).

We recently compared several models of neuropathy in rats (Shi et al. 1999): photochemically induced lesions (based on the model of Gazelius et al. 1996), total nerve transection (performed according to Wall and Gutnick 1979; Wall et al. 1979), nerve constriction (according to Bennett and Xie 1988), and partial ligation of the sciatic nerve (slightly modified from Seltzer et al. 1990). We introduced lesions at mid-thigh level on one hindlimb and then tested the animals for tactile hypersensitivity using calibrated von Frey nylon filaments. No rats with total nerve transection showed tactile hypersensitivity, compared to virtually all those processed according to the Gazelius model and about half those treated according to the Seltzer and Bennett models. We assigned the rats to six groups for immunohistochemical analysis: (1) rats with total nerve transection, (2) allodynic and (3) nonallodynic Bennett model rats, (4) allodynic and (5) nonallodynic Seltzer model rats, and (6) allodynic Gazelius model rats. Two markers, galanin and NPY, were used (Shi et al. 1999).

Rats with allodynia displayed a less pronounced galanin upregulation than did those with relatively normal sensitivity. In the Bennett model the difference was significant; 23% of all neuron profiles were galanin positive in the allodynic rats versus 43% in the nonallodynic ones. A similar tendency was observed in the Seltzer rat (29% versus 35%), but this difference was not statistically significant. The Gazelius rats, where all except one animal exhibited allodynia, showed the lowest percentage of galanin-positive profiles (13%). NPY was strongly upregulated in all four models; nonallodynic Bennett and Seltzer rats exhibited a more pronounced NPY upregulation than did allodynic ones, although these differences were not significant (22% versus 30% in the Bennett model; 22% versus 27% in the Seltzer model).

We also performed an in situ hybridization analysis with only four experimental groups not separated by allodynic status. Only small numbers of DRG neurons were galanin positive on the contralateral limb. The percentage of galanin-mRNA-positive neurons increased markedly in all four models 2 weeks after the lesion. These neurons were mainly small, but we also observed medium and large neurons.

The role of galanin in dorsal horn transmission, particularly in pain processing, has been debated over the last 10 years. Several stimuli can cause upregulation of galanin, including axotomy, nerve compression (Villar et al. 1989), local application of vinblastine sulfate (Kashiba et al. 1992), herpes simplex infection (Henken and Martin 1992a,b), and stimuli used in the various neuropathic pain models described above.

Using the nociceptive flexor reflex model, Wiesenfeld-Hallin and collaborators (1992a) have shown that local application of galanin onto the dorsal horn of the spinal cord causes a biphasic response, with facilitation at low doses and inhibition at higher doses (see also Cridland and Henry 1988). After nerve injury the inhibitory component is enhanced (Wiesenfeld-Hallin et al. 1992b). Interestingly, a low dose of galanin, which by itself causes facilitation, markedly increases the morphine-induced inhibition of the reflex, an effect that is even more pronounced when a CCK_B antagonist is also administered (Wiesenfeld-Hallin et al. 1990a, 1991). Galanin also enhances the effect of morphine in the tail-flick model (Wiesenfeld-Hallin et al. 1990b).

Given the dramatic upregulation of galanin synthesis after nerve injury, we have advanced the hypothesis that galanin counteracts pain after nerve injury and thus represents an endogenous analgesic (Wiesenfeld-Hallin et al. 1992a; Hökfelt et al. 1997). The analgesic effect of galanin is supported by investigations of a putative galanin antagonist (Verge et al. 1993) and by studies using antisense probes against galanin mRNA (Ji et al. 1994) and against GAL-R1 receptor mRNA (Pooga et al. 1998). However, others have expressed opposing views, based on the facilitatory effect of galanin in the nociceptive reflex at low concentrations. Kuraishi et al. (1991) reported that intrathecal injection of antiserum against porcine galanin reverses the decrease in nociceptive threshold for mechanical but not thermal stimulation in rat hindpaws treated with carrageenan, and that intrathecal injection of porcine galanin decreases the mechanical nociceptive threshold. Furthermore, in a partial nerve injury model, Kerr et al. (1998) have shown that galanin-deficient mice are hypoalgesic.

Ma and Bisby (1997) revealed new aspects relevant to galanin function in the dorsal horn, although we dispute some of their conclusions. They observed that in neuropathic pain models, such as the Bennett model, the percentages of galanin-positive DRG neurons were significantly higher than after complete nerve transection. They also found a higher proportion of medium and large galanin-positive neurons in the neuropathic pain models than after complete nerve transection, and a marked increase in galanin-positive fibers, not only in laminae I and II but also in deeper laminae into which the large DRG neurons project. They proposed two possible explanations, one being that "partial nerve injury causes more severe neuropathic pain than complete nerve injury, thus leading to a higher level of galanin expression or a compensatory response." However, they also suggested that the increased galanin expression "actually facilitates transmission and nociceptive information in the pain pathways," showing a possible correlation with degree of pain (i.e., more pain and more galanin in allodynic than in totally nerve-transected rats). However, Ma and Bisby did not differentiate between allodynic and nonallodynic rats. In our study (Shi et al. 1999), the Gazelius model had the *lowest upregulation of galanin and the highest degree of allodynia*; in the Bennett model, galanin upregulation occurred in *almost twice as many DRG neurons in the nonallodynic rats as in the allodynic ones.* These results are difficult to reconcile with the view that galanin has an algesic effect. A further difference is the dramatic increase in galanin fibers in laminae III and IV noted by Ma and Bisby. We observed an increase in galanin fibers in the ipsilateral dorsal horn, but it was mainly confined to the superficial laminae, although it extended somewhat into lamina III, but by no means as extensively as found by Ma and Bisby. One difference between the two studies seems to be that Ma and Bisby made lesions in the upper thigh, whereas our lesions were at mid-thigh level, further away from the DRG. It is possible that the upregulation is stronger when the lesion is closer to the cell bodies.

In summary, after more than 10 years of study it is still unclear whether the main effect of galanin at the dorsal horn level is analgesic or algesic. Thus, further studies are needed to clarify this point. Galanin is expressed early during embryogenesis and is downregulated postnatally (Xu et al. 1996a). These findings suggest changes during development and possible trophic effects, and correlate with the axotomy-induced upregulation of galanin. In fact, regeneration in galanin knock-out mice may be attenuated compared to wild-type mice, indicating that galanin enhances neurite outgrowth (D. Wynick, personal communication).

CONCLUDING REMARKS

The results of the studies by Tong et al. (1999) and Shi et al. (1999) emphasize the profound changes in phenotype induced by axotomy, including not only messenger molecules and their receptors, but also uptake properties for lectins, such as CTB and B4. These findings can enhance our understanding of the mechanisms underlying neuropathic pain, and suggest that galanin and/or galanin agonists can be used alone or in combination with morphine to attenuate such pain.

ACKNOWLEDGMENTS

These studies have been supported by the Swedish MRC (04X-2887), Marianne and Marcus Wallenberg's Foundation, Knut and Alice Wallenberg's Foundation, a European Community Grant (BMH4CT95-0172), a Bristol-Myers Squibb Unrestricted Neuroscience Grant, and the Natural Science Foundation of China (3952501, 39500045).

REFERENCES

Ahmad S, Shen SH, Walker P, Wahlestedt C. Molecular cloning of a novel widely distributed galanin receptor subtype (GALR2). In: *Abstracts, 8th World Congress on Pain*. Seattle: IASP Press, 1996, p 134.

Arvidsson F, Piehl H, Johnson H, et al. The peptidergic motoneurone. *Neuroreport* 1993; 4:849–856.

Arvidsson U, Dado RJ, Riedl M, et al. δ-opioid receptor immunoreactivity: distribution in brainstem and spinal cord, and relationship to biogenic amines and enkephalin. *J Neurosci* 1995a; 15:3328–3341.

Arvidsson U, Riedl M, Chakrabarti S, et al. Distribution and targeting of a μ-opioid receptor (MOR1) in brain and spinal cord. *J Neurosci* 1995b; 15:1215–1235.

Arvidsson U, Riedl M, Chakrabarti S, et al. The κ-opioid receptor (KOR1) is primarily postsynaptic: combined immunohistochemical localization of the receptor and endogenous opioids. *Proc Natl Acad Sci USA* 1995c; 92:5062–5066.

Bennett GJ, Xie Y-K. A peripheral mononeuropathy in rat that produces disorders of pain sensation like those seen in man. *Pain* 1988; 33:87–107.

Besse D, Lombard MC, Perrot S, Besson JM. Regulation of opioid binding sites in the superficial dorsal horn of the rat spinal cord following loose ligation of the sciatic nerve: comparison with sciatic nerve section and lumbar dorsal rhizotomy. *Neuroscience* 1992; 50:921–933.

Betancur C, Azzi M, Rostène W. Nonpeptide antagonists of neuropeptide receptors: tools for research and therapy. *Trends Physiol Sci* 1997; 18:372–386.

Burgevin M-C, Loquet I, Quarteronet D, Habert-Ortoli E. Cloning, pharmacological characterization, and anatomical distribution of a rat cDNA encoding for a galanin receptor. *J Mol Neurosci* 1995; 6:33–41.

Cheng PY, Svingos AL, Wang H, et al. Ultrastructural immunolabeling shows prominent presynaptic vesicular localization of δ-opioid receptor within both enkephalin- and nonenkephalin-containing axon terminals in the superficial layers of the rat cervical spinal cord. *J Neurosci* 1995; 15:5976–5988.

Cridland RA, Henry JL. Effects of intrathecal administration of neuropeptides on a spinal nociceptive reflex in the rat: VIP, galanin, CGRP, TRH, somatostatin and angiotensin II. *Neuropeptides* 1988; 11:23–32.

Cuatrecacas P. Gangliosides and membrane receptors for cholera toxin. *Biochemistry* 1973; 12:3558–3566.

Dado RJ, Law PY, Loh HH, Elde R. Immunofluorescent identification of a delta (δ)-opioid receptor on primary afferent nerve terminals. *Neuroreport* 1993; 5:341–344.

Dumoulin FL, Raivich G, Streit WJ, Kreutzberg GW. Differential regulation of calcitonin gene-related peptide (CGRP) in regenerating rat facial nucleus and dorsal root ganglion. *Eur J Neurosci* 1991; 3:338–342.

Fathi Z, Cunningham AM, Iben LG, et al. Cloning, pharmacological characterization and distribution of a novel galanin receptor. *Mol Brain Res* 1997; 51:49–59.

Fields HL, Emson PC, Leigh BK, et al. Multiple opiate receptors on primary afferent fibers. *Nature* 1980; 284:351–353.

Florence SL, Garraghty PE, Carlson M, Kaas JH. Sprouting of peripheral nerve axons in the spinal cord of monkeys. *Brain Res* 1993; 601:343–348.

Gazelius B, Cui J-G, Svensson M, et al. Photochemically induced ischaemic lesion of the rat sciatic nerve. A novel method providing high incidence of mononeuropathy. *Neuroreport* 1996; 7:2619–2623.

Habert-Ortoli E, Amiranoff B, Loquet I, et al. Molecular cloning of a functional human galanin receptor. *Proc Natl Acad Sci USA* 1994; 91:9780–9783.

Hao J-X, Shi T-J, Xu IS, et al. Intrathecal galanin alleviates allodynia-like behavior in rats after partial peripheral nerve injury. *Eur J Neurosci* 1999; 11:427–432.

Henken DB, Martin JR. Herpes simplex virus infection induces a selective increase in the proportion of galanin-positive neurons in mouse sensory ganglia. *Exp Neurol* 1992a; 118:195–203.

Henken DB, Martin JR. The proportion of galanin-immunoreactive neurons in mouse trigeminal ganglia is transiently increased following corneal inoculation of herpes simplex virus type-1. *Neurosci Lett* 1992b; 140:177–180.

Hökfelt T, Wiesenfeld-Hallin Z, Villar MJ, Melander T. Increase of galanin-like immunoreactivity in rat dorsal root ganglion cells after peripheral axotomy. *Neurosci Lett* 1987; 83:217–220.

Hökfelt T, Zhang X, Wiesenfeld-Hallin Z. Messenger plasticity in primary sensory neurons following axotomy and its functional implications. *Trends Neurosci* 1994; 17:22–30.

Hökfelt T, Zhang X, Xu Z-Q, et al. Phenotype regulation in dorsal root ganglion neurons after nerve injury: focus on peptides and their receptors. In: Borsook D (Ed). *Molecular Neurobiology of Pain*. Seattle: IASP Press, 1997, pp 115–143.

Holmgren J, Lönnroth I, Svennerholm L. Tissue receptor for cholera exotoxin: postulated structure from studies with GM1 ganglioside and related glycolipids. *Infec Immun* 1973; 8:889–890.

Honda CN, Arvidsson U. Immunohistochemical localization of delta- and mu-opioid receptors in primate spinal cord. *Neuroreport* 1995; 6:1025–1028.

Howard AD, Tan C, Shiao LL, et al. Molecular cloning and characterization of a new receptor for galanin. *FEBS Lett* 1997; 405:285–290.

Jessell T, Tsunoo A, Kanazawa I, Otsuka M. Substance P: depletion in the dorsal horn of the rat spinal cord after section of the peripheral processes of primary sensory neurons. *Brain Res* 1979; 168:247–259.

Ji RR, Zhang Q, Bedecs K, et al. Galanin antisense oligonucleotides reduce galanin levels in dorsal root ganglia and induce autotomy in rats after axotomy. *Proc Natl Acad Sci USA* 1994; 91:12540–12543.

Ji R-R, Zhang Q, Law P-Y, et al. Expression of μ-, δ-, and κ-opioid receptor-like immunoreactivities in rat dorsal root ganglia after carrageenan-induced inflammation. *J Neurosci* 1995; 15:8156–8166.

Jonakait GM. Cytokines in neuronal development. *Adv Pharmacol* 1997; 37:35–67.

Kashiba H, Senba E, Kawai Y, et al. Axonal blockade induces the expression of vasoactive intestinal polypeptide and galanin in rat dorsal root ganglion neurons. *Brain Res* 1992; 577:19–28.

Kerr BJ, Thompson SWN, Wynick D, McMahon SB. Galanin mutant mice are hypoalgesic in a partial nerve injury model. *Soc Neurosci Abstr* 1998; 24:1391.

King CA, van Heyningen WE. Deactivation of cholera toxin by sialidase-resistant mono-sialosylganglioside. *J Infec Dis* 1973; 127:639–647.

Koerber HR, Mirnics K, Brown PB, Mendell LM. Central sprouting and functional plasticity of regenerated primary afferents. *J Neurosci* 1994; 14:3655–3671.

Kopin AS, Lee YM, McBride EW, et al. Expression cloning and characterization of the canine parietal cell gastrin receptor. *Proc Natl Acad Sci USA* 1992; 89:3605–3609.

Kreutzberg GW. Microglia: a sensor for pathological events in the CNS. *Trends Neurosci* 1996; 19:312–318.

Kupers RC, Wei Y, Persson JKE, et al. Photochemically-induced ischemia of the rat sciatic nerve produces a dose-dependent and highly reproducible mechanical, heat and cold allodynia, and signs of spontaneous pain. *Pain* 1998; 76:45–59.

Kuraishi Y, Kawamura M, Yamaguchi T, et al. Intrathecal injections of galanin and its antiserum affect nociceptive response of rat to mechanical, but not thermal, stimuli. *Pain* 1991; 44:321–324.

Ma W, Bisby M. Differential expression of galanin immunoreactivities in the primary sensory neurons following partial and complete sciatic nerve injuries. *Neuroscience* 1997; 79:1183–1195.

Maekawa K, Minami M, Yabuuchi K, et al. In situ hybridization of µ- and κ-opioid receptor mRNAs in the rat spinal cord and dorsal root ganglia. *Neurosci Lett* 1994; 168:97–100.

Maekawa K, Minami M, Masuda T, Satoh M. Expression of µ- and κ-, but not δ-, opioid receptor mRNAs is enhanced in the spinal dorsal horn of the arthritic rats. *Pain* 1995; 64:365–371.

Mansour A, Fox CA, Burke S, et al. Mu, delta, and kappa opioid receptor mRNA expression in the rat CNS: An in situ hybridization study. *J Comp Neurol* 1994; 350:412–438.

Mansour A, Fox CA, Akil H, Watson SJ. Opioid-receptor mRNA expression in the rat CNS: anatomical and functional implications. *Trends Neurosci* 1995; 18:22–29.

Mansour A, Burke S, Pavlic RJ, et al. Immunohistochemical localization of the cloned κ₁ receptor in the rat CNS and pituitary. *Neuroscience* 1996; 71:671–690.

Meyerhof W, Darlison MG, Richter D. The elucidation of neuropeptide receptors and their subtypes through the application of molecular biology. In: Hucho F (Ed). *New Comprehensive Biochemistry*. Amsterdam: Elsevier, 1993, pp 335–353.

Minami M, Satoh M. Molecular biology of the opioid receptors: structures, functions and distribution. *Neurosci Res* 1995; 23:121–145.

Minami M, Onogi T, Toya T, et al. Molecular cloning and in situ hybridization histochemistry for rat µ-opioid receptor. *Neurosci Res* 1994; 18:315–322.

Minami M, Maekawa K, Yabuuchi K, Satoh M. Double in situ hybridization study on coexistence of µ-, δ-, and κ-opioid receptor mRNAs with preprotachykinin A mRNA in the rat dorsal root ganglia. *Mol Brain Res* 1995; 30:203–210.

Molander C, Grant G. Cutaneous projections from the rat hindlimb foot to the substantia gelatinosa of the spinal cord studied by transganglionic transport of WGA-HRP conjugate. *J Comp Neurol* 1985; 237:476–484.

Nahin RL, Ren K, de León M, Ruda M. Primary sensory neurons exhibit altered gene expression in a rat model of neuropathic pain. *Pain* 1994; 58:95–108.

Nielsch V, Bisby MA, Keen P. Effect of cutting or crushing the rat sciatic nerve on synthesis of substance P by isolated L5 dorsal root ganglia. *Neuropeptides* 1987; 10:137–145.

Noguchi K, Senba E, Morita Y, et al. α-CGRP and β-CGRP mRNAs are differentially regulated in the rat spinal cord and dorsal root ganglion. *Mol Brain Res* 1990; 7:299–304.

Parker EM, Izzarelli DG, Nowak HP, et al. Cloning and characterization of rat GALR1 galanin receptor from RIN14B insulinoma cells. *Mol Brain Res* 1995; 34:179–189.

Pooga M, Soomets U, Hällbrink M, et al. Cell penetrating PNA constructs regulate galanin receptor levels and modify pain transmission in vivo. *Nature Biotech* 1998; 16:857–861.

Raivich G, Bluethmann H, Kreutzberg GW. Signaling molecules and neuroglial activation in the injured central nervous system. *Keio J Med* 1996; 45:239–247.

Réthelyi M. Preterminal and terminal axon arborization in the substantia gelatinosa of cat's spinal cord. *J Comp Neurol* 1977; 172:511–528.

Schwartz TW, U.G, Schambye HT, Hjorth SA. Molecular mechanism of action of non-peptide ligands for peptide receptors. *Current Pharm Design* [Not in IM]1995; 1:325–342.

Seltzer Z, Dubner R, Shir Y. A novel behavioural model of neuropathic pain disorders produced in rats by partial sciatic nerve injury. *Pain* 1990; 43:205–218.

Shehab SA, Atkinson ME. Vasoactive intestinal polypeptide (VIP) increases in the spinal cord after peripheral axotomy of the sciatic nerve originate from primary afferent neurons. *Brain Res* 1986; 372:37–44.

Shi T-JS, Zhang X, Holmberg K, et al. Expression and regulation of galanin-R2 receptors in rat primary sensory neurons: effect of axotomy and inflammation. *Neurosci Lett* 1997; 237:57–60.

Shi T-J, Cui J-G, Meyerson BA, et al. Regulation of galanin and neuropeptide Y in dorsal root ganglia and dorsal horn in rat mononeuropathic models: possible relation to tactile hypersensitivity. *Neuroscience* 1999, in press.

Smith KE, Forray C, Walker MW, et al. Expression cloning of a rat hypothalamic galanin receptor coupled to phosphoinositide turnover. *J Biol Chem* 1997; 272:24612–24616.

Stoeckel K, Schwab M, Thoenen H. Role of gangliosides in the uptake and retrograde transport of cholera and tetanus toxin as compared to nerve growth factor and wheat germ agglutinin. *Brain Res* 1977; 132:273–285.

Streit WJ, Schulte BA, Balentine JD, Spicer SS. Histochemical localization of galactose-containing glycoconjugates in sensory neurons and their processes in the central and peripheral nervous system of the rat. *J Histochem Cytochem* 1985; 33:1042–1052.

Streit WJ, Schulte BA, Balentine JD, Spicer SS. Evidence for glycoconjugate in nociceptive primary sensory neurons and its origin from the Golgi complex. *Brain Res* 1986; 377:1–17.

Tanaka K, Masu M, Nakanishi S. Structure and functional expression of the cloned rat neurotensin receptor. *Neuron* 1990; 4:847–854.

Tong Y-G, Wang HF, Ju G, et al. Increased uptake and transport of cholera toxin B-subunit in dorsal root ganglion neurons after peripheral axotomy: possible implications for sensory sprouting. *J Comp Neurol* 1999; 404:143–158.

Verge VMK, Xu X-J, Langel Ü, et al. Evidence for an endogenous inhibitory control on autotomy, a behavioral sign of neuropathic pain, by galanin in the rat after sciatic nerve section: demonstrated by chronic intrathecal infusion of M-35, a newly developed high affinity galanin receptor antagonist. *Neurosci Lett* 1993; 149:193–197.

Villar MJ, Cortés R, Theodorsson E, et al. Neuropeptide expression in rat dorsal root ganglion cells and spinal cord after peripheral nerve injury with special reference to galanin. *Neuroscience* 1989; 33:587–604.

Villar MJ, Ceccatelli S, Bedecs K, et al. Upregulation of nitric oxide synthase and galanin message-associated peptide in hypothalamic magnocellular neurons after hypophysectomy. Immunohistochemical and in situ hybridization studies. *Brain Res* 1994; 650:219–228.

Wakisaka S, Kajander KC, Bennett GJ. Increased neuropeptide (NPY)-like immunoreactivity in rat sensory neurons following peripheral axotomy. *Neurosci Lett* 1991; 124:200–203.

Wakisaka S, Kajander KC, Bennett GJ. Effects of peripheral nerve injuries and tissue inflammation on the levels of neuropeptide Y-like immunoreactivity in rat primary afferent neurons. *Brain Res* 1992; 598:349–352.

Wall M, Gutnick M. Ongoing activity in peripheral nerves: the physiology and pharmacology of impulses originating from a neuroma. *Exp Neurol* 1979; 43:580–593.

Wall PD, Devor M, Inbal R, et al. Autotomy following peripheral nerve lesions: experimental anaesthesia dolorosa. *Pain* 1979; 7:103–113.

Wang S, Hashemi T, He C, et al. Molecular cloning and pharmacological characterization of a new galanin receptor subtype. *Mol Pharmacol* 1997; 52:337–343.

Wiesenfeld-Hallin Z, Xu XJ, Hughes J, et al. PD134308, a selective antagonist of cholecystokinin type B receptor, enhances the analgesic effect of morphine and synergistically interacts with intrathecal galanin to depress spinal nociceptive reflexes. *Proc Natl Acad Sci USA* 1990a; 87:7105–7109.

Wiesenfeld-Hallin Z, Xu XJ, Villar MJ, Hökfelt T. Intrathecal galanin potentiates the spinal analgesic effect of morphine: electrophysiological and behavioural studies. *Neurosci Lett* 1990b; 109:217–221.

Wiesenfeld-Hallin Z, Xu XJ, Hughes J, et al. Studies on the effect of systemic PD134308 (CAM 958) in spinal reflex and pain models with special reference to interaction with morphine and intrathecal galanin. *Neuropeptides* 1991; 19:79–84.

Wiesenfeld-Hallin Z, Bartfai T, Hökfelt T. Galanin in sensory neurons in the spinal cord. *Front Neuroendocrinol* 1992a; 13:319–343.

Wiesenfeld-Hallin Z, Xu X-J, Langel Ü, et al. Galanin-mediated control of pain: enhanced role after nerve injury. *Proc Natl Acad Sci USA* 1992b; 89:3334–3337.

Woolf CJ. Molecular signals responsible for the reorganization of the synaptic circuitry of the dorsal horn after peripheral nerve injury: the mechanisms of tactile allodynia. In: Borsook D (Ed). *Molecular Neurobiology of Pain*. Seattle: IASP Press, 1997, pp 171–200.

Woolf CJ, Shortland P, Coggeshall RE. Peripheral nerve injury triggers central sprouting of myelinated afferents. *Nature* 1992; 355:75–79.

Woolf CJ, Shortland P, Reynolds M, et al. Reorganization of central terminals of myelinated primary afferents in the rat dorsal horn following peripheral axotomy. *J Comp Neurol* 1995; 360:121–134.

Xu Z-Q, Shi T-J, Hökfelt T. Expression of galanin and a galanin receptor in several sensory systems and bone anlage of rat embryos. *Proc Natl Acad Sci USA* 1996a; 93:14901–14905.

Xu Z-Q, Shi T-J, Landry M, Hökfelt T. Evidence for galanin receptors in primary sensory neurones and effect of axotomy and inflammation. *Neuroreport* 1996b; 8:237–242.

Ygge J, Grant G. The organization of the thoracic spinal nerve projection in the rat dorsal horn demonstrated with transganglionic transport of horseradish peroxidase. *J Comp Neurol* 1983; 216:1–9.

Zhang Q, Shi T-J, Ji R-R, et al. Expression of pituitary adenylate cyclase-activating polypeptide in dorsal root ganglia following axotomy: time course and coexistence. *Brain Res* 1995; 705:149–158.

Zhang X, Dagerlind Å, Elde RP, et al. Marked increase in cholecystokinin B receptor messenger RNA levels in rat dorsal root ganglia after peripheral axotomy. *Neuroscience* 1993a; 57:227–233.

Zhang X, Ju G, Elde R, Hökfelt T. Effect of peripheral nerve cut on neuropeptides in dorsal root ganglia and the spinal cord of monkey with special reference to galanin. *J Neurocytol* 1993b; 22:342–381.

Zhang X, Xu Z-Q, Bao L, et al. Complementary distribution of receptors for neurotensin and NPY in small neurons in rat lumbar DRGs and regulation of the receptors and peptides after peripheral axotomy. *J Neurosci* 1995; 15:2733–2747.

Zhang X, Bao L, Shi T-J, et al. Down-regulation of μ opiate receptors in rat and monkey dorsal root ganglion neurons and spinal cord after peripheral axotomy. *Neuroscience* 1998; 82:223–240.

Zhang Y-Z, Hannibal J, Zhao Q, et al. Pituitary adenylate cyclase activating peptide (PACAP) expression in the rat dorsal root ganglia: up-regulation after peripheral nerve injury. *Neuroscience* 1996; 74:1099–1110.

Zigmond RE, Hyatt-Sachs H, Mohney RP, et al. Changes in neuropeptide phenotype after axotomy of adult peripheral neurons and the role of leukemia inhibitor factor. *Perspect Dev Neurobiol* 1996; 4:75–90.

Correspondence to: Tomas Hökfelt, Department of Neuroscience, Section of Chemical Neurotransmission, Berzelius Laboratory, Karolinska Institute, S-17177 Stockholm, Sweden. Tel: 46-8-728-7070/7065; Fax: 46-8-331692; email: tomas.hokfelt@neuro.ki.se.

Opioid Sensitivity of Chronic Noncancer Pain,
Progress in Pain Research and Management,
Vol. 14, edited by Eija Kalso, Henry J. McQuay,
and Zsuzsanna Wiesenfeld-Hallin, IASP Press,
Seattle, © 1999.

10

Opioid Analgesic Activity in Neuropathic Pain States

Michael H. Ossipov,[a] Josephine Lai,[b] T. Philip Malan, Jr.,[a,b] and Frank Porreca[a,b]

Departments of [a]Pharmacology and [b]Anesthesiology, Health Sciences Center, University of Arizona, Tucson, Arizona, USA

Nerve damage arising from either trauma or disease affecting peripheral nerves can lead to abnormal pain states. Such pain may continue for long periods after the initial injury has healed or in the absence of observable tissue damage. Persons afflicted with neuropathic pain often have an exaggerated sensitivity to nociceptive stimuli (hyperalgesia) or may perceive normally innocuous stimuli as painful (allodynia) (Payne 1986). Causes of neuropathic pain may include diabetic neuropathy, herpes zoster, nerve traction or compression, radiation therapy for lung and other cancers, complex regional pain syndrome, type I (reflex sympathetic dystrophy), and complications from acquired immune deficiency syndrome (AIDS). Neuropathic dysesthesias are frequently characterized by burning or shooting pains along with sensations often described as "tingling," "crawling," or "electrical" in quality. Painful neuropathy represents a seriously debilitating syndrome that affects millions of people and significantly impairs their quality of life.

The efficacy of opioids as analgesics in conditions of acute pain is well established. Opioid analgesics are routinely used in postoperative pain and in the treatment of many short-term painful conditions. However, pain states differ greatly in their sensitivity to opioids. For example, pain of inflammatory origin is effectively suppressed by opioids, and experimental data suggest enhanced activity of opioids under such conditions. In contrast, pain of neuropathic origin is generally perceived to be resistant to treatment with opioids. Several factors may influence the lack of opioid activity in neuropathic pain, including the nature of the afferent stimulus and the neurochemical and neuroanatomical changes that occur in the central nervous system (CNS) and in the periphery. Such changes may include alterations in spinal dynorphin or cholecystokinin levels, increased release of neuropeptide and excitatory amino acid transmitters leading to states of "central sensitization," sprouting of axons to enlarge the receptive fields, and phenotypic changes of primary afferent neurons. Of particular interest as it relates to the loss of activity of spinal morphine following experimental nerve injury is the increased expression of spinal dynorphin and the possible interaction between this peptide, or its fragments, and the NMDA receptor complex.

PAIN STATES AND OPIOID ACTIVITY

The perception that neuropathic pain is resistant to treatment by opioids may lie partly in the doses and levels of efficacy of the opioids employed. For example, in one study of postherpetic neuralgia, codeine (120 mg) was reported to be no different from placebo control (Max et al. 1988). Such results might have been simply due to an insufficient dose (Rowbotham et al. 1991). It has been suggested that opioid dosing should be titrated until adequate analgesia is achieved or side effects are intolerable and untreatable (Portenoy et al. 1990). In a double-blind, placebo-controlled study, intravenous (i.v.) morphine infusions successfully treated both spontaneous pain and allodynia caused by postherpetic neuralgia (Rowbotham et al. 1991). Data from experimental studies in animals support the view that systemic administration of opioids can block hyperalgesia and allodynia resulting from peripheral nerve injury. However, the route of administration and probable site of opioid action seem especially significant to the effectiveness of the treatment. In an interesting comparison, it was found that bolus intrathecal (i.t.) morphine failed to reduce the incidence of autotomy in rats following sciatic nerve section (Xu et al. 1993), whereas the same group found that a chronic (14-day) i.t. infusion of morphine prevented autotomy (Wiesenfeld-Hallin 1984). Such studies suggest that determination of the clinical utility of opioids must consider the pain modality, route of administration, dosage, and specific opioid in the formulation of opioid treatment protocols for neuropathic pain.

An important factor in determining the utility of opioids in the treatment of neuropathic pain, either experimentally or clinically, is the particular aspect of the dysesthesia being considered. Notably, i.t. injection of morphine, even at doses well beyond the antinociceptive range in sham-operated rats (e.g., 100 μg), to rats with L5/L6 spinal nerve ligation did not alleviate tactile allodynia (Bian et al. 1995, Lee et al. 1995). In contrast, in both the chronic constriction injury (CCI) (Yamamoto and Yaksh 1991;

Mao et al. 1995a,b) and the L5/L6 ligation model (Wegert et al. 1997) of neuropathic pain, i.t. morphine reversed thermal hyperalgesia produced by applying radiant heat to the plantar aspect of the hindpaw ipsilateral to the injury. Additionally, i.t. morphine produced dose-dependent antinociception (elevation of the response above threshold in sham-operated rats) in the same models, although at significantly (about five- to six-fold) reduced potency (Yamamoto and Yaksh 1991; Mao et al. 1995a,b; Wegert et al. 1997). Observations such as these strongly suggest that the mechanisms underlying allodynia and hyperalgesia differ, and that the effect, or lack of effect, of i.t. opioids is dependent on the nature of the stimulus. A surprising observation was the loss of antinociceptive efficacy and potency of i.t. morphine against the tail-flick response following L5/L6 nerve injury (Ossipov et al. 1995b). This observation suggests that in addition to the nature of the afferent input, plasticity in the spinal cord across multiple spinal segments (i.e., sacral to lumbar) is likely to influence resistance to opioid actions.

NEUROANATOMICAL CONSIDERATIONS

The hypothesis that thermal hyperalgesia and tactile allodynia arising from nerve injury may be mechanistically distinguished arises from observations that these dysesthesias are differentially sensitive to i.t. morphine and to other manipulations such as lesions of the spinal cord. Such differences suggest the involvement of separate spinal and supraspinal neuronal circuitries for these abnormal pains. Complete midthoracic transection (Bian et al. 1998) or hemisection (Sung et al. 1998) of the spinal cord abolishes tactile allodynia in rats with ligations of the L5/L6 or sacral (S1 or S2) spinal nerves. This loss of responsiveness to tactile stimuli is not the result of hindlimb paralysis, as spinal nociceptive reflexes to noxious pinch are still present. In contrast to tactile allodynia, spinal transection increases the differences in response latencies between sham-operated and L5/L6-ligated rats to thermal stimuli applied to the paw (Bian et al. 1998). A separate study showed that spinal nerve ligation or carrageenan injection produced allodynia to mechanical and cold stimuli that was abolished by midthoracic spinal transection, while this procedure increased hyperalgesia to radiant heat (Kauppila et al. 1998). Studies involving electrophysiologic recording of wide-dynamic range (WDR) neurons of the spinal dorsal horn found that spinal transection abolished facilitated responses to mechanical stimuli caused by neurogenic inflammation induced by mustard oil (Pertovaara 1998). The conclusion was that brain-stem spinal pathways not only suppress nociception, but that under some pathophysiological conditions concurrent facilitatory influences may predominate and enhance mechanical hyperexcitability. These observations also indicate significant differences in the processing of thermal and mechanical stimuli in the nerve-injured state.

Another study used a different approach and assessed tactile allodynia and three measures of thermal nociception (tail-flick, paw-flick, and hot-plate responses) after L5/L6 ligation injury or sham surgery for an extended time after a single systemic injection of resiniferatoxin (RTX), an ultrapotent analogue of the C-fiber-specific neurotoxin, capsaicin (Ossipov et al. 1999). Treatment with RTX resulted in a significant and long-lasting (i.e., apparently irreversible) increase in threshold to noxious thermal stimuli in both sham-operated and nerve-injured rats. Nerve-injury-induced thermal hyperalgesia was abolished in both sham-operated and nerve-injured rats, and RTX produced thermal antinociception. However, RTX treatment did not affect the tactile allodynia seen in the same nerve-injured rats (Ossipov et al. 1999). These data support the concept that thermal hyperalgesia after nerve ligation, as well as noxious thermal stimuli, are likely to be mediated by capsaicin-sensitive C-fiber afferents. In contrast, nerve-injury-related tactile allodynia is insensitive to RTX treatment, which clearly desensitizes C fibers, so such responses are not likely to be mediated through C-fiber afferents. The hypothesis that tactile allodynia may be due to inputs from large (i.e., Aβ) afferents offers a mechanistic basis for the observed insensitivity of this endpoint to i.t. morphine in the nerve-injury model.

Non-noxious tactile stimulation is thought to be transmitted chiefly through low-threshold, large-diameter, myelinated Aβ fibers, while noxious thermal stimuli are believed to be transmitted to the spinal cord through high-threshold, thin, unmyelinated primary afferent fibers (e.g., Yeomans et al. 1996). After peripheral nerve axotomy (Woolf et al. 1995) or L5/L6 spinal nerve ligation (Lekan et al. 1996), the large-diameter, low-threshold fibers that normally terminate in lamina III of the dorsal horn sprout into the superficial laminae and perhaps form novel physiopathic synapses with transmission neurons. These second-order neurons, which normally code for nociceptive input, now appear to receive non-noxious input from the low-threshold fibers; thus, innocuous tactile input might be interpreted as nociceptive. This is one mechanism believed to be responsible for the development of tactile allodynia (Woolf et al. 1995; Lekan et al. 1996). A corresponding sprouting of C fibers has not been reported. In contrast to tactile allodynia, spinal receptor systems involved with processing of noxious thermal afferent stimuli are believed to be similarly active in "normal" and nerve-injured animals (Yamamoto and Yaksh 1991).

ROLE OF SPINAL OPIOID RECEPTORS

If the hypothesis is correct that non-noxious stimuli are transmitted via non-C-fiber afferents, then the lack of spinal morphine activity against tactile allodynia seems reasonable. Activation of opioid receptors located on the presynaptic terminals of unmyelinated nociceptor C fibers is believed to prevent calcium influx necessary for synaptic transmission and thus to inhibit the release of nociceptive transmitters (e.g., substance P; Aimone and Yaksh 1989). Additionally, activation of opioid receptors located postsynaptically on cell bodies of projection neurons can lead to the hyperpolarization of the second-order neurons and inhibit the ascending transmission of nociceptive input to supraspinal centers. Besse et al. (1990) found that dorsal rhizotomy produced an approximate 70% loss of δ-opioid receptors and 60% loss of spinal μ-opioid receptors, which suggests that though opioid receptor populations exist both on primary afferent nerve terminals and on cell bodies of neurons in the dorsal horn of the spinal cord, the predominant population is presynaptic. In situ hybridization techniques have revealed the existence of mRNA for μ- and κ-opioid receptors in soma of the dorsal root ganglia (DRG), which have axonal projections both to the spinal cord and to the periphery (Maekawa et al. 1994). Mansour and colleagues (1994, 1995) have described the distribution of mRNA for opioid receptors in cells of the DRG. Opioid-receptor-binding sites are found predominantly in the DRG and the superficial layers of the dorsal horn (Mansour et al. 1995), which correspond with terminals of C fibers rather than the terminal region of larger-diameter fibers (e.g., laminae III and IV). Finally, Taddese and colleagues (1995), using patch-clamp techniques on isolated nociceptors, found that activation of μ-opioid receptors predictably inhibited Ca^{++} channels of small-diameter nociceptors but not of large-diameter cells, which suggests that μ-receptor activation selectively inhibits the activity of C fibers.

Other evidence supports the view that the δ-opioid receptors of the spinal dorsal horn are located presynaptically on the terminals of primary afferents (C fibers) or on descending modulatory fibers (Dado et al. 1993; Arvidsson et al. 1995). In the neuropathic state, it is reasonable to suggest that tactile allodynia is transmitted to the spinal cord through the large-diameter Aβ fibers, which do not appear to express opioid receptors on the nerve terminals (Taddese et al. 1995). Under such conditions, spinal morphine or other spinal opioids would exert their activity only at the minority population of postsynaptic opioid receptors. We would predict that this situation would result in a rightward displacement of the dose-response curve, with decreased efficacy due to a loss of available (in this case, relevant postsynaptic) opioid receptors, a situation analogous to blockade of a fraction of the opioid receptors with an irreversible antagonist or the loss of opioid activity in the tolerant state. Under such circumstances, high-efficacy opioids with a large receptor reserve, but not low-efficacy opioids, might be expected to show significant antiallodynic action following spinal administration. Indeed, i.t. [D-Ala^2,NMePhe^4,Gly-ol]enkephalin (DAMGO), a high-efficacy opioid, produced dose-dependent antiallodynic activity in rats with L5/L6 spinal nerve ligation (Nichols et al. 1995), although at doses higher than those required to block acute nociceptive inputs. In contrast, morphine as a low-efficacy partial μ-opioid agonist was completely inactive (up to 100 μg i.t.) against tactile allodynia.

Many reported clinical studies of opioid efficacy against neuropathic pain have employed morphine or opioids of lesser efficacy (see Arner and Meyerson 1988), and the use of compounds with greater analgesic efficacy should be considered. Fentanyl given spinally to patients with postamputation stump pain provided immediate, long-lasting (8 hours), and complete pain relief that was considered to be superior to that of spinal lidocaine (Jacobson et al. 1990). In a randomized, double-blind, active-placebo-controlled crossover study, i.v. fentanyl was superior to morphine in alleviating neuropathic pain (Dellemijn and Vanneste 1997). Similar observations were made regarding fentanyl given either subcutaneously or transdermally (Paix et al. 1995; Ahmedzai 1997a, b). Reports have also indicated that infusions of i.v. hydromorphone have achieved adequate analgesia in neuropathic pain patients (Portenoy et al. 1990), but the dose-response curve was shifted to the right, possibly beyond what are normally considered to be "usual" doses for the treatment of pain of non-neuropathic origins. Additionally, some investigators have suggested that opioids may alleviate neuropathic pain, but at "higher than normal doses" (Portenoy and Foley 1986; Jadad et al. 1992). Such findings appear to be consistent with preclinical studies and may reflect a lack of involvement of a population of (possibly presynaptic) opioid receptors in the observed effects. Additionally, other factors, such as the expected synergistic interaction between different areas of the CNS for pain relief, also appear to be important in the ultimate efficacy demonstrated by a systemically administered opioid.

LOSS OF SPINAL/SUPRASPINAL SYNERGY

In contrast to spinal morphine, the systemic or intracerebroventricular (i.c.v.) injection of morphine has produced an antiallodynic effect in L5/L6-

ligated rats (Bian et al. 1995; Lee et al. 1995). However, the doses required tend to be greater than expected when compared to antinociceptive doses in noninjured animals. The clinical situation also suggests a loss of morphine activity, as described in detail above and extensively reviewed (Twycross 1982; Tasker et al. 1983). It has been demonstrated that a spinal/supraspinal synergistic antinociceptive interaction is produced by morphine against acute noxious stimuli (Yeung and Rudy 1980a,b). Without such synergy among sites, it is unlikely that systemic morphine would be sufficiently potent for clinical utility. The lack of spinal efficacy of morphine against tactile allodynia, as demonstrated in rats with experimental nerve injury, presumably for the reasons described above, would obviously appear to contribute to a loss of spinal/supraspinal synergy.

Previous studies have demonstrated that one consequence of nerve-ligation injury in rats is a significant reduction in the antinociceptive potency and efficacy of i.t. morphine and a complete loss of i.t. antiallodynic efficacy (Bian et al. 1995; Ossipov et al. 1995a,b). The finding of reasonable antiallodynic actions of systemic and supraspinal morphine, though at higher doses than needed to alter acute nociceptive stimuli (Bian et al. 1995), was puzzling in that the clinical experience of morphine activity in neuropathic pain states is one of poor, or reduced, activity. In response to this observation, Bian et al. (1999) explored the synergistic interaction of morphine given simultaneously in the spine and i.c.v. in L5/L6-ligated and sham-operated rats by using the tail-flick test and probing with von Frey filaments. In these studies, i.t. morphine failed to produce an antiallodynic effect, and while the compound was active against noxious inputs, its effect was significantly less potent than it was in sham-operated rats. Further, the spinal/supraspinal interaction in nerve-injured rats was not synergistic against either thermal nociception to the tail or tactile allodynia of the hindpaw. In contrast, sham-operated rats demonstrated a robust synergistic interaction in the tail-flick test. These findings suggest that the observed antiallodynic actions of systemic morphine may be the result of actions only at supraspinal sites. Without the normally expected spinal/supraspinal synergy, there is a need for higher systemic doses to achieve the same level of activity.

EXTRATERRITORIAL NEUROPATHIC PAIN

Convergent evidence shows that peripheral nerve injury produces a generalized central sensitization of spinal neurons such that central second-order projection neurons demonstrate increased responsivity to intact, adjacent afferents as well as to the injured nerve, resulting in extraterritorial hyperesthesias. Using the chronic constriction injury (CCI) model of neuro-pathic pain, Tal and Bennett (1994) showed that rats exhibited exaggerated withdrawal reflexes to pinprick stimulation, indicative of mechano-hyperalgesia, in the hindpaw territories of both the injured sciatic nerve and the uninjured saphenous nerve. Likewise, the withdrawal responses to von Frey hair stimulation on the nerve-injured side occurred at a significantly lower threshold, indicating the presence of mechano-allodynia. The severity and time course of the tactile allodynia were similar in both nerve territo-ries. Complete section of the neighboring saphenous, but not of the sciatic, nerve abolished tactile allodynia in the saphenous territory. Conversely, complete section of the sciatic, but not of the saphenous, nerve abolished allodynia arising from the mid-plantar sciatic territory. The authors sug-gested that extraterritorial pain may be due to a peripheral nerve injury-evoked dysfunction of pain-processing neurons in the CNS.

A clinical study that applied local anesthetic block to an injured nerve achieved relief of hyperalgesia and allodynia in the region of an adjacent, intact nerve (Gracely et al. 1992). It is probable that sustained afferent drive from the injured nerve is needed to maintain the abnormal, heightened sen-sitivity of adjacent territory. Corroborative evidence is found in electro-physiological studies where baseline discharge frequencies from the spinal cord segment (L5 and L6) corresponding to the sciatic nerve of rats with CCI were abnormally high, as were responses of these same neurons to electrical and mechanical noxious stimulation of the neighboring saphenous nerve, whereas responses in the saphenous segment (L2) of the cord were within normal ranges (Sotgiu et al. 1996). Application of lidocaine to the sciatic nerve significantly attenuated the abnormal baseline discharges in the sciatic segment of the cord and reduced its sensitivity to noxious stimu-lation of the saphenous nerve. The authors concluded that excessive dis-charge of injured afferents drive central sensitization, and that afferent in-put from the uninjured nerve extends beyond the normal spinal segment innervated by the adjacent nerve to cause hyperresponsivity.

Extraterritorial effects were also demonstrated where tight ligation of the L5/L6 afferents produced an unexpected loss of i.t. morphine activity against thermal nociception applied to the tail (Ossipov et al. 1995a,b). The dose-response curve for spinal morphine in the hot-water (55°C) tail-flick test was displaced significantly four-fold to the right and downward when compared to that of sham-operated rats (Ossipov et al. 1995a). Afferent sensory fibers from the paw and the tail terminate in the lumbar and sacral spinal cord, respectively, without any significant overlap (Swett and Woolf 1985), so the observed loss of activity of spinal morphine is probably due to multisegmental changes that may occur after peripheral nerve injury. The application of bupivacaine at doses that produced no motor or paralytic effects directly at the site of L5/L6 injury restored the potency and efficacy of i.t. morphine against the hot-water tail-flick test, which further suggests that sustained afferent drive from the injured nerve serves to maintain the neuropathic pain state at extraterritorial sites (Ossipov et al. 1995b).

SACRAL NERVE LIGATION PRODUCES EXTRASEGMENTAL EFFECTS

Intriguing observations made after tight ligation of the S2 sacral spinal nerve strongly support the hypothesis that peripheral nerve injury leads to extrasegmental changes in the spinal cord. Tight ligation of the S2 sacral nerve has produced a robust tactile allodynia and thermal hyperalgesia in both hindpaws within 3 days of surgery and extending beyond 40 days after nerve ligation (Bian et al. 1998b; Ibrahim et al. 1998). Importantly, because the sacral nerves do not innervate the lumbar segments of the spinal cord, and the afferents from the hindpaw do not terminate in the sacral cord (Swett and Woolf 1985), the bilateral allodynia and hyperalgesia of the paws must derive from extrasegmental changes induced by injury to the sacral nerves. The application of lidocaine directly at the site of injury to the sacral spinal nerves blocked both tactile allodynia and thermal hyperalgesia of the hindpaws, which also suggests that sustained afferent drive from the injured nerve serves to maintain this abnormal hyperesthetic state (Bian et al. 1998b; Ibrahim et al. 1998). No motor disturbances or paralysis after local anesthetic were observed in these studies, which rules out an inhibition of motor activity. The animals still maintained a robust nociceptive reflex to radiant heat after the "normal" baseline was reached, indicating that loss of afferent drive from the S2 spinal nerve blocked extrasegmental tactile allodynia and thermal hyperalgesia without producing an additional antinociception (Bian et al. 1998b; Ibrahim et al. 1998).

DYNORPHIN IS ELEVATED ACROSS MULTIPLE SEGMENTS

Extrasegmental manifestations of neuropathic pain may be partly related to an elevated dynorphin content in the spinal cord. Considerable evidence indicates that elevated spinal dynorphin is associated with neuropathic pain (see Dubner 1991 for review), and possibly with the loss of morphine activity. A role of dynorphin in chronic pain is indicated by observations that spinal dynorphin is elevated after hindpaw inflammation (Riley et al. 1996). In situ hybridization revealed increased prodynorphin mRNA in laminae I, II, V, and VI after peripheral inflammation (Ruda et al. 1988). Dubner and Ruda (1992) demonstrated elevated spinal dynorphin mRNA after nerve injury. Studies using radioimmunoassay and immunocytochemical techniques found elevated dynorphin levels ipsilateral to the site of injury in the superficial (I–II) and deeper (V–VII) laminae of the spinal cord within 5 days of CCI, with a peak occurring 10 days after the injury and continuing for 20 days (Kajander et al. 1990). Immunostaining techniques revealed dynorphin in both lamina I projection and interneurons, which suggests both local spinal and supraspinal functions of dynorphin (Lima et al. 1993). Spinothalamic tract neurons with terminations in the medial thalamus also contain dynorphin (Nahin 1988). It is generally suggested that interneurons of the dorsal horn are the predominant source of spinal dynorphin (Botticelli et al. 1981; Takahashi et al. 1990). While evidence for the presence of dynorphin in primary afferent neurons is controversial, the consensus is that spinal dynorphin is not of primary afferent origin (Nahin et al. 1992).

More recently, we determined that peripheral nerve injury induces multisegmental and time-dependent increases in spinal dynorphin content (Bian et al. 1998b, 1999; Ibrahim et al. 1998). Rats that had ligations of the L5 and L6 spinal nerves or sham surgery demonstrated tactile allodynia and thermal hyperalgesia of the ipsilateral hindpaw 10 days after surgery. At that time point, we used immunoassay to determine the spinal dynorphin content of the ipsilateral dorsal quadrant of the spinal cord. Rats with L5/L6 spinal nerve ligation demonstrated significantly greater dynorphin content in the ipsilateral dorsal quadrant of the L4–L6 segment of the lumbar cord when compared to sham-operated rats (Bian et al. 1998b, 1999; Ibrahim et al. 1998). Importantly, the adjacent lumbar (L1–L3) and sacral segments also demonstrated significant elevations in dynorphin content, whereas there were no significant differences in dynorphin content between ligated and sham-operated rats in the thoracic and cervical segments of the cord. A time-course study indicated that the content of dynorphin in the ipsilateral dorsal quadrant of the spinal cord significantly increased within 2 days of L5/L6 spinal nerve ligation, reached a peak level 10 days after surgery, and returned to baseline levels by day 55; these findings correlate with the development of tactile allodynia (Ibrahim et al. 1998). This time course is similar to that observed after CCI (Kajander et al. 1990). As expected, tight ligation of the S2 spinal nerve also resulted in significant elevation of dynorphin content in the sacral cord (Ibrahim et al. 1998). Furthermore, significant elevations in dynorphin content occurred in the dorsal quadrants of the L3–L6 segment both ipsilateral and contralateral to the S2 ligation (Bian et al. 1998b; Ibrahim et al. 1998). These results clearly indicate that peripheral nerve ligation produces a significant elevation of spinal dynorphin content. Importantly, the elevation occurs across multiple spinal segments relative to the site of the nerve injury, but not at all spinal cord segments, such as those distant from the injured nerve (i.e., thoracic or cervical). The time and place of elevated dynorphin content correlates well with the appearance of signs of neuropathic pain, and such elevated dynorphin appears to be functionally relevant.

ANTISERUM TO DYNORPHIN BLOCKS THERMAL HYPERALGESIA

Studies with antiserum to dynorphin have suggested that elevated or pathological levels of spinal dynorphin contribute to the consequences of the nerve-injured state. The i.t. treatment with antiserum to dynorphin reduces neurological impairment after nerve injury (Cox et al. 1985; Faden 1990), which suggests an involvement of endogenous dynorphin in the pathogenesis of traumatic spinal cord injury. A more recent study showed that thermal hyperalgesia elicited by peripheral nerve injury is amenable to treatment with dynorphin antiserum (Nichols et al. 1997). While the i.t. injection of antiserum to dynorphin $A_{(1-17)}$ did not alter paw withdrawal responses to noxious radiant heat in sham-operated rats, dynorphin antiserum reversed established thermal hyperalgesia resulting from L5/L6 ligation injury and produced withdrawal thresholds in these rats up to, but not beyond, the baseline withdrawal latencies of the sham-operated rats (Nichols et al. 1997). Similar observations following i.t. administration of MK-801 suggest that the thermal hyperalgesia associated with peripheral nerve injury may be partly due to an excitatory, pronociceptive effect of the elevated spinal dynorphin content observed after peripheral nerve injury (Nichols et al. 1997). In contrast, the spinal application of antiserum to dynorphin $A_{(1-17)}$ did not reverse tactile allodynia after L5/L6 spinal nerve ligation (Nichols et al. 1997), nor did systemic injection of antiserum prevent tactile allodynia after cryoneurolysis (Wagner and DeLeo 1996). Again, similar results were obtained with MK-801 in both studies. Finally, i.t. dynorphin antiserum attenuated facilitation of the flexor reflex induced by a conditioning stimulus to the sciatic nerve in L5/L6-ligated, but not in sham-operated rats, which suggests that dynorphin may participate in establishing central sensitization after peripheral nerve injury (Bian et al. 1997). These studies strongly indicate that at least some consequences of peripheral nerve injury may be partly due to an excitatory, pronociceptive effect of the elevated spinal dynorphin content observed after peripheral nerve injury. This effect is probably mediated through direct, or indirect, activation of the NMDA-receptor complex.

Similar observations were made with regard to extrasegmental neuro-pathic pain. Tight ligation of the S2 sacral nerve established tactile allodynia and thermal hyperalgesia of the hindpaws (Bian et al. 1998b; Ibrahim et al. 1998). As with L5/L6 ligations, the i.t. injection of antiserum to dynorphin $A_{(1-17)}$ significantly reversed thermal hyperalgesia and elevated paw-with-drawal latencies up to, but not beyond, those of the sham-operated rats (Bian et al. 1998b; Ibrahim et al. 1998). In contrast, the tactile allodynia of the hindpaws produced by S2 ligation was unaffected by i.t. antiserum to dynorphin $A_{(1-17)}$ (Bian et al. 1998b; Ibrahim et al. 1998). Dynorphin antise-rum had no effect in sham-operated rats. In the same study, the application of lidocaine at the site of injury reversed both tactile allodynia and thermal hyperalgesia. Motor activity and gait were normal, and withdrawal reflexes of the paws and tail to nociceptive pinch indicated that the increased paw-withdrawal thresholds were not attributed to paralysis or lumbar sensory blockade. These data indicate that injury of a single peripheral nerve can produce signs of neuropathic pain, tactile allodynia, and thermal hyperalge-sia at sites not associated with the injured nerve. Afferent drive from the injured nerve may evoke extrasegmental changes that drive extraterritorial dysesthesias (e.g., Kauppila et al. 1998; Pertovaara 1998). Given the obser-vations presented here, where signs of neuropathic pain are associated with corresponding elevations in spinal dynorphin content, this peptide is a likely candidate to mediate segmental and extrasegmental changes associated with peripheral nerve injury.

DYNORPHIN ANTISERUM RESTORES
SPINAL/SUPRASPINAL SYNERGY

As discussed in detail above, it is well established that peripheral nerve injury is accompanied by a loss of efficacy and potency of i.t. morphine against tactile allodynia and thermal hyperalgesia (Bian et al. 1995; Lee et al. 1995, Ossipov et al. 1995a,b). Additionally, the well-established spinal/ supraspinal synergy of morphine is also lost after peripheral nerve injury (Bian et al. 1999). The hypothesis that the loss of spinal morphine activity was related to the elevated spinal dynorphin content observed after nerve injury was confirmed by i.t. injection of antiserum to dynorphin $A_{(1-17)}$. Al-though it did not reverse tactile allodynia directly, the antiserum was able to restore the activity of spinal morphine against tactile allodynia of the hindpaws following L5/L6 ligation (Nichols et al. 1997). A more recent study observed that the spinal injection of antiserum to dynorphin $A_{(1-17)}$

restored the spinal/supraspinal synergy of morphine against thermal nociception (tail-flick test) and against tactile allodynia of the hindpaws without
affecting the normal synergistic interaction of spinal and supraspinal morphine in sham-operated rats (Bian et al. 1999). The noncompetitive NMDA-
receptor antagonist MK-801 produced remarkably similar effects to antiserum to dynorphin $A_{(1-17)}$ in several studies. Like dynorphin antiserum, MK-801
restored the spinal/supraspinal synergy of morphine against the tail-flick
and tactile allodynia in L5/L6-ligated rats (Bian et al. 1999). Additionally,
MK-801 reversed thermal hyperalgesia in rats with L5/L6 (Wegert et al.
1997) or S2 (Bian et al. 1998b) ligations, but did not alter tactile allodynia
or the responses of sham-operated animals to thermal nociception, and it
restored the antinociceptive potency and efficacy of spinal morphine against
the tail-flick in L5/L6-ligated rats (Ossipov et al. 1995b).

DYNORPHIN ACTING AT THE NMDA RECEPTOR COMPLEX

These observations support the hypothesis that the pathological role of
elevated spinal dynorphin during conditions of neuropathic pain may be
due to interactions of elevated, pathological concentrations of dynorphin
with the NMDA receptor complex and that such interactions drive central
sensitization. Consistent with this hypothesis, a binding site for dynorphin
was identified on the NMDA receptor (Lai et al. 1997), although it appears
to modulate the NMDA site negatively. Studies showing dynorphin-medi-
ated inhibition of NMDA current at micromolar concentrations suggest that
this inhibitory effect may not be physiologically relevant (Chen et al.
1995a,b); however, such concentrations might be achieved at the synapse
(Chen and Huang 1998). Some studies in vitro have demonstrated excitatory
effects of dynorphin $A_{(2-17)}$ that are revealed by low glycine concentrations,
which suggests that dynorphin may act as a co-agonist at the NMDA-receptor complex to potentiate NMDA-mediated currents (Zhang et al. 1997).
While dynorphin/NMDA interactions in vitro have generally suggested an
inhibitory modulation (Chen et al. 1995a,b; Lai et al. 1997), even more
recent studies show that dynorphin $A_{(1-17)}$ or dynorphin $A_{(2-17)}$ can potentiate NMDA-activated currents in some cells in a nonopioid-mediated, rapid,
and reversible fashion in the periaqueductal gray (Lai et al. 1998). Lai and
colleagues (1998) proposed that dynorphin may either potentiate or inhibit
NMDA-mediated currents, depending on the composition of the subunits
making up the NMDA receptor complex. While a high-affinity specific binding site for des-tyr-dynorphin on the NMDA receptor has been identified,
the functional significance of this site is unclear (Lai et al. 1997).

Aside from the possibility of a direct interaction of dynorphin with the NMDA receptor, considerable in vivo evidence favors the interpretation that spinal dynorphin may act as a functional NMDA agonist (Walker et al. 1980, 1982). Both i.t. dynorphin $A_{(1-13)}$ and dynorphin fragments that do not interact with opioid receptors (e.g., dynorphin $A_{(2-17)}$, dynorphin $A_{(2-13)}$, and dynorphin $A_{(3-13)}$) produce hindlimb paralysis through nonopioid mechanisms (Przewlocki et al. 1983, Faden and Jacobs 1984; Stevens and Yaksh 1986). Further, both i.t. dynorphin $A_{(1-13)}$ and dynorphin fragments deplete cell bodies of interneurons and sensory and motor neurons in the spinal cord (Long et al. 1988). Protection against dynorphin-induced hindlimb paralysis (Bakshi and Faden 1990a,b; Long et al 1994; Long and Skolnick 1995), loss of tail-flick reflex (Caudle and Isaac 1988; Stewart and Isaac 1991), and loss of neuronal cell bodies (Long et al. 1994; Long and Skolnick 1995) is afforded by both NMDA antagonists and agents that modulate the NMDA–glycine receptor complex. Finally, single i.t. injections of subparalytic doses of dynorphin $A_{(1-17)}$, dynorphin $A_{(1-13)}$, or the corresponding des-tyr fragments, which act at NMDA but not opioid receptors, produced a long-lasting tactile allodynia (Vanderah et al. 1996). This effect was blocked by the prior i.t. administration of MK-801, but not naloxone. Based on such observations, it seems reasonable to conclude that dynorphin, or its fragments, may directly or indirectly produce a positive modulation of the NMDA-receptor complex.

SUMMARY AND CONCLUSIONS

The information presented in this chapter demonstrates that L5/L6 nerve-ligation injury produces a complete loss of activity of i.t. morphine against tactile allodynia and a significant loss of efficacy against an acute thermal nociceptive stimulus. Critically, this loss of spinal activity correlates with a loss of spinal/supraspinal synergy of morphine. The development of allodynia and hyperalgesia also correlates with elevations in spinal dynorphin content, both at the segment associated with the injured nerve and in the adjacent segments. This extrasegmental elevation in spinal dynorphin may account, at least in part, for the extraterritorial tactile allodynia and thermal hyperalgesia observed after peripheral nerve injury. We suggest that the pathological role of elevated spinal dynorphin across multiple segments during conditions of neuropathic pain is due to direct or indirect interactions with the NMDA-receptor complex that drive central sensitization. This effect in turn leads to a loss of spinal morphine activity and of the spinal/supraspinal synergy of morphine. We suspect that this synergistic interaction may account for the remarkable clinical analgesic effect of morphine, and its loss may explain the relative lack of clinical utility of morphine against neuropathic pain.

Despite the commonalities in the mechanisms for tactile allodynia and thermal hyperalgesia, some important differences exist between these dysesthetic states. Thermal hyperalgesia is readily reversed by either antiserum to dynorphin $A_{(1-17)}$ or MK-801 given spinally, whereas tactile allodynia is not. Allodynia is likely mediated by large-diameter, low-threshold Aβ fibers and appears dependent on a spinal/supraspinal loop, because it is abolished by spinal transection and not by RTX. In contrast, thermal hyperalgesia may be processed by local spinal circuitries, and appears to be mediated by high-threshold, small-diameter (C-fiber) afferents, since it is abolished by RTX but not affected by spinal transection. In the case of spinal administration of opioids, mediation of tactile allodynia by large-diameter afferents means that the relevant fraction of opioid receptors are postsynaptic. This allows agonists with large receptor reserves (i.e., full- or high-efficacy agonists) to be effective against non-noxious stimulation, while low-efficacy, partial agonists (such as morphine) show no activity against such stimuli. Nonetheless, elevated spinal dynorphin, probably acting as a functional agonist at the NMDA-receptor complex, is also important to tactile allodynia, because the time course of elevation correlates with the appearance of allodynia and spinal dynorphin antiserum restores the antiallodynic activity of spinal morphine and reestablishes its spinal/supraspinal synergy. Thus, it is clear that the efficacy of the individual opioid, the nature of the dysesthesia, and the plasticity of the spinal cord following nerve injury (resulting in a maintained state of sensitization, due in part to afferent input) are all critical in the determination of opioid actions in the neuropathic situation.

REFERENCES

Ahmedzai S. New approaches to pain control in patients with cancer. *Eur J Can* 1997a; 33(Suppl 6):S8–14.

Ahmedzai S. Current strategies for pain control. *Ann Oncol* 1997b; 8 (Suppl 3):S21–24.

Aimone LD, Yaksh TL. Opioid modulation of capsaicin-evoked release of substance P from rat spinal cord in vivo. *Peptides* 1989; 10:1127–1131.

Arner S, Meyerson BA. Lack of analgesic effect on neuropathic and idiopathic forms of pain. *Pain* 1988; 33:11–23.

Arvidsson U, Dado RJ, Riedl M, et al. δ-Opioid receptor immunoreactivity: distribution in brainstem and spinal cord, and relationship to biogenic amines and enkephalin. *J Neurosci* 1995; 15:1215–1235.

Bakshi R, Faden AI. Blockade of the glycine modulatory site of NMDA receptors modifies dynorphin-induced behavioral effects. *Neurosci Lett* 1990a; 110:113–117.

Bakshi R, Faden AI. Competitive and non-competitive NMDA antagonists limit dynorphin A-induced rat hindlimb paralysis. *Brain Res* 1990b; 507:1–5.

Besse D, Lombard MC, Zajac JM, Roques BP, Besson JM. Pre- and postsynaptic distribution of μ, δ and κ opioid receptors in the superficial layers of the cervical dorsal horn of the rat spinal cord. *Brain Res* 1990; 521:15–22.

Bian D, Nichols ML, Ossipov MH, Lai J, Porreca F. Characterization of the antiallodynic efficacy of morphine in a model of neuropathic pain in rats. *Neuroreport* 1995; 6:1981–1984.

Bian D, Wegert S, Zhong C, Ossipov MH, Porreca F. Antisera to dynorphin $A_{(1-13)}$ prevents facilitation of the flexor reflex in L5/L6 nerve injured, but not in sham-operated, rats. *Soc Neurosci Abstr* 1997; 23:164.

Bian D, Ossipov MH, Malan TP, Porreca F. Tactile allodynia, but not thermal hyperalgesia, of the hindlimbs is blocked by spinal transection in rats with nerve injury. *Neurosci Lett* 1998a; 241:79–82.

Bian D, Malan TP, Ossipov MH, Zhong C, Porreca F. Differential sensitivity of thermal hyperalgesia and tactile allodynia to dynorphin antiserum after S2 ligation. *Soc Neurosci Abstr* 1998b; 24:383.

Bian D, Ossipov MH, Ibrahim M, et al. Loss of antiallodynic and antinociceptive spinal/supraspinal morphine synergy in nerve-injured rats: restoration by MK-801 or dynorphin antiserum. *Brain Res* 1999, in press.

Botticelli LJ, Cox BM, Goldstein A. Immunoreactive dynorphin in mammalian spinal cord and dorsal root ganglia. *Proc Natl Acad Sci USA* 1981; 78:7783–7786.

Caudle RM, Isaac L. A novel interaction between dynorphin(1–13) and N-methyl-D-aspartate. *Brain Res* 1988; 443:329–332.

Chen L, Huang LY. Dynorphin block of N-methyl-D-aspartate channels increases with the peptide length. *J Pharmacol Exp Ther* 1998; 284:826–831.

Chen L, Gu Y, Huang L-Y M. The mechanism of action of for the block of NMDA receptor channels by the opioid peptide dynorphin. *J Neurosci* 1995a; 15:4602–4611.

Chen L, Gu Y, Huang LY. The opioid peptide dynorphin directly blocks NMDA receptor channels in the rat. *J Physiol* 1995b; 482(Pt 3):575–581.

Cox BM, Molineaux CJ, Jacobs TP, Rossenberger JG, Faden AI. Effects of traumatic injury on dynorphin immunoreactivity in spinal cord. *Neuropeptides* 1985; 5:571–574.

Dado RJ, Law PY, Loh HH, Elde R. Immunofluorescent identification of a delta (δ)-opioid receptor on primary afferent nerve terminals. *Neuroreport* 1993; 5:341–344.

Dellemijn PL. Vanneste JA. Randomised double-blind active-placebo-controlled crossover trial of intravenous fentanyl in neuropathic pain. *Lancet* 1997; 349:753–758.

Dubner R. Neuronal plasticity and pain following peripheral tissue inflammation or nerve injury. In: Bond MR, Charlton JE, Woolf CJ (Eds). *Proceedings of the 6th World Congress on Pain.* Amsterdam: Elsevier Science Publishers BV, 1991, pp 263–276.

Dubner R, Ruda MA. Activity-dependent neuronal plasticity following tissue injury and inflammation. *Trends Neurosci* 1992; 15:96–103.

Faden AI. Opioid and nonopioid mechanisms may contribute to dynorphin's pathophysiological actions in spinal cord injury. *Ann Neurol* 1990; 27:67–74.

Faden AI, Jacobs TP. Dynorphin-related peptides cause motor dysfunction in the rat through a non-opiate action. *Br J Pharmacol* 1984; 81:271–276.

Gracely RH, Lynch SA, Bennett GJ. Painful neuropathy: altered central processing maintained dynamically by peripheral input. *Pain* 1992; 51:175–194.

Ibrahim M, Chawla MK, Chengmin Z, et al. Spatial and temporal correlation of spinal dynorphin content with behavioral signs of nerve injury. *Soc Neurosci Abstr* 1998; 24:892.

Jacobson L, Chabal C, Brody MC, Mariano AJ, Chaney EF. A comparison of the effects of intrathecal fentanyl and lidocaine on established postamputation stump pain. *Pain* 1990; 40:137–141.

Jadad AR, Carroll D, Glynn CJ, Moore RA, McQuay HJ. Morphine responsiveness of chronic pain: double blind randomized cross-over study with patient-controlled analgesia. *Lancet* 1992; 339:1367–1371.

Kajander KC, Sahara Y, Iadarola MJ, Bennett GJ. Dynorphin increases in the dorsal spinal cord in rats with a painful peripheral neuropathy. *Peptides* 1990; 11:719–728.

Kauppila T, Kontinen VK, Pertovaara A. Influence of spinalization on spinal withdrawal reflex responses varies depending on the submodality of the test stimulus and the experimental pathophysiological condition in the rat. *Brain Res* 1998; 797:234–242.

Lai J, Tang Q, Porreca F. High affinity binding of *des-Tyr*-Dynorphin A_{2-17} to the NMDA receptor complex. *Soc Neurosci Abstracts* 1997; 23:941.

Lai SL, Gu Y, Huang LY. Dynorphin uses a non-opioid mechanism to potentiate N-methyl-D-aspartate currents in single rat periaqueductal gray neurons. *Neurosci Lett* 1998; 247:115–118.

Lee Y-W, Chaplan SR, Yaksh TL. Systemic and supraspinal but not spinal opiates suppress allodynia in a rat neuropathic pain model. *Neurosci Lett* 1995; 199:111–114.

Lekan HA, Carlton SM, Coggeshall RE. Sprouting of A beta fibers into lamina II of the rat dorsal horn in peripheral neuropathy. *Neurosci Lett* 1996; 208:147–150.

Lima D, Avelino A, Coimbra A. Morphological characterization of marginal (lamina I) neurons immunoreactive for substance P, enkephalin, dynorphin and gamma-aminobutyric acid in the rat spinal cord. *J Chem Neuroanat* 1993; 6:43–52.

Long JB, Petras JM, Mobley WC, Holaday JW. Neurological dysfunction after intrathecal injection of dynorphin A(1–13) in the rat. II. Nonopioid mechanisms mediate loss of motor sensory and autonomic function. *J Pharmacol Exp Ther* 1988; 246:1167–1174.

Long JB, Rigamonti DD, Oleshansky MA, Wingfield CP, Martinez-Arizala A. Dynorphin A-induced rat spinal cord injury: evidence for excitatory amino acid involvement in a pharmacological model of ischemic spinal cord injury. *J Pharmacol Exp Ther* 1994; 269:358–366.

Long JB, Skolnick P. 1-Aminocyclopropanecarboxylic acid protects against dynorphin A-induced spinal injury. *Eur J Pharmacol* 1995; 261:295–301.

Maekawa K, Minami M, Masuda T, Satoh M. Expression of μ- and κ-, but not δ-, opioid receptor mRNAs is enhanced in the spinal dorsal horn of the arthritic rats. *Pain* 1994; 64:365–371.

Mansour A, Fox CA, Thompson RC, Akil H, Watson SJ. μ-Opioid receptor mRNA expression in the rat CNS: comparison to μ-receptor binding. *Brain Res* 1994; 643:245–265.

Mansour A, Fox CA, Akil H, Watson SJ. Opioid-receptor mRNA expression in the rat CNS: anatomical and functional implications. *Trends Neurosci* 1995;18:22–29.

Mao J, Price DD, Mayer DJ. Experimental mononeuropathy reduces the antinociceptive effects of morphine: implications for common intracellular mechanisms involved in morphine tolerance and neuropathic pain. *Pain* 1995a; 61:353–364.

Mao J, Price DD, Mayer DJ. Mechanisms of hyperalgesia and morphine tolerance: a current view of their possible interactions. *Pain* 1995b; 62:259–274.

Max MB, Schafer SC, Culnane M. Association of pain relief with drug side-effects in postherpetic neuralgia: a single dose study of clonidine codeine ibuprofen and placebo. *Clin Pharmacol Ther* 1988; 43:363–371.

Nahin RL. Immunocytochemical identification of long ascending, peptidergic lumbar spinal neurons terminating in either the medial or lateral thalamus of the rat. *Brain Res* 1988; 443:345–349.

Nahin RL, Hylden JL, Humphey E. Demonstration of dynorphin A_{1-8} immunoreactive axons contacting spinal cord projection neurons in a rat model of peripheral inflammation and hyperalgesia. *Pain* 1992; 5113–5143.

Nichols ML, Bian D, Ossipov MH, Porreca F. Evidence for regulation of opioid activity by CCK in a model of neuropathic pain. *J Pharmacol Exp Ther* 1995; 275:1337–1345.

Nichols ML, Lopez Y, Ossipov MH, Bian D, Porreca F. Enhancement of the antiallodynic and antinociceptive efficacy of spinal morphine by antisera to dynorphin $A_{(1-13)}$ or MK-801 in a nerve-ligation model of peripheral neuropathy. *Pain* 1997; 69:317–322.

Ossipov MH, Nichols ML, Bian D, Porreca F. Inhibition by spinal morphine of the tail-flick response is attenuated in rats with nerve ligation injury. *Neurosci Lett* 1995a; 199:83–86.

Ossipov MH, Lopez Y, Nichols ML, Bian D, Porreca F. The loss of antinociceptive efficacy of spinal morphine in rats with nerve ligation injury is prevented by reducing spinal afferent drive *Neurosci Lett* 1995b:199:87–90.

Ossipov MH, Bian D, Malan TP, Lai J, Porreca F. Lack of involvement of capsaicin-sensitive primary afferents in nerve-ligation injury induced tactile allodynia in rats. *Pain* 1999; 79:127–133.

Paix A, Coleman A, Lees J, et al. Subcutaneous fentanyl and sufentanil infusion substitution for morphine intolerance in cancer pain management. *Pain* 1995; 63:263–269.

Payne R. Neuropathic pain syndromes with special reference to causalgia and reflex sympathetic dystrophy. *Clin J Pain* 1986; 2:59–73.

Pertovaara A. A neuronal correlate of secondary hyperalgesia in the rat spinal dorsal horn is submodality selective and facilitated by supraspinal influence. *Exp Neurol* 1998; 149:193–202.

Portenoy RK, Foley KM. Chronic use of opioid analgesics in non-malignant pain: report of 38 cases. *Pain* 1986; 25:171–186.

Portenoy RK, Foley KM, Inturrisi CE. The nature of opioid responsiveness and its implications for neuropathic pain: new hypotheses derived from studies of opioid infusions. *Pain* 1990; 43:273–286.

Przewlocki R, Shearman GT, Herz A. Mixed opioid/nonopioid effects of dynorphin and dynorphin related peptides after their intrathecal injection in rats. *Neuropeptides* 1983; 3:233–240.

Riley RC, Zhao ZQ, Duggan AW. Spinal release of immunoreactive dynorphin A(1–8) with the development of peripheral inflammation in the rat. *Brain Res* 1996; 710:131–142.

Rowbotham MC, Reisner-Keller LA, Fields HL. Both intravenous lidocaine and morphine reduce the pain of postherpetic neuralgia. *Neurology* 1991; 41:1024–1028.

Ruda MA, Iadarola MJ, Cohen LV, Young WS. In situ hybridization histochemistry and immunocytochemistry reveal an increase in spinal dynorphin biosynthesis in a rat model of peripheral inflammation and hyperalgesia. *Proc Natl Acad Sci USA* 1988; 85:622–626.

Sotgiu ML, Biella G, Lacerenza M. Injured nerve block alters adjacent nerves spinal interaction in neuropathic rats. *Neuroreport* 1996; 7:1385–1388.

Stevens CW, Yaksh TL. Dynorphin A and related peptides administered intrathecally in the rat: a search for putative kappa opiate receptor activity. *J Pharmacol Exp Ther* 1986; 238:833–838.

Stewart P, Isaac L. A strychnine-sensitive site is involved in dynorphin-induced paralysis and loss of the tail-flick reflex. *Brain Res* 1991; 543:322–326.

Sung B, Na HS, Kim YI, et al. Supraspinal involvement in the production of mechanical allodynia by spinal nerve injury in rats. *Neurosci Lett* 1998; 246:117–119.

Swett JE, Woolf CJ. The somatotopic organization of primary afferent terminals in the superficial laminae of the dorsal horn of the rat spinal cord. *J Comp Neurol* 1985; 231:66–77.

Taddese A, Nah S-Y, McCleskey EW. Selective opioid inhibition of small nociceptive neurons. *Science* 1995; 270:1366–1369.

Takahashi O, Shiosaka S, Traub RJ, Ruda MA. Ultrastructural demonstration of synaptic connections between calcitonin gene-related peptide immunoreactive axons and dynorphin A(1–8) immunoreactive dorsal horn neurons in a rat model of peripheral inflammation and hyperalgesia. *Peptides* 1990; 11:1133–1137.

Tal M, Bennett GJ. Extra-territorial pain in rats with a peripheral mononeuropathy: mechano-hyperalgesia and mechano-allodynia in the territory of the uninjured nerve. *Pain* 1994; 57:375–382.

Tasker RR, Buda T, Hawrylyshyn P. Clinical neurophysiological investigation of deafferentation pain. In: Bonica JJ, Lindblom U, Iggo A (Eds). *Advances in Pain Research and Therapy,* Vol. 5. New York: Raven Press, 1983, pp 713–738.

Twycross RG. Morphine and diamorphine in the terminally ill patient. *Acta Anesthesiol Scand* 1982; (Suppl)74:128–134.

Vanderah TW, Laughlin T, Lashbrook JM, et al. Single intrathecal injections of dynorphin A or *des*-tyr-dynorphins produce long-lasting allodynia in rats: blockade by MK-801 but not naloxone. *Pain* 1996; 68:275–281.

Wagner R, DeLeo JA. Pre-emptive dynorphin and N-methyl-D-aspartate glutamate receptor antagonism alters spinal immunocytochemistry but not allodynia following complete peripheral nerve injury. *Neuroscience* 1996; 72:527–534.

Walker JM, Katz RJ, Akil H. Behavioral effects of dynorphin 1–13 in the mouse and rat: initial observations. *Peptides* 1980; 1:341–345.

Walker JM, Moises HC, Coy DH, Baldrighi G, Akil H. Nonopiate effects of dynorphin and des-tyr-dynorphin. *Science* 1982; 218:1136–1138.

Wegert S, Ossipov MH, Nichols ML, et al. Differential activities of intrathecal MK-801 or morphine to alter responses to thermal and mechanical stimuli in normal or nerve-injured rats. *Pain* 1997; 71:57–64.

Wiesenfeld-Hallin Z. The effects of intrathecal morphine and naltrexone on autotomy in sciatic nerve sectioned rats. *Pain* 1984; 18:267–278.

Woolf CJ, Shortland P, Reynolds M, et al. Reorganization of central terminals of myelinated primary afferents in the rat dorsal horn following peripheral axotomy. *J Comp Neurol* 1995; 360:121–134.

Xu X-J, Puke MJC, Verge VMK, et al. Up-regulation of cholecystokinin in primary sensory neurons is associated with morphine insensitivity in experimental neuropathic pain in the rat. *Neurosci Lett* 1993; 152:129–132.

Yamamoto T, Yaksh TL. Spinal pharmacology of thermal hyperesthesia induced by incomplete ligation of sciatic nerve. I. Opioid and nonopioid receptors. *Anesthesiology* 1991; 75:817–826.

Yeomans DC, Pirec V, Proudfit HK. Nociceptive responses to high and low rates of noxious cutaneous heating are mediated by different nociceptors in the rat: behavioral evidence. *Pain* 1996; 68:133–140.

Yeung JC, Rudy TA. Sites of antinociceptive action of systemically injected morphine: involvement of supraspinal loci as revealed by intracerebroventricular injection of naloxone. *J Pharmacol Exp Ther* 1980a; 626–632.

Yeung JC, Rudy TA. Multiplicative interaction between narcotic agonisms expressed at spinal and supraspinal sites of antinociceptive action as revealed by concurrent intrathecal and intracerebroventricular injection of morphine. *J Pharmacol Exp Ther* 1980b; 215:633–642.

Zhang L, Peoples RW, Oz M, et al. Potentiation of NMDA receptor-mediated responses by dynorphin at low extracellular glycine concentrations. *J Neurophysiol* 1997; 78:582–590.

Correspondence to: Frank Porreca, PhD, Departments of Pharmacology and Anesthesiology, Health Sciences Center, University of Arizona, Tucson, AZ 85724, USA. Tel: 520-626-7421; Fax: 520-626-4182; email: frankp@u.arizona.edu.

Opioid Sensitivity of Chronic Noncancer Pain,
Progress in Pain Research and Management,
Vol. 14, edited by Eija Kalso, Henry J. McQuay,
and Zsuzsanna Wiesenfeld-Hallin, IASP Press,
Seattle, © 1999.

11

Opioid Sensitivity in Experimental Central Pain after Spinal Cord Injury in Rats

Xiao-Jun Xu,[a] Wei Yu,[a] Jing-Xia Hao,[a] Tomas Hökfelt,[b] and Zsuzsanna Wiesenfeld-Hallin[a]

[a]Department of Medical Laboratory Sciences and Technology, Division of Clinical Neurophysiology, Huddinge University Hospital, Huddinge, Sweden; and [b]Department of Neuroscience, Karolinska Institute, Stockholm, Sweden

CENTRAL PAIN AND ITS CLINICAL MANAGEMENT

Central pain is caused by a primary lesion or dysfunction of the central nervous system (CNS). Although the concept of central pain originated from cases involving stroke in the thalamus, lesions along the entire neuroaxis in the CNS may be associated with central pain (Tasker 1990; Boivie 1994). Clinically, major causes include vascular lesions, traumatic spinal cord injury, multiple sclerosis, and tumors (Tasker 1990; Boivie 1994). The reported incidence of central pain varies widely due to differences in criteria used, selection and size of the patient group, timing of the observation, and duration of follow-up (Tasker 1990; Bonica 1991; Boivie 1994). The clinical significance of central pain has become increasingly important because of the increased rate of survival and longer life expectancy among patients with CNS injury due to improved medical care.

Traumatic spinal cord injury is associated with a high incidence of central pain (Beric et al. 1988; Cohen et al. 1988; Davidoff and Roth 1991; Boivie 1994). Patients with multiple sclerosis, syringomyelia, vascular diseases, tumors, and metastases also may have central pain of spinal origin. The incidence of central pain after spinal cord injury varies in different studies, ranging from 7.5% to 94% (Nepomuceno et al. 1979; Beric et al. 1988; Bonica 1991; Davidoff and Roth 1991).

Central pain shares common characteristics despite various etiologies, although its severity and pattern can vary. It is usually associated with other neurological problems, including sensory deficits, but sometimes pain is the only symptom. The onset of pain after the original injury varies from immediate onset to a delay of days to years (Nepomuceno et al. 1979; Boivie 1994). The pain can be continuous or intermittent, and the intensity varies from a discomforting or unpleasant sensation to unbearable suffering. The characteristics of central pain include burning, pricking, and lancinating sensations and dysesthesia. In addition to spontaneous pain, allodynia (pain evoked by normally non-noxious touch or temperature stimuli) is common in these patients (Davidoff and Roth 1991; Boivie 1994; Eide et al. 1996).

Central pain is among the most difficult pain conditions to treat. Numerous strategies have been attempted with limited success. Pharmacological treatments include antidepressants, anticonvulsants, and systemically administered local anesthetics (Leijon and Boivie 1991; Bowsher and Nurmikko 1996). Opioids are believed to have little effect in most cases of central pain, although definitive studies are lacking (Hammond 1991; Leijon and Boivie 1991; Bowsher and Nurmikko 1996). The sensitivity of opioids in treating neuropathic pain has been a matter of controversy (Arnér and Meyerson 1988; Portenoy et al. 1990). Researchers have suggested that neuropathic pain of central origin may respond more poorly to opioids than does pain following peripheral nerve injury (see Chapter 18).

ANIMAL MODELS OF CENTRAL PAIN

Animal models for specific human pain conditions have been developed to explore underlying mechanisms and find effective new treatments. These models may also be useful in addressing controversial clinical issues such as opioid sensitivity in neuropathic pain. Animal models for central pain have only recently become available (Yezierski 1996; Wiesenfeld-Hallin et al. 1997). These mainly involve injury to the spinal cord and observation of pain-related behaviors that develop after the injury.

Our laboratory used a photochemical technique to produce graded spinal cord ischemia in rats. In addition to spinal tissue damage and motor impairment that were the expected consequences of spinal injury, we observed that the animals also exhibited pain-like behaviors. Thus, after both transient and irreversible ischemia, an acute phase of mechanical allodynia started within 24 hours and lasted 4–5 days (Hao et al. 1991, 1992a). After irreversible ischemia, chronic allodynia developed with a delay of days to months (Xu et al. 1992). Table I summarizes the characteristics of both acute and chronic allodynia models. Extensive behavioral, electrophysiologi-

Table I
Characteristics of acute and chronic allodynia-like behaviors after
spinal cord ischemic injury in rats

	Acute Allodynia	Chronic Allodynia
Irradiation duration	1–10 min	10 min
Degree of ischemia	Transient to irreversible	Irreversible
Morphological damage	Not critical	Dorsal columns, dorsolateral funiculi, laminae I–V
Motor deficit	Not critical	Present
Percentage of animals	90%	Minority
Time of onset	Within 24 h	1 wk–3 mo
Duration	4–5 d	Months to years
Mechanical allodynia	Present	Present
Cold hypersensitivity	Present	Present
Tactile allodynia	Present	Present
Allodynic area detected	Diffuse	Discrete

cal, and morphological studies conducted in our laboratory have presented multiple lines of evidence indicating that these two animal models may represent central pain after spinal cord injury (Wiesenfeld-Hallin et al. 1997).

THE EFFECT OF MORPHINE IN CENTRAL PAIN

EFFECT OF MORPHINE ON ACUTE ALLODYNIA-LIKE BEHAVIOR

Acute allodynia-like behaviors, which consist of tactile and punctate allodynia to mechanical stimulation, are primarily a result of hyperexcitability of dorsal horn wide dynamic range neurons (Hao et al. 1992b). Dysfunction of spinal GABAergic inhibitory control as a consequence of ischemia appears to play a crucial role. Thus, behavioral allodynia and neuronal hyperexcitability can be reversed by the GABA$_B$-receptor agonist baclofen (Hao et al. 1991, 1992c). Moreover, the number of dorsal horn neurons containing GABA-like immunoreactivity (GABA-LI) was substantially reduced after spinal ischemia (Zhang et al. 1994).

A moderate dose of systemic morphine (2 mg/kg) totally alleviated transient mechanical allodynia in an area surrounding the surgical wound in sham-operated rats (Hao et al. 1991). Systemic morphine at 2 mg/kg also had some anti-allodynic effect in the spinally injured rats a few hours after ischemia, indicating that allodynia at this time primarily reflected postoperative pain. However, morphine up to 5 mg/kg did not produce an anti-allodynic effect 1–2 days after spinal ischemia when the pain was likely to have a central origin. We have also recently studied the effect of intrathecal (i.t.) morphine by injecting cumulative doses of morphine 2 days after spinal cord ischemia was induced (Yu et al. 1999). The vocalization threshold to stimulation with von Frey hairs was not significantly reduced by i.t. morphine up to a 10-μg cumulative dose (Fig. 1A). In a few rats, however, the vocalization threshold was normalized at this dose. Intrathecal morphine also did not significantly reduce the allodynia-like responses to stroking the skin at a 10-μg cumulative dose (Fig. 1B). In contrast, i.t. morphine dose-dependently prolonged the tail-flick latency in the allodynic rats, as in normal controls (Fig. 1C).

EFFECTS OF SPINAL CORD ISCHEMIA ON MU-OPIOID RECEPTORS IN THE DORSAL HORN

Several studies have shown that after peripheral nerve injury in rats, where morphine may have a reduced effect, the level of opioid receptors decreases in dorsal root ganglia and in the dorsal horn (Besse et al 1992: Zhang et al. 1998). To explore the underlying mechanisms of opioid insensitivity during acute allodynia, we conducted an immunohistochemical study to examine the level of μ-opioid receptors in the spinal cord in normal rats and rats with spinal cord ischemia induced by laser irradiation (Yu et al. 1999). Normal rats had a dense distribution of μ-opioid-receptor-like immunoreactivity (MOR-LI) in the superficial laminae of the dorsal spinal cord, including fibers, dendrites, and cell bodies. However, 2 days after laser irradiation we observed a marked bilateral decrease in MOR-LI one spinal segment rostral to the epicenter of the ischemia. The expression of MOR-LI at cervical and sacral segments was normal, and 2 weeks after the irradiation MOR-LI had returned to normal levels.

MECHANISMS OF MORPHINE INSENSITIVITY DURING ACUTE ALLODYNIA

Several features suggest that the reduction in MOR-LI during acute allodynia is due to decreased synthesis of the receptors as a direct or indirect result of localized ischemia, rather than to nonspecific factors such as tissue damage, poor fixation by insufficient perfusion, or generalized effects (Yu et al. 1999). As the area of acute allodynia is fairly large, covering dermatomes of several spinal segments, it is likely that the segments rostral to the epicenter of the ischemia are located in the pathways related to the transmission of allodynic signals. Thus, a reduction of μ-opioid receptors may underlie the apparent lack of anti-allodynic effect by systemic or i.t. morphine.

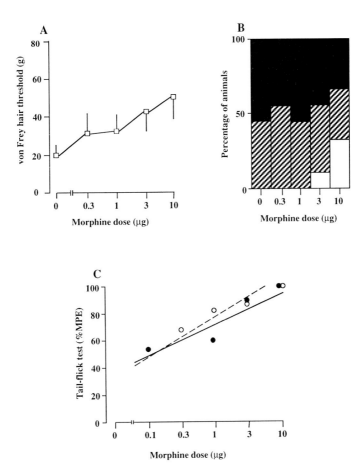

Fig. 1. Effects of cumulative doses of intrathecal (i.t.) morphine on responses to pressure/touch stimulation with (A) von Frey hairs or (B) stroking in allodynic rats (n = 10), and (C) on tail-flick latency in normal and acute allodynic rats. (A) Intrathecal morphine had no significant effect on the vocalization response threshold to stimulation with von Frey hairs. (B) Percentage of animals that responded to tactile stimulation, scored as described in Yu et al. (1998). Open areas represent a score of 0, hatched areas a score of 1, and black areas a score of 2. Intrathecal morphine did not significantly influence the response to tactile stimulation. (C) Data are expressed as percentage of MPE (maximum possible effect), which was calculated based according to the formula: MPE = ([post-morphine response] – [predrug response]/[maximal response] – [predrug response]) × 100, where maximal response is 10 seconds. ANOVA was highly significant for both regressions, but no significant difference was found between normal (open circles) and acute allodynic (filled circles) rats.

Other mechanisms may be also involved in morphine insensitivity during acute allodynia. For example, morphine has a relatively selective inhibitory effect on C-fiber input (Le Bars et al. 1975; Zieglgänsberger and Bayerl 1976; Yaksh 1978). Since the mechanical allodynia-like responses, particularly to tactile stimulation, are likely to be mediated by large-diameter myelinated afferent fibers, morphine may have limited effect. This argument is, however, contradicted by findings that morphine (particularly when administered i.t.) had an anti-allodynic effect in chronic allodynia, which is also likely to be mediated by capsaicin-insensitive Aβ fibers (Yu et al. 1997a).

EFFECT OF MORPHINE ON CHRONIC
ALLODYNIA-LIKE BEHAVIOR

Although acute allodynia represents a special form of central hypersensitivity as a result of spinal disinhibition, chronic allodynia more closely mimics clinical central pain in patients with spinal cord injury (Xu et al. 1992, Wiesenfeld-Hallin et al. 1997). We therefore studied the effect of morphine via different routes of administration on chronic allodynia-like behaviors in rats (Yu et al. 1997a). Systemic morphine given either subcutaneously (s.c.) or intraperitoneally (i.p.) did not significantly alleviate allodynia up to a 3 mg/kg cumulative dose (Fig. 2). The rats were somewhat sedated at this dose, and the activity level tested with the open field test was decreased by nearly 50%. A cumulative dose of 10 mg/kg systemic morphine markedly increased the vocalization threshold to von Frey hair stimulation in all rats, which was accompanied by heavy sedation and profound ataxia (Fig. 2). In contrast to the lack of effect of systemic morphine, i.t. morphine dose-dependently alleviated the mechanical allodynia-like behaviors, with significant effect observed after a 3-μg cumulative dose (Fig. 2). Intrathecal morphine produced no sedation up to a 10-μg cumulative dose (Fig. 2). Anti-allodynic effect was also observed after a single i.t. injection of morphine.

Intracerebroventricular (i.c.v.) morphine produced differential effects on different components of the response to von Frey hair stimulation. The vocalization component of the response was abolished by 0.1 μg i.c.v. morphine (Fig. 2). However, other components of the abnormal reaction remained, such as agitation, jumping, and avoidance. The threshold for evoking these responses was slightly increased after a 3 μg i.c.v. dose (Fig. 2). Only at the highest dose of 10 μg were the abnormal pain-like reactions totally abolished and the response threshold raised to 270 g (Fig. 2). However, both 3 and 10 μg i.c.v. morphine produced severe sedation.

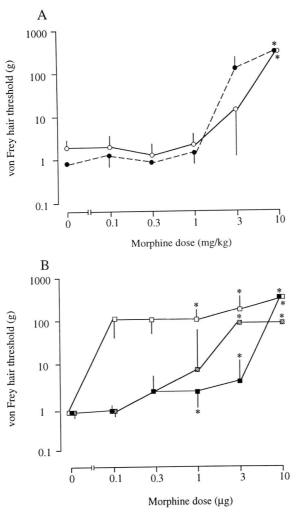

Fig. 2. Effects of cumulative doses of (A) systemic or (B) i.t. or i.c.v. morphine on nocifensive reactions to innocuous mechanical stimulation with von Frey hairs in allodynic rats. Note the logarithmic scale on both axes. (A) Morphine was administered either s.c. (filled circles) or i.p. (open circles). A significant increase in response threshold (referring to both vocalization and other responses) was seen at the highest dose, with no difference between the two routes of administration. (B) Morphine was administered either i.t. (hatched squares) or i.c.v (filled or open squares). Since i.c.v. morphine affected differentially vocalization and other components of the response, they are presented separately (open squares for vocalization, filled squares for other reactions). For i.t. morphine, a significantly overall increase in vocalization threshold was observed. For i.c.v. morphine, a significant overall changes in thresholds for both vocalization and other responses was seen. (From Yu et al. 1997a).

EFFECT OF MORPHINE ON TAIL-FLICK LATENCY IN NORMAL AND ALLODYNIC RATS

The tail-flick latency was increased dose-dependently by systemic morphine in normal rats. There was no difference between the effect of s.c. and i.p. routes. A similar dose-dependent antinociceptive effect of morphine was observed in normal rats after i.t. or i.c.v. administration. Morphine also produced dose-dependent antinociception after systemic or i.t. administration in the allodynic rats in the tail-flick test. In contrast, i.c.v. morphine produced no significant antinociception in the allodynic rats (Yu et al. 1997a).

To compare the potency of morphine to different stimulus modalities, we converted the von Frey hair threshold and the tail-flick latency to percentage of maximum possible effect (MPE) (Table II). The ED_{50} (median effective dose) of systemic, i.t., and i.c.v morphine in the von Frey hair test was compared to the respective ED_{50} in the tail-flick test in the allodynic rats (Table II). The anti-allodynic potency of morphine was significantly less than its antinociceptive effect in allodynic animals.

MECHANISMS OF MORPHINE SENSITIVITY IN TREATING CHRONIC ALLODYNIA-LIKE BEHAVIORS

We have shown that systemic morphine at low to moderate doses did not suppress allodynia, while at high doses it induced severe sedation. It is unclear whether the effect of sedative doses of morphine on allodynia re-

Table II

Comparison of the antinociceptive and antiallodynic effects of systemic (s.c. and i.p.), i.t., and i.c.v. morphine in normal and allodynic rats

ED_{50} of %MPE	Route of Administration*			
	s.c.	i.p.	i.t.	i.c.v.
Tail-flick, normal rats	0.9 mg/kg	0.7 mg/kg	0.1 μg	0.8 μg
Tail-flick, allodynic rats	1.6 mg/kg	2.2 mg/kg	0.9 μg	No effect
von Frey hair test	4.8 mg/kg	4.5 mg/kg	3.1 μg	0.3 μg[a]
Threshold				5.1 μg[b]

Source: Yu et al. (1997a).
Note: Percentage maximum possible effort (MPE) is calculated with 10 s as cut-off time in the tail-flick (TF) test and 73 g (response threshold in normal rats) in the von Frey hair test. Median effective dose (ED_{50}) is obtained from the regression line constructed from the effects of multiple doses of morphine administration following different routes of administration. The ED_{50} for the tail-flick test could not be obtained in the allodynic rats after i.c.v. morphine as %MPE did not exceed 50%.
(a) Vocalization, (b) other reactions.
* s.c. = subcutaneous; i.p. = intraperitoneal; i.t. = intrathecal; i.c.v. = intracerebroventricular.

flected a genuine anti-allodynic effect, as the behavioral assessment in our model was an integrated response. In contrast, i.t. morphine dose-dependently and fully alleviated chronic allodynia without causing sedation at any dose. The anti-allodynic effect of i.t. morphine as judged by ED_{50} is, however, less potent than its antinociceptive effect. This would suggest that a relatively high spinal concentration of morphine is required to obtain the anti-allodynic effect, which may not be reached by systemic administration before morphine starts to exert its supraspinal sedative effect.

We have recently observed that in rats with chronic (unlike acute) allodynia, the level of MOR-LI in spinal segments rostral to the lesion is comparable to normal controls (W. Yu et al., unpublished observations). Thus, the relative morphine insensitivity in chronic allodynia is unlikely to be due to changes in μ-receptor levels. In the spinal cord, 50–75% of μ receptors are located on terminals of unmyelinated fibers (Besse et al. 1990; Arvidsson et al. 1995). Opioids preferentially inhibit input from unmyelinated C fibers (Le Bars et al. 1975; Zieglgänsberger and Bayerl 1976; Yaksh 1978), which are unlikely to be involved in mediating mechanical allodynia-like behaviors in our model (Hao et al. 1996). Thus, morphine probably exerts its anti-allodynic effect postsynaptically, and with decreased potency in comparison to its powerful antinociception through a combined pre- and postsynaptic mechanism.

Our results differ from several studies where no effect of i.t. morphine on mechanical allodynia was observed after peripheral nerve injury (Bian et al. 1995; Lee et al. 1995). The results obtained with models of peripheral nerve injury cannot be fully explained by the ineffectiveness of morphine on myelinated fiber input. Additional mechanisms such as reduction in opioid receptors (Besse et al. 1992; Zhang et al. 1998), upregulation of antiopioid peptides (Xu et al. 1993; Nichols et al. 1995), and increased activity of excitatory amino acids (Mao et al. 1995) may also play important roles. These changes may occur primarily at the spinal level after peripheral nerve injury, making i.t. morphine ineffective. We do not know, however, whether and to what extent these changes occur after spinal cord injury.

Intrathecal morphine reduced all components of the reaction to stimulation with von Frey hairs. In contrast, i.c.v. morphine selectively reduced the vocalization component of the reaction. It is unlikely that suppression of vocalization was due to sedation, as doses that reduced vocalization (below 1 μg) did not cause sedation. Other pain-related behaviors were suppressed after high doses of i.c.v. morphine (3–10 μg), which caused sedation. Vocalization in response to noxious stimuli may reflect the affective component of pain in rodents (Levine et al. 1984; Borszcz 1995). It is thus possible that supraspinal morphine influenced the affective components of the allodynia-like behavior without influencing its sensory components. This may resemble the clinical situation where patients report disassociation of the affective and sensory aspects of neuropathic pain following systemic morphine (Kupers et al. 1991).

TOLERANCE TO THE ANTI-ALLODYNIC EFFECT OF INTRATHECAL MORPHINE

Repeated application of opioids induces the development of tolerance and dependence. It is unclear whether significant tolerance develops when opioids are used to treat chronic pain in the clinic. Although the need for dose escalation has been observed in several studies when opioids are used chronically in cancer patients (Ventafridda et al. 1987; Onofrio and Yaksh 1990; Sallerin et al. 1998), it is unclear whether this reflects the development of tolerance or the progression of the disease and associated increase in anxiety (Foley 1991; Portenoy 1996). Outcomes of studies using animal models are also unclear. Some results indicate that the presence of tonic or chronic inflammatory pain may delay the development of tolerance (Colpaert et al. 1978; Abbott et al. 1981; Vaccarino et al. 1993), whereas others suggest that it may accelerate its process (Kayser 1985; Connell et al. 1994; Detweiler et al. 1995; Gutstein et al. 1995).

We examined whether tolerance and dependence develop to 10 μg i.t. morphine administered twice daily to spinally injured rats with chronic allodynia (Yu et al. 1997b). While morphine totally reversed the mechanical allodynia for 2 days, the anti-allodynic effect of i.t. morphine was significantly reduced from day 3 and decreased further thereafter (Fig. 3). The baseline vocalization threshold to stimulation with von Frey hairs prior to drug administration also successively decreased on days 3–8 compared to day 1 (Fig. 3). The effect of i.t. morphine on tail-flick latency in the same rats was also reduced during the course of chronic treatment, but with a somewhat slower time course (Fig. 3). No decrease in baseline tail-flick latency was observed (Fig. 3). Tolerance to the antinociceptive effect of i.t. morphine in the tail-flick and paw-pressure tests developed similarly in allodynic and normal rats (Fig. 3).

After 21 days of 10 μg i.t. morphine twice daily, naloxone (1 mg/kg, i.p.) rapidly elicited signs of withdrawal in both normal and allodynic rats, primarily involving caudal body parts, such as scratching the lower trunk, biting the hind paws, tail trembling, hindpaw lifting, wet dog shakes, ataxia, and spasms of the lower back. The allodynic rats showed significantly more scratching and biting, but there was no overall significant difference between the two groups. We noted no signs of systemic withdrawal, such as ptosis, diarrhea, or irritation.

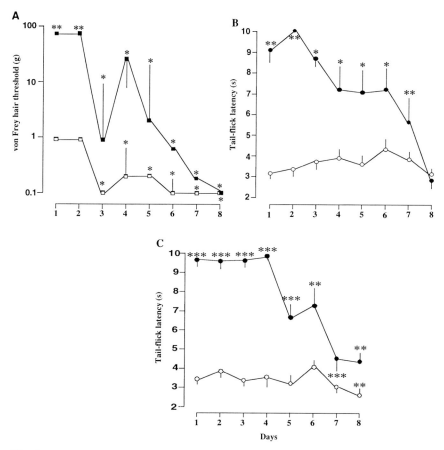

Fig. 3. Development of tolerance to the effects of i.t. morphine in (A, B) allodynic and (C) normal rats. (A) Vocalization threshold of allodynic rats to von Frey hairs before (open squares) and 30 minutes after (filled squares) the morning dose of 10 μg i.t. morphine. A significant elevation of vocalization threshold was observed compared to baseline response on days 1 and 2, with no significant effect on days 3–8 (compared to morphine's effect on day 1). Hyperalgesia of the predrug response compared to day 1 was observed on days 3–8, which was not reversed by morphine. Note that the y-axis is logarithmic. (B) Tail-flick latency in allodynic rats before (open circles) and 30 minutes after (filled circles) the morning dose of morphine. Significant antinociception compared to predrug response latency was observed on days 1–6, with tolerance on days 7 and 8. A significant reduction of the antinociceptive effect of morphine was observed on days 6–8 compared to day 1. (C) Tail-flick latency before (open circles) and 30 minutes after (filled circles) the morning dose of morphine in normal controls. Significant antinociception compared to pre-drug response latency was observed on days 1–6. A significant reduction of the antinociceptive effect of morphine compared to day 1 was observed on days 5–8. The predrug response was reduced on day 8 compared to day 1, which was reversed by morphine. Asterisks indicate statistical significance: * $P < 0.05$; ** $P < 0.01$; *** $P < 0.001$.

These data showed unequivocally that the anti-allodynic effect of i.t. morphine was diminished following chronic administration and that dependence also developed. As the chronic allodynia-like behavior was usually stable in the absence of morphine treatment, the reduced effect of chronic morphine more likely reflects the development of tolerance rather than increased pain level. The rate of tolerance development to the anti-allodynic effect of i.t. morphine was similar to that for the antinociceptive effect in normal and allodynic rats. Thus, we obtained no evidence that the presence of chronic pain influences the rate of tolerance development, even when morphine is used to treat pain. Moreover, chronic i.t. morphine also induced physical dependence in the spinally injured rats similarly to normal rats.

It must be emphasized that a constant dose of i.t. morphine was used in our study, which is unlikely to occur in a clinical setting. Thus, it is possible that the development of tolerance to opioids would be different if morphine were administered in increasing doses. Also, in order to rapidly produce pharmacological tolerance, the dose of morphine employed in our study was high, whereas in the clinical situation the dose is usually titrated to match the level of pain (Foley 1991; Portenoy 1996). Thus, the individual regime of administration of opioids and other analgesics for patients may have contributed to the controversial clinical observations. Intrathecal or systemic naloxone aggravated chronic allodynia (Hao et al., unpublished observations), indicating that endogenous opioidergic control is still active in these rats, although with reduced strength. The development of tolerance to exogenous morphine may also reduce the effectiveness of endogenous opioid control, resulting in the aggravation of chronic pain.

SELECTIVE OPIOID-RECEPTOR AGONISTS IN ANIMAL MODELS OF CHRONIC ALLODYNIA

In addition to the well-established subtypes of opioid receptors, μ, δ, and κ, an additional orphan opioid-receptor-like (ORL1) receptor was cloned a few years ago for which orphanin FQ (OFQ) or nociceptin has been identified as an endogenous ligand (Meunier et al. 1995; Reinscheid et al. 1995). Compounds that selectively activate opioid-receptor subtypes may be clinically useful as analgesics with reduced side effects. We tested the effects of i.t. DAMGO, DPDPE, U50488H, and OFQ, selective agonists of μ, δ, κ, and ORL1 receptors, respectively, on chronic allodynia-like behaviors in spinally injured rats (Hao et al. 1998a,b).

Intrathecal DAMGO, DPDPE, and OFQ dose-dependently alleviated mechanical allodynia and cold allodynia in spinally injured rats with no noticeable side effects. These three compounds also induced antinociception. The potency for the anti-allodynic and antinociceptive effect of DAMGO, DPDPE, and OFQ did not differ significantly. The anti-allodynic effects of DAMGO and DPDPE were reversed by the selective μ- and δ-receptor antagonists CTOP and naltrindole, respectively. Intrathecal administration of the selective κ-receptor agonist U50488H significantly increased mechanical and cold allodynia-like behaviors in spinally injured rats in a dose-dependent fashion. Moreover, the anti-allodynic and antinociceptive effect of DAMGO was blocked by U50488H. Intrathecal U50488H did not produce an anti-allodynic effect even at high doses, and did not significantly alter tail-flick latency. Thus, i.t. administration of selective agonists of μ or δ receptors dose-dependently alleviated the mechanical allodynia-like behavior in spinally injured rats. The doses of the two agonists were comparable to or lower than those used in previous studies (Drower et al. 1991; Miaskowski et al. 1991; Guirimand et al. 1994). The effects of the agonists were reversed by respective antagonists, indicating receptor specificity of the anti-allodynic effects of the μ and δ agonists. In contrast, the κ agonist U50488H further decreased the vocalization threshold of the rats to von Frey hairs, increased the cold response, and also triggered and enhanced tactile allodynia. Intrathecal dynorphin and related peptides have complex effects on spinal cord function, including excitation, depression, and neurotoxicity. Although some of the spinal effects of dynorphin are nonopioid in nature (Steward and Isaac 1991; Vanderah et al. 1996), activation of spinal κ receptors may increase the excitability of dorsal horn neurons (Knox and Dickenson 1987; Hylden et al. 1991). Moreover, numerous laboratories have reported that spinal administration of dynorphin and U50488H antagonized antinociception induced by morphine or other μ-receptor agonists (see Pan 1998 for review). We also observed that the anti-allodynic effect of DAMGO was markedly reduced by U50488H, indicating an antianalgesic action of κ-receptor agonists in spinally injured rats. Such a μ-receptor blocking effect of U50488H may account for the enhancement of the allodynia-like behavior, as naloxone exerted similar effects (Hao et al., unpublished observations).

Of particular interest is the potent anti-allodynic effect of i.t. OFQ in the model of chronic allodynia (Hao et al. 1998b). Thus, although earlier studies have shown that OFQ may induce hyperalgesia, we and others have provided strong evidence that spinal administration of OFQ produced antinociception (for review see Henderson and McKnight 1997; Darland et al. 1998). Intrathecal OFQ also reversed abnormal pain-like behaviors in animal models of inflammation or partial peripheral nerve injury (Yamamoto et al. 1997a,b; Hao et al. 1998b). The spinal inhibitory effect of OFQ was not reversed by naloxone (Xu et al. 1996). It is thus likely that OFQ-induced antinociception is mediated by an unknown mechanism independent of classical opioid receptors. This may raise the possibility that OFQ or its receptor agonists may represent a new class of analgesics with therapeutic potential.

CONCLUSIONS AND CLINICAL IMPLICATIONS

Our experimental studies using animal models of central pain indicated that morphine is relatively ineffective in alleviating pain-like behaviors in spinally injured rats. This is particularly clear in acute allodynia, where morphine upon both systemic and i.t. administration produced no significant effect. During chronic allodynia, however, i.t. morphine appeared to provide significant pain relief with no side effects. Morphine is less potent in alleviating allodynia than in producing antinociception. Thus, high spinal concentrations of morphine are needed, which are unlikely to be reached by systemic morphine before the sedative effect of the drug becomes apparent. Several mechanisms may explain the relative morphine insensitivity in treating central pain. These involve reduction in the density of opioid receptors in the spinal cord in spinally injured rats, plasticity leading to increased activity of antiopioid systems, and the reduced ability of opioids to alleviate pain mediated by large-diameter afferent fibers.

Although spinal administration of morphine was initially effective in our model of chronic central pain, it is unclear whether monotherapy with i.t. morphine could provide long-term relief in patients with pain following spinally cord injury, as tolerance may present a serious problem. Thus, combination therapy with, for example, α_2-adrenoceptor agonists or alternative approaches such as i.t. implantation of chromaffin cells may represent better choices. Moreover, receptor-selective opioids may be developed that have fewer side effects and a reduced rate of tolerance development. Finally, new drugs such as gabapentin or OFQ-receptor agonists may also provide alternative treatment for central pain patients.

ACKNOWLEDGMENTS

The studies conducted in the authors' laboratory were supported by the Swedish Medical Research Council, Astra Pain Control, the European Commission, and the Clinical Research Center at Huddinge University Hospital, Sweden.

REFERENCES

Abbott FV, Franklin KBJ, Ludwick RJ, Melzack R. Apparent lack of tolerance in the formalin test suggests different mechanisms for morphine analgesia in different types of pain. *Pharmacol Biochem Behav* 1981; 15:637–640.

Arnér S, Meyerson B. Lack of analgesic effect of opioids on neuropathic and idiopathic forms of pain. *Pain* 1988; 33:11–23.

Arvidsson U, Riedl M, Chakrabarti S, et al. Distribution and targeting of a μ-opioid receptor (MOR1) in brain and spinal cord. *J Neurosci* 1995; 15:3328–3341.

Beric A, Dimitrijevic MR, Lindblom U. Central dysesthesia syndrome in spinal cord injury patients. *Pain* 1988; 34:109–116.

Besse D, Lombard MC, Zajac JM, Roques BP, Besson JM. Pre- and postsynaptic distribution of mu, delta and kappa opioid receptors in the superficial layers of the cervical dorsal horn of the rat spinal cord. *Brain Res* 1990; 521:15–22.

Besse D, Lombard MC, Perrot S, Besson JM. Regulation of opioid binding sites in the superficial dorsal horn of the rat spinal cord following loose ligation of the sciatic nerve: comparison with sciatic nerve section and lumbar dorsal rhizotomy. *Neuroscience* 1992; 50:921–933.

Bian D, Nichols ML, Ossipov MH, Lai J, Porreca F. Characterization of the anti-allodynic efficacy of morphine in a model of neuropathic pain in rats. *Neuroreport* 1995; 6:1981–1984.

Boivie J. Central pain. In: Wall PD, Melzack R (Eds). *Textbook of Pain.* London: Churchill Livingstone, 1994, pp 871–892.

Bonica JJ. Introduction: semantic, epidemiologic, and educational issues. In: Casey KL (Ed). *Pain and Central Nervous System Disease: The Central Pain Syndromes.* New York: Raven Press, 1991, pp 13–30.

Borszcz G. Increases in vocalization and motor reflex thresholds are influenced by the site of morphine microinjection: comparisons following administration into the periaqueductal gray, ventral medulla, and spinal subarachnoid space. *Behav Neurosci* 1995; 109:502–522.

Bowsher D, Nurmikko T. Central post-stroke pain—drug treatment options. *CNS Drugs* 1996; 5:160–165.

Cohen M, McArthur D, Vulpe M, Schandler S, Gerber K. Comparing chronic pain from spinal cord injury to chronic pain of other origins. *Pain* 1988; 35:57–63.

Colpaert FC, Niemegeers CJE, Janssen PAJ. Nociceptive stimulation prevents development of tolerance to narcotic analgesia. *Eur J Pharmacol* 1978; 49:335–336.

Connell BG, Barnes J, Blatt T, Tasker RA. Rapid development of tolerance to morphine in the formalin test. *Neuroreport* 1994; 5:817–820.

Darland T, Heinricher MM, Grandy DK. Orphanin FQ/nociceptin—a role in pain and analgesia, but so much more. *Trends Neurosci* 1998; 21:215–221.

Davidoff G, Roth EJ. Clinical characteristics of central (dysesthetic) pain in spinal cord injury patients. In: Casey KL (Ed). *Pain and Central Nervous System Disease: The Central Pain Syndromes.* New York: Raven Press, 1991, pp 77–84.

Detweiler DJ, Rohde DS, Basbaum AI. The development of opioid tolerance in the formalin test in the rat. *Pain* 1995; 63:251–254.

Drower EJ, Stapelfeld A, Rafferty MF, et al. Selective antagonism by naltrindole of the antinociceptive effects of the delta opioid agonist cyclic [D-penicillamine2-D-penicillamine5]enkephalin in the rat. *J Pharmacol Exp Ther* 1991; 259:725–731.

Eide PK, Jorum E, Stenehjem AI. Somatosensory findings in patients with spinal cord injury and central dysaesthesia pain. *J Neurol Neuro Psych* 1996; 60:411–415.

Foley KM. Clinical tolerance to opioids. In: Basbaum AI, Besson JM (Eds). *Towards a New Pharmacotherapy of Pain.* New York: Wiley, 1991, pp 181–203.

Guirimand F, Strimbu-Gozariu M, Willer JC, Le Bars D. Effects of mu, delta and kappa opioid antagonists on the depression of a C-fiber reflex by intrathecal morphine and DAGO in the rat. *J Pharmacol Exp Ther* 1994; 269:1007–1020.

Gutstein HB, Trujillo KA, Akil H. Dose chronic nociceptive stimulation alter the development of morphine tolerance? *Brain Res* 1995; 680:173–179.

Hammond D. Do opioids relieve central pain. In: Casey KL (Ed). *Pain and Central Nervous System Disease: The Central Pain Syndromes.* New York: Raven Press, 1991, pp 233–242.

Hao J-X, Xu X-J, Aldskogius H, Seiger Å, Wiesenfeld-Hallin Z. Allodynia-like effects in rat after ischemic spinal cord injury photochemically induce by laser irradiation. *Pain* 1991; 45:175–185.

Hao J-X, Xu X-J, Aldskogius H, Seiger Å, Wiesenfeld-Hallin Z. Photochemically induced transient spinal ischemia induces behavioral hypersensitivity to mechanical and cold stimuli, but not to noxious-heat stimuli, in the rat. *Exp Neurol* 1992a; 118:187–194.

Hao J-X, Xu X-J, Yu Y-X, Seiger Å, Wiesenfeld-Hallin Z. Transient spinal cord ischemia induces temporary hypersensitivity of dorsal horn wide dynamic range neurons to myelinated, but not unmyelinated, fiber input. *J Neurophysiol* 1992b; 68:384–391.

Hao J-X, Xu X-J, Yu Y-X, Seiger Å, Wiesenfeld-Hallin Z. Baclofen reverses the hypersensitivity of dorsal horn wide dynamic range neurons to mechanical stimulation after transient spinal cord ischemia; implications for a tonic GABAergic inhibitory control of myelinated fiber input. *J Neurophysiol* 1992c; 68:392–396.

Hao J-X, Yu W, Xu X-J, Wiesenfeld-Hallin Z. Capsaicin-sensitive afferents mediate chronic cold, but not mechanical, allodynia-like behavior in spinally injured rats. *Brain Res* 1996; 722:177–180.

Hao J-X, Yu W, Wiesenfeld-Hallin Z, Xu X-J. Treatment of chronic allodynia in spinally injured rats: effects of intrathecal selective opioid receptor agonists. *Pain* 1998a; 75:209–217.

Hao J-X, Xu IS, Wiesenfeld-Hallin Z, Xu X-J. Anti-allodynic and anti-hyperalgesic effect of intrathecal orphanin FQ/nociceptin in rats after spinal cord injury, peripheral nerve injury and inflammation. *Pain* 1998b; 76:387–396.

Henderson G, McKnight AT. The orphan opioid receptor and its endogenous ligand—orphanin FQ/nociceptin. *Trends Pharmacol Sci* 1997; 18:293–300.

Hylden JL, Nahin RL, Traub RJ, Dubner R. Effects of spinal kappa-opioid receptor agonists on the responsiveness of nociceptive superficial dorsal horn neurons. *Pain* 1991; 44:187–193.

Kayser V. Can tolerance to morphine be induced in arthritic rats? *Brain Res* 1985; 334:335–338.

Knox RJ, Dickenson AH. Effects of selective and non-selective kappa-opioid receptor agonists on cutaneous C-fibre-evoked responses of rat dorsal horn neurones. *Brain Res* 1987; 415:21–29.

Kupers RC, Konings H, Adriaemsen H, Gybels JM. Morphine differentially affects the sensory and affective pain ratings in neurogenic and idiopathic forms of pain. *Pain* 1991; 47:5–12.

Le Bars D, Menetrey D, Conseiller C, Besson JM. Depressive effects of morphine upon lamina V cells activities in the dorsal horn of the spinal cat. *Brain Res* 1975; 98:261–277.

Lee YW, Chaplan SR, Yaksh TL. Systemic and supraspinal, but not spinal, opiates suppress allodynia in a rat neuropathic pain model. *Neurosci Lett* 1995; 199:111–114.

Leijon G, Boivie J. Pharmacological treatment of central pain. In: Casey KL (Ed). *Pain and Central Nervous System Disease: The Central Pain Syndromes.* New York: Raven Press, 1991, pp 257–266.

Levine J, Feldmesser M, Tecott L, Gordon N, Izdebski K. Pain-induced vocalization in the rat and its modification by pharmacological agents. *Brain Res* 1984; 296:121–127.

Mao J, Price DD. Mayer DJ. Experimental mononeuropathy reduces the antinociceptive effects of morphine: implications for common intracellular mechanisms involved in morphine tolerance and neuropathic pain. *Pain* 1995; 61:353–364.

Meunier J-C, Mollereau C, Toll L, et al. Isolation and structure of the endogenous agonist of opioid receptor-like ORL1 receptor. *Nature* 1995; 377:532–535.

Miaskowski C, Sutters KA, Taiwo YO, Levine JD. Comparison of the antinociceptive and motor effects of intrathecal opioid agonists in the rat. *Brain Res* 1991; 553:105–109.

Nepomuceno C, Fine PR, Richards JS. Pain in patients with spinal cord injury. *Arch Physical Med Rehab* 1979; 60:605–609.

Nichols ML, Bian D, Ossipov MH, Lai J, Porreca F. Regulation of morphine anti-allodynic efficacy by cholecystokinin in a model of neuropathic pain in rats. *J Pharmacol Exp Ther* 1995; 275:1339–1345.

Onofrio BM, Yaksh TL. Long-term pain relief produced by intrathecal morphine infusion in 53 patients. *J Neurosurg* 1990; 72:200–209.

Pan ZZ. Mu-opposing actions of the kappa-opioid receptor. *Trends Pharmacol Sci* 1998; 19:94–98.

Portenoy RK. Opioid therapy for chronic nonmalignant pain: a review of the critical issues. *J Pain Symptom Manage* 1996; 11:203–217.

Portenoy RK, Foley KM, Inturrisi CE. The nature of opioid responsiveness and its implications for neuropathic pain: new hypotheses derived from studies of opioid infusions. *Pain* 1990; 43:273–286.

Reinscheid RK, Nothacker HP, Bourson A, et al. Orphanin FQ: a neuropeptide that activates an opioid-like G protein-coupled receptor. *Science* 1995; 270:792–794.

Sallerin CB, Lazorthes Y, Deguine O, et al. Does intrathecal morphine in the treatment of cancer pain induce the development of tolerance? *Neurosurgery* 1998; 42:44–49.

Stewart P, Isaac L. Dynorphin-induced depression of the dorsal root potential in rat spinal cord: a possible mechanism for potentiation of the C-fiber reflex. *J Pharmacol Exp Ther* 1991; 259:608–613.

Tasker RR. Pain resulting from central nervous system pathology (central pain). In: Bonica JJ (Ed). *The Management of Pain.* Philadelphia: Lea and Febiger, 1990, pp 264–283.

Vaccarino AL, Marek P, Kest B, et al. Morphine fails to produce tolerance when administered in the presence of formalin pain in rats. *Brain Res* 1993; 627:287–290.

Vanderah TW, Laughlin T, Lashbrook JM, et al. Single intrathecal injections of dynorphin A or des-Tyr-dynorphins produce long-lasting allodynia in rats: blockade by MK-801 but not naloxone. *Pain* 1996; 68:275–281.

Ventafridda V, Spoldi E, Carageni A, De Conno F. Intraspinal morphine for cancer pain. *Acta Anaesth Scand* 1987; 31(Suppl 85):47–53.

Wiesenfeld-Hallin Z, Hao J-X, Xu X-J. Mechanisms of central pain. In: Jensen TS, Turner JA, Wiesenfeld-Hallin Z. (Eds). *Proceedings of the 8th World Congress on Pain*, Progress in Pain Research and Management, Vol. 8. Seattle: IASP Press, 1997, pp 575–589.

Xu X-J, Hao J-X, Aldskogius H, Seiger Å, Wiesenfeld-Hallin Z. Chronic pain-related syndrome in rats after ischemic spinal cord lesion: a possible animal model for pain in patients with spinal cord injury. *Pain* 1992; 48:279–290.

Xu X-J, Puke MJC, Verge VMK, et al. Up-regulation of cholecystokinin in primary sensory neurons is associated with morphine insensitivity in experimental neuropathic pain. *Neurosci Lett* 1993; 152:129–132.

Xu X-J, Hao J-X, Wiesenfeld-Hallin Z. Orphanin FQ or antiorphanin FQ: potent spinal antinociceptive effect of orphanin FQ/nociceptin in the rat. *Neuroreport* 1996; 7:2092–2094.

Yaksh TL. Inhibition by etorphine of the discharge of dorsal horn neurons: effects on the neuronal response to both high- and low-threshold sensory input in the decerebrate spinal cat. *Exp Neurol* 1978; 60:23–40.

Yamamoto T, Nozaki-Taguchi N, Kimura S. Effects of intrathecally administered orphanin FQ, an opioid receptor-like 1 (ORL1) receptor agonist, on the thermal hyperalgesia induced by carrageenan injection into the rat paw. *Brain Res* 1997a; 754:329–332.

Yamamoto T, Nozaki-Taguchi N, Kimura S. Effects of intrathecally administered orphanin FQ, an opioid receptor-like 1 (ORL1) receptor agonist, on the thermal hyperalgesia induced by unilateral constriction injury to the sciatic nerve in the rat. *Neurosci Lett* 1997b; 224:107–110.

Yezierski RP. Pain following spinal cord injury: the clinical problem and experimental studies. *Pain* 1996; 68:185–192.

Yu W, Hao J-X, Xu X-J, Wiesenfeld-Hallin Z. Comparison of the anti-allodynic and antinociceptive effects of systemic, intrathecal and intracerebroventricular morphine in a rat model of central neuropathic pain. *Eur J Pain* 1997a; 1:17–29.

Yu W, Hao J-X, Xu X-J, Wiesenfeld-Hallin Z. The development of morphine tolerance and dependence in rats with chronic pain. *Brain Res* 1997b; 756:141–146.

Yu W, Hao J-X, Xu X-J, et al. Spinal ischemia reduces μ-opioid receptors in rats: correlation with morphine insensitivity. *Neuroreport* 1999, in press.

Zhang AL, Hao J-X, Seiger Å, et al. Decreased GABA immunoreactivity in spinal cord dorsal horn neurons after transient spinal cord ischemia in the rat. *Brain Res* 1994; 656:187–190.

Zhang X, Bao L, Shi T-J, et al. Down-regulation of mu-opioid receptors in rat and monkey dorsal root ganglion neurons and spinal cord after peripheral axotomy. *Neuroscience* 1998; 82:223–240.

Zieglgänsberger W, Bayerl H. The mechanism of inhibition of neuronal activity by opiates in the spinal cord of cat. *Brain Res* 1976; 115:111–128.

Correspondence to: Xiao-Jun Xu, Division of Clinical Neurophysiology, Huddinge University Hospital, S-141 86 Huddinge, Sweden. Tel: 46-8-58582213; Fax: 46-8-7748856; email: xiao-jun.xu@neurophys.hs.sll.se.

Opioid Sensitivity of Chronic Noncancer Pain,
Progress in Pain Research and Management,
Vol. 14, edited by Eija Kalso, Henry J. McQuay,
and Zsuzsanna Wiesenfeld-Hallin, IASP Press,
Seattle, © 1999.

12

Antinociceptive Effect of Opioid Substances in Different Models of Inflammatory Pain

G. Guilbaud, V. Kayser, S. Perrot, and H. Keita

*Research Unit on the Physiopharmacology
of the Nervous System, INSERM, Paris, France*

The antinociceptive action of opioids in models of clinical pain was one of the main concerns of various groups conducting research in this field at the end of the seventies. Studies were first performed in rats rendered polyarthritic by injection of Freund's adjuvant into the tail (Pircio et al. 1975; Colpaert 1979, 1987; Colpaert et al. 1980; De Castro-Costa et al. 1981; Kayser and Guilbaud 1983; Millan 1986; Millan et al. 1987), while later studies used rats with a localized inflammatory process induced in one hindpaw by Freund's adjuvant (Millan et al. 1988; Hylden et al. 1989) or carrageenan (Kayser and Guilbaud 1987; Hargreaves et al. 1988; Kayser et al. 1991b). For a description of the models see Kayser and Guilbaud (1987, 1997) and Besson and Guilbaud (1988). Since then, rat models of inflammatory pain have been extensively validated and widely studied with different classical and modern approaches (see references in Besson and Guilbaud 1988; Abbadie and Besson 1993; Honoré et al. 1996a,b,c; Chapman and Besson 1997; Dickenson and Besson 1997; MacArthur et al. 1999). They are still used to analyze the basic mechanisms of the different actions of opioids and appear to be useful tools for preclinical studies (see several chapters of this volume). This chapter reports old and new data obtained by using behavioral tests to assess the antinociceptive efficacy of opioids in rats with inflammation. In addition to the "classical" models, this chapter will consider a more recent model consisting of repeated carrageenan injections.

EFFECT OF OPIOIDS IN INFLAMMATORY PAIN MODELS

RATS WITH POLYARTHRITIS

Nociceptive tests using intravenous and intrathecal morphine

At the end of the seventies and at the beginning of the eighties, several studies showed evidence of more potent antinociceptive action of morphine in arthritic than in normal rats. Studies used both intravenous (i.v.) and intrathecal (i.t.) administration in tests that evaluated spontaneous behavior or nociceptive reactions to mechanical, thermal, and electrical stimuli (Pircio et al. 1978; Colpaert 1979; Oliveras et al. 1979; De Castro-Costa et al. 1981; Kayser and Guilbaud 1983; Przewloski et al. 1984; Millan et al. 1987). However, in a range of relatively low doses (0.1–1 mg/kg i.v.) Kayser and Guilbaud (1990) have demonstrated that this increase in the antinociceptive effect was highly related to the test used to assess antinociception. No significant difference in the antinociceptive effect of morphine between arthritic and normal rats was found when using the paw withdrawal threshold, in contrast to the dramatic difference in the vocalization threshold to paw pressure (VTPP) (Kayser and Guilbaud 1983, 1990). The VTTP, greatly reduced in arthritic animals as compared to normal animals before morphine injection (around 120–160 g versus 275–300 g according to various studies), was increased 2–3 times more in arthritic than in normal animals after morphine administration. For example, in arthritic rats a normal VTPP was reestablished with 0.3 mg/kg i.v. of morphine, and a higher value of up to 300 g or more was attained with a dose of 1 mg/kg, according to replication studies conducted since 1983 (Fig. 1).

This potent action of opioids is linked to the presence of pain-related behaviors. All the studies describing this increase in potency have been carried out 3–4 weeks following the Freund's adjuvant, when the pain behaviors are at their maximum. The increase was not found later, at 8 weeks, when the VTPP had recovered to normal values.

Effect of specific agonists and inhibitors of enkephalin-degrading enzymes

The dramatic effect of morphine on the VTPP in arthritic rats has also been observed with other opioids such as buprenorphine, nalbuphine, tramadol (an analgesic substance with both opioid and noradrenergic components) (Kayser et al. 1991a), and with more specific agonists, such as DAMGO (a μ-opioid receptor agonist), several κ-opioid receptor agonists, and a δ-opioid agonist (BUBU, but not DTLET) (Neil et al. 1986; Desmeules et al. 1993).

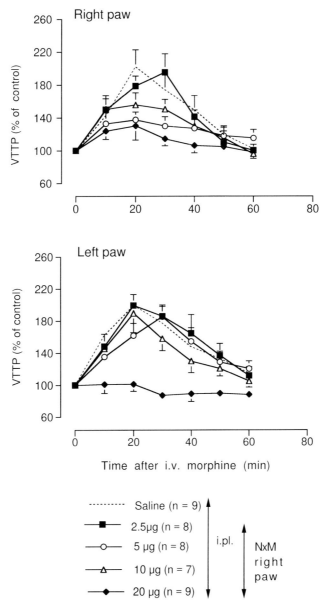

Fig. 1. Curves of mean values illustrating the potent effect of morphine 1 mg/kg i.v. on the vocalization threshold to paw pressure (VTPP) of polyarthritic rats. The local injection of naloxone methiodide in the right plantar paw reduced, but did not suppress, the morphine effect obtained in this paw and did not influence the antinociceptive action observed from the left paw (H. Keita et al., unpublished data). Error bars indicate SEM.

Antinociceptive effects have been elicited using low doses devoid of obvious side effects, such as drowsiness or locomotor deficit.

Different inhibitors of the enkephalin-degrading enzymes (Fournié-Zaluski et al. 1992) have also been studied in both normal and arthritic animals using the VTPP test after i.v. administration. Either a selective inhibitor of neutral endopeptidase (NEP) (acetorphan), or mixed inhibitors of both NEP and the aminopeptidase (kelatorphan, and a prodrug PC12) elicited a potent antinociceptive effect in both normal and arthritic rats (Kayser and Guilbaud 1983; Kayser et al. 1989; Perrot et al. 1993). A potent antinociceptive dose-dependent effect was obtained with low doses. As an example, after the injection of kelatorphan 2.5–10 mg/kg i.v., the maximum increase of the VTPP was 100–300%, but a ceiling effect was observed for higher doses. The intensity of antinociceptive effects of the inhibitors of the enkephalin-degrading enzymes seems to be dependent on the tests used and on their bioavailability or pharmacokinetic properties (references in Kayser et al. 1989; Perrot et al. 1993). In any case, the interesting point is that their administration can reestablish the VTPP of arthritic rats to or beyond the normal values.

"Tolerance-like" phenomena

The potent antinociceptive effect measured in arthritic rats (at least with the VTPP) ceased rapidly after morphine pretreatment, not only after progressively increasing doses over 4 days (40–160 mg/kg subcutaneously [s.c.]; method adapted from Collier et al. 1972) but also with lower doses (0.3, 0.9, or 3 mg/kg s.c. twice daily for 4 days). In arthritic rats pretreated with low doses of morphine for 4 days, the antinociceptive effect of a single injection of morphine (0.1, 0.3, or 1 mg/kg i.v.) on day 5 was dramatically and dose-dependently reduced (Kayser et al. 1986). In addition, the antinociceptive effect of 1 mg/kg of morphine was reduced by 50% as early as 24 hours after the first morphine pretreatment. Unlike other opioids such as nalbuphine, buprenorphine, or a κ agonist (U-50,488H), only the δ agonists (DTLET, BUBU) and tramadol could maintain their antinociceptive action in arthritic rats pretreated with morphine (Neil et al. 1986; Kayser et al. 1991b; Desmeules et al. 1993). Although these "tolerance-like" phenomena cannot be directly linked to human tolerance, their occurrence might be useful in improving our understanding of the mechanisms involved.

Although antinociceptive effects of opioids in the arthritic rat were observed after i.t. morphine, the fact that polyarthritic rats exhibit a general disease in which several physiological functions can be altered raises several questions about the significance of the great efficacy of morphine in these animals. In fact, liver function and the permeability of the blood–brain barrier, altered in the first stage of the disease, had been described as normal at the time of the studies, i.e., 3–4 weeks after the inoculation of the arthritic agent (Pearson and Wood 1959; Pearson et al. 1961; Quevauviller et al. 1968; Reiber et al. 1984). Nevertheless, for a clear interpretation of the data without any caveats, we considered it necessary to study the antinociceptive effect of opioids in rats with more localized inflammation.

RATS WITH A LOCALIZED INFLAMMATORY PROCESS

The most commonly used models involve injection of carrageenan or Freund's adjuvant into a hindpaw and testing paw withdrawal to pressure or VTPP. In all models, an increased antinociceptive action of opioids was observed in the inflamed compared to the non-inflamed paw (Joris et al. 1987; Hargreaves et al. 1988; Stein et al. 1988a; Kayser et al. 1991b). For instance, in carrageenan-injected rats the VTPP was about 190 g in the inflamed paw and 270 g in the non-inflamed paw before morphine injection, and reached nearly identical values for the two paws (420 and 430 g, respectively) 30 minutes after i.v. morphine 1 mg/kg. This effect was totally reversed by i.v. naloxone 0.1 mg/kg (Kayser et al. 1991a) (Fig. 2).

This increased effect of opioids in localized inflammation seemed to be related to the presence of an hyperalgesic state (also observed in mononeuropathic rats; Neil et al. 1990; Attal et al. 1991), and several studies have sought to understand the reasons for these changes. Were they linked to changes in the endogenous opioid systems (substances and receptors) or to changes in the peripheral sites of action of the opioids?

CHANGES IN THE ENDOGENOUS OPIOID SYSTEMS

Biosynthesis and release

Early in the eighties, the increase in the level of the endogenous opioid peptides in the dorsal horn of the spinal cord was described for met-enkephalin, dynorphin, and their precursors in conditions of both diffuse and localized inflammation (Cesselin et al. 1980; Faccini et al. 1984; Przewloski et al. 1984; Millan 1986; Höllt et al. 1987; Millan et al. 1987; Iadarola et al. 1988; Draisci et al. 1991; Dubner and Ruda 1992). These studies emphasized the increase in the expression of preprodynorphin and preproenkephalin. In addition, in agreement with a previous study showing an increase of descending inhibitory controls in monoarthritic rats (Schaible et al. 1991), recent research has shown that the dramatic upregulation of preprodynorphin and preproenkephalin mRNA at the spinal level following

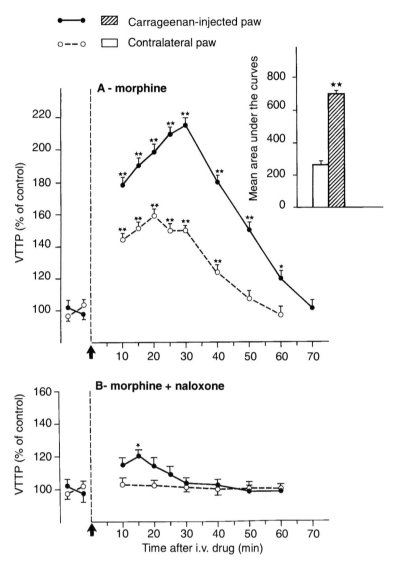

Fig. 2. Curves of mean values and mean areas under the curves. (A) The effect of morphine 1 mg/kg i.v. on the VTPP of rats, injected with carrageenan in one plantar paw 4 hours previously. The increase in threshold is much more pronounced for the inflamed than for the noninflamed paw. (B) Naloxone injected i.v. at 0.1 mg/kg totally suppressed the morphine effect (see Kayser et al. 1991b for details). Error bars indicate SEM; asterisks show statistical significance ($*P < 0.05$, $**P < 0.01$).

unilateral peripheral inflammation is modulated by descending axons (MacArthur et al. 1999).

From other studies, it appeared that NEP (Van Veldhoven and Carton

1982; Delay-Goyet et al. 1989) was unmodified in polyarthritic rats, but complex changes in the release of endogenous opioids have been suggested (Cesselin et al. 1988; Hamon et al. 1988; Bourgoin et al. 1994). Finally, biochemical data suggest that these endogenous opioid substances could control their own release by negative biofeedback mechanisms (references in Kayser 1994 and Cesselin 1997).

Behavioral studies

Polyarthritic and carrageenan-injected rats given a high dose of naloxone (1 mg/kg i.v.) exhibited a further decrease of their VTTP and appeared very sensitive to handling, which indicated the existence of tonic inhibitory controls exerted by endogenous opioid substances. According to many studies between 1981 and 1994 (Kayser and Guilbaud 1981; references in Kayser 1994), this effect appeared to be mediated via δ-opioid receptors as it was blocked by a specific antagonist of this receptor subtype. By progressively decreasing the i.v. naloxone doses down to 1 µg/kg, a paradoxical antinociceptive effect was revealed: the VTPP was increased and the animals appeared quiet and peaceful, almost drowsy. This antinociceptive effect of naloxone peaked at 3 µg/kg and was comparable to that of 1 mg/kg of morphine. From several experimental series using various specific opioid-receptor antagonists, enough consistent data have been accumulated to suggest that the biphasic effect of naloxone occurs because the endogenous opioids control their own release via negative feedback mechanisms, which could be mediated via µ and κ autoreceptors (references in Kayser 1994). The additional putative interaction of the endogenous opioid and cholecysto-kininergic systems will be discussed below (see *Modulation of opioid antinociception by the CCK system*). Whatever the mechanisms and the functional significance of the different interactions, which tend to be involved in a vicious cycle, reinforcing pain-related behaviors, it is clear that endogenous opioids are profoundly modified in animals with experimental inflammatory pain.

CHANGES IN OPIOID RECEPTORS

Several studies found no significant modification in the number of opioid binding sites in the spinal cord and in the brain of arthritic rats (Cesselin et al. 1980;Yonehara et al. 1983). This was confirmed for µ- and δ-opioid receptor subtypes by Delay-Goyet et al. (1989), and more recently for µ-opioid receptors by Kar et al. (1994). However, when using bremazocine as a κ-opioid receptor ligand, Millan et al. (1987) found a discrete increase in κ-opioid receptor subtypes in the periaqueductal gray matter. More recently, two studies found an increase in μ and κ sites in the spinal dorsal horn ipsilateral to an inflamed paw (Besse et al 1992; Maekawa et al. 1996), but the techniques used did not allow distinction between the labeling of opioid receptors localized on the afferent fiber terminals and on the spinal neurons themselves. In fact, Ohta et al. (1997) did not find any change in the three receptor subtypes in homogenates of the whole brain or of the spinal cord from rats with carrageenan-induced inflammation. Thus, it is difficult to conclude whether the number of central opioid receptors truly increased. In contrast, changes in the peripheral opioid receptors have been well documented in the last decade.

ANTINOCICEPTIVE ACTION OF OPIOIDS
VIA PERIPHERAL SITES OF ACTION

In an initial study, Ferreira and Nakamura (1979) used paw withdrawal to assess the antinociceptive effect of intraplantar morphine or met-enkephalin. They found an antinociceptive effect in rats with prostaglandin-induced hyperalgesia that was not considered to be due to opioid receptors because it was not clearly reversed by naloxone. Then, studies by Joris et al. (1987) and Hargreaves et al. (1988) that used carrageenan inflammation and by Stein et al. (1988a,b) that used localized injection of Freund's adjuvant observed potent antinociceptive effects of local fentanyl or ethylketocyclazocine in the inflamed but not in the contralateral paw. Finally, Stein et al. (1988b, 1989), with the same inflammatory model, also clearly observed a potent antinociceptive effect of several opioid agonists, which was reversed by their specific antagonists.

Other researchers investigated the involvement of peripheral blockade in the antinociceptive effect of systemic opioids. Studies with carrageenan-injected (Kayser et al. 1991b; Kayser and Guilbaud 1994) and polyarthritic rats (H. Keita et al., unpublished manuscript) attempted to reverse the antinociceptive effect of systemic morphine by an intraplantar injection of low doses of naloxone or naloxone methiodide (which has limited access to the central nervous system and is considered to have the properties of a local antagonist). It is clear that in the two models it was possible to reduce the effect of i.v. morphine 1 mg/kg on the VTPP of the inflamed but not of the noninflamed paw (Fig. 3); intraplantar naloxone 0.25–1 μg decreased the morphine effect (only by about 40% with 1 μg). Higher doses were not tested in these inflammatory conditions because doses of 2.5 μg have a central effect in normal rats due to systemic diffusion (Kayser et al. 1990).

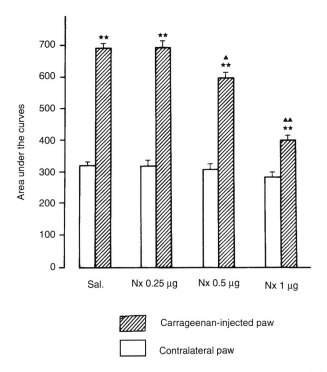

Fig. 3. Mean areas under the curves of the time course of VTPP, obtained for each paw in carrageenan-injected rats (as in Fig. 2) after injection of a combination of morphine 1 mg/kg i.v. and naloxone (0.25, 0.5, and 1 µg) or saline administered locally into the inflamed paw in the same volume (0.1 mL) (see Kayser et al. 1991b for details). Error bars indicate SEM; asterisks show statistical significance ($*P < 0.05$, $**P < 0.01$).

Interestingly, in polyarthritic rats, the maximum reduction of the morphine effect by local naloxone methiodide (2.5 µg) did not exceed 39% (Fig. 1). Higher doses of 5, 10, or 20 µg were no more potent, while a central effect was suspected for 20 µg .

Thus, the effect of the antagonist injected locally strongly contrasts with the complete reversal observed with the i.v. injection of 0.1 mg/kg (Fig. 2). Nevertheless, all the animal experimental studies confirmed that opioids can induce an antinociceptive action when injected locally, and that the peripheral effect, although limited, can also contribute to the effect observed after a systemic injection (see also data obtained in neuropathic rats by Kayser et al. 1995).

Many studies have confirmed previous observations (Fields et al. 1980; Young et al 1980; Laduron 1984) and have clearly demonstrated that peripheral opioid receptors are located on primary afferent neurons (Stein 1988a, 1989; Schäfer et al. 1994, 1998; Coggeshall et al. 1997; Zhou et al.

1998). Several basic mechanisms have been suggested to explain the involvement of opioid receptors in inflammatory states, including interaction of endogenous opioids from immune cells with peripheral opioid receptors on peripheral sensory nerves (Czlonkowski et al. 1987; Stein et al. 1990), leakage of the perineural barrier facilitating access to opioid receptors on peripheral nerves (Antonijevic et al. 1995), increased transport of opioid receptors to peripheral nerve terminals (Hassan et al. 1993; Jeanjean et al. 1994; Ji et al. 1995), and enhanced coupling of opioid receptors to G proteins (Selley et al. 1993). Whatever the mechanism(s) involved, even if the κ receptors do play a major role as some studies suggest (Wilson et al. 1996; Ho et al. 1997), there is general agreement about the peripheral effect of morphine, which has also been confirmed by other techniques such as C-*fos* expression at the spinal level after intraplantar injection of morphine (Honoré et al. 1996a). This is not the case for the data obtained in clinical studies, and the analgesic efficacy and usefulness of local opioid administration is still highly controversial (references in Kalso et al. 1997).

To seek a solution to these clinical controversies, we explored the hypothesis that local opioid efficacy might differ under varied experimental conditions, such as during different phases of inflammation. For this purpose we used a variant of the carrageenan-injected model, which can at least partially mimic recurrent inflammatory pain encountered in clinical situations. In rats that had recovered from a first carrageenan injection, a second injection 7 days later induced a greater inflammatory state with significantly more hyperalgesia and edema compared to the response to the first injection (Fletcher et al 1997b; Kayser et al. 1998). This finding led us to reconsider the antinociceptive efficacy of local morphine in initial and recurrent inflammatory phases.

LOCAL INJECTION OF MORPHINE IN A RECURRENT VERSUS AN INITIAL INFLAMMATORY PROCESS

Antinociceptive action

Three hours after the onset of the first inflammatory state, the intraplantar injection of 50–150 µg morphine dose-dependently increased the VTPP of the injected and inflamed paw, while the contralateral paw was unaffected. With 150 µg the VTPP was increased by approximately 60% for 70 minutes. This effect was completely blocked by 40 µg of naloxone methiodide and roughly fits that obtained with morphine 1 mg/kg i.v. (Fig. 4). In contrast, after the second carrageenan injection in rats that had recovered from their first inflammatory state and were still opioid naïve, the local intraplantar

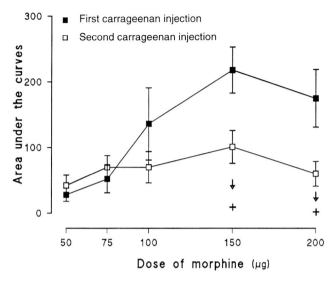

Fig. 4. Mean area under the curves of the time course of VTPP, obtained for the carrageenan-injected paw after the intraplantar (i.pl.) injection of morphine (50–200 µg) 3 hours after a first or a second inflammation (S. Perrot et al., unpublished data). Error bars indicate SEM.

administration of morphine induced a much weaker and shorter increase of the VTPP. This response was especially striking for the high doses (S. Perrot et al., unpublished data).

Preemptive action

Local opioid injections could be used in chronic articular diseases (references in Kalso et al. 1997; see also Chapters 3 and 20 of this volume), so we wondered to what extent the preemptive local administration of opioid before a first carrageenan injection could be beneficial for a second inflammation. Morphine injected locally 10 minutes before the first carrageenan injection prevented the decrease of the VTPP for 2 hours, but then it reached progressively the same value as in saline-pretreated controls 3 hours after the carrageenan injection (Fig. 5). This temporary analgesic effect was weaker than that obtained with a bupivacaine block, which maintained the VTPP at cut-off, above 600 g (Fletcher et al. 1996). In addition, contrasting with this anesthetic block (Fletcher et al. 1997b), local pretreatment with morphine had no influence on the degree of hyperalgesia and edema when the second inflammation was induced.

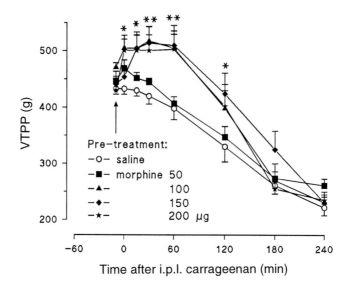

Fig. 5. Mean maximum values of the VTPP obtained for the carrageenan-injected paw after pretreatment with local morphine (50–200 μg), and followed for 4 hours after the carrageenan injection (S. Perrot et al., unpublished data). Error bars indicate SEM.

COMBINATION OF LOW DOSES OF OPIOIDS WITH OTHER SUBSTANCES

Despite the great efficacy of opioid substances in inducing antinociceptive effect in these rat models of inflammatory pain, it was important to decrease side effects by decreasing the doses used without losing antinociceptive action. Many combinations of opioids and other substances are commonly used in humans, particularly in the management of postoperative pain, but most of the animal studies have not been performed with relevant models of clinical inflammatory pain and appropriate behavioral tests (references in Chapman and Besson 1997).

We will consider some data obtained by the combination of two substances, administered i.v. in polyarthritic or carrageenan-injected rats in two different situations: (1) One of the substances has its own antinociceptive effect, but this effect is limited by an endogenous product. Can combination with an antagonist remove this limitation, and under what conditions? (2) Each substance has its own antinociceptive effect. Does the combination still have a beneficial action, and does it reflect an additive or a synergistic effect?

MODULATION OF OPIOID ANTINOCICEPTION
BY THE CCK SYSTEM

The antinociceptive effect of morphine may be modulated by an endogenous neuropeptide and neurotransmitter, e.g., cholecystokinin (CCK). There
is considerable evidence that CCK modulates pain transmission, and the
anti-opioid effects of this peptide are well documented (Itoh et al. 1982;
Faris et al. 1983; O'Neil et al. 1989; Dourish et al. 1990; Valverde et al.
1994; Nichols et al. 1995, 1996). It has already been demonstrated that in
carrageenan-injected rats CCK is able to attenuate the antinociceptive effect
of i.t. morphine (Stanfa and Dickenson 1993). This effect was not reversed
by the CCK_B-receptor antagonist L-365,260. In contrast, this same antagonist enhanced the ability of a low dose of systemic morphine to reduce C-*fos*
expression in the spinal cord of carrageenan-injected rats (Chapman et al.
1995). In fact, in these rats we found that the injection of the CCK_B antagonist made a low dose of morphine (0.1 mg/kg i.v.) effective, but did not
enhance the antinociceptive effect elicited by higher doses (0.3–1 mg/kg)
(Perrot et al. 1998) (Fig. 6). After pretreatment with the CCK_B-receptor antagonist, morphine 0.1 mg/kg i.v. induced an antinociceptive effect equal to
that seen with 0.3 mg/kg injected alone. In addition, this beneficial action
was limited according to the phase of the inflammation, observed at 3 hours
but not at 24 hours following the carrageenan injection. Finally, this beneficial effect was also dependent on the degree of the pain-related behavior

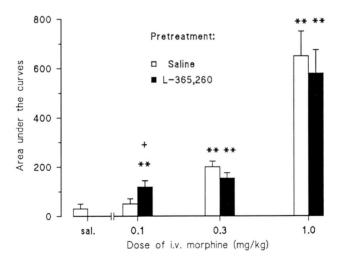

Fig. 6. Mean area under the curves of the time course of VTPP, obtained for the inflamed
paw after i.v. morphine, in rats pretreated with saline or L-365,260 (a CCK_B-receptor
antagonist), 3 hours after the carrageenin injection (from data in Perrot et al. 1998).
Error bars indicate SEM; asterisks show statistical significance (*P < 0.05, **P < 0.01).

(more potent for rats with a more pronounced decrease of the VTPP). These two limitations (timing and intensity of the pain-related behavior) suggest that in the rats in which the decrease of the VTPP was more pronounced and the CCK_B-receptor antagonist more effective, inhibition of the release of endogenous opioid substances by endogenous CCK might in turn reinforce the intensity of the abnormal nociceptive responses. Comparable results have been observed in a neuropathic rat model (Idänpään-Heikkilä et al. 1997).

It is thus possible to reveal a beneficial effect of the combination of these two drugs, but the effect depends on the phase of inflammation, on the dose of morphine used, and on the degree of the allodynia-like behavior.

MORPHINE COMBINED WITH OTHER ANALGESIC SUBSTANCES: ANTAGONISM? ADDITIVITY? SYNERGY?

Association with clonidine

The combination of morphine and clonidine, an α_2-adrenoceptor agonist, is routinely used in clinical situations, but the data from systematic studies are sometimes contradictory and show that the analgesic benefit is often associated with sedation (Motsh et al. 1990; Vercauteren et al. 1990; Rostaing et al. 1991; Van Essen et al. 1991; references in McQuay 1992). Several animal studies also suggest that this combination is effective (references in Yaksh 1985; Loomis et al. 1987; Sullivan et al. 1987; Ossipov et al. 1989, 1990; Monasky et al. 1990; Meert et al. 1994; Naguib and Yaksh 1994; references in Chapman and Besson 1997), but in experimental conditions that do not mimic clinical situations. The effect of the combination on C-*fos* expression at the spinal cord level has also been studied (Honoré et al. 1996b). In polyarthritic rats, clonidine injected alone was similar to morphine in exhibiting a potent antinociceptive effect that was dose dependent (at least for 30, 50, and 100 μg/kg i.v.) and reversed by the antagonists yohimbine or idazoxan (Honoré et al. 1996b; previously reported by Kayser et al. 1992). The effect was more pronounced in these rats than in normal animals: with 30 μg/kg i.v. the VTPP reached 160% compared to a control value of 124%. The highest dose, 100 μg/kg, had secondary effects on general behavior as the rats were particularly quiet in their cages. We then tried low doses of clonidine in combination with morphine. Using isobolographic representation (Tallarida 1992) in two novel experimental series ($n = 120$) (V. Kayser et al., unpublished data), we first studied the effect on the VTPP of the combination of morphine (87%) plus clonidine (13%) in a range of total doses from 60 to 300 μg/kg i.v. We then used a combination of morphine 100 μg/kg plus clonidine 15 μg/kg i.v. to study antagonism by naloxone (10 μg/kg i.v.) or the α_2-adrenoceptor blocker, idazoxan (100 μg/kg i.v.). Both antagonists had no effect when injected alone, but did reverse the effect of their respective agonist. Finally, a significant antinociceptive synergy was found for combinations of 115–300 µg/kg of morphine plus clonidine, but the supra-additivity was especially significant for the highest doses (Fig. 7). Although the combination of morphine 100 µg /kg plus clonidine 15 µg/kg only induced a potentiation, it was possible to increase the VTPP to 155% of the control value for 70 minutes, a potent antinociceptive effect, with doses of each substance low enough to substantially reduce the risk of side effects. Interestingly, in arthritic rats the depressive effect of this combination on thalamic neuronal responses to pressure on the inflamed joints was much more pronounced (mean response = 22% of the control, over 70 minutes) than that produced by either 100 µg or 15 µg clonidine injected alone. By using a higher total dose, equal to 400 µg, (i.e., 348 µg morphine plus 52 µg clonidine, doses devoid of secondary effect), it was possible to induce an antinociceptive effect roughly equivalent to that of 1 mg/kg morphine i.v.

Association with NSAIDs

The association of morphine with nonsteroidal anti-inflammatory drugs (NSAIDs), described by Dahl and Kehlet (1991), has been examined in both clinical and basic studies (Pircio et al. 1978; Kehlet and Dahl 1993; Malberg

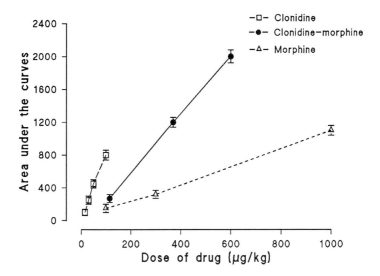

Fig. 7. Dose-response curves of morphine, clonidine, and morphine plus clonidine at a dose ratio of 87% morphine:13% clonidine (values are expressed as means ± SEM) (V. Kayser et al., unpublished data).

and Yaksh 1993). Synergy between ketorolac and morphine has been described after intrathecal injection, but this route of administration is not commonly used for the management of pain. The result of the combination of butorphanol and acetaminophen on the writhing test in mice seemed complex and variable according to the ratio of the two substances. We tested morphine in combination with NSAIDs in carrageenan-injected rats, using i.v. injections of the drugs and several combination ratios. The analgesic potencies of the combinations of morphine and diclofenac (in ratios of 1:5.66 and 1:10), and morphine and propacetamol (in a ratio of 1:250) were evaluated and compared with the effects of each drug injected alone, as recommended by Tallarida (1992). The effects of propacetamol and morphine were additive for all the tested doses (Fletcher et al. 1997a). In contrast, synergy between intravenous morphine and diclofenac was observed with the higher doses for both ratios tested (Fig. 8). We obtained an antinociceptive effect roughly equal to that of 1 mg/kg i.v. of morphine with a total dose of 2.2 mg/kg (i.e., 0.35 mg morphine + 1.85 mg diclofenac) without side effects.

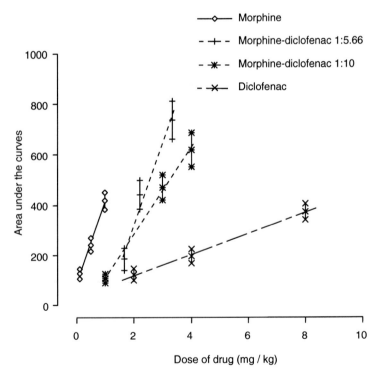

Fig. 8. Dose-response curves of morphine, diclofenac, and morphine plus diclofenac combination at two different dose ratios (values are expressed as means ± SEM) (from Fletcher et al. 1997a).

Results for diclofenac plus propacetamol were reported by Fletcher et al. (1997a).

Although incomplete, this approach clearly shows that it is valuable to look at different combinations of drugs and determine whether the combination results in an additive or a synergistic effect, or is limited by the dose or the timing of the inflammation, as in the case of morphine plus anti-CCK_B.

CONCLUSIONS

The antinociceptive effects of opioids in animal models of inflammatory pain have been investigated in numerous studies that have provided interesting data concerning the validation, development, and design of reproducible models of inflammatory pain. These studies have enhanced our understanding of the mechanisms of opioids, from both a basic and a clinical perspective, and have clearly emphasized the dramatic modification of the endogenous opioid systems in inflammatory conditions and in painful situations in general, and their role in the balance between anti- and pronociception. Due to the potent antinociceptive effect of opioids in animal models of clinical pain, the use of these models is recommended when assessing the activity of newly designed analgesic substances. The animal models also appear to be a good tool to determine the optimal use of peripheral versus systemic administration of opioids, or for combining opioids with other substances, the final goal being to reduce drug dosages and achieve better analgesia without any side effects.

ACKNOWLEDGMENTS

The authors wish to thank all those who participated in the studies reported in the manuscript, and those who assisted in the preparation of the figures and in translation.

REFERENCES

Abbadie C, Besson JM. Effects of morphine and naloxone on basal and evoked fos-like immunoreactivity in lumbar spinal cord neurones in arthritic rats. *Pain* 1993; 52:29–39.

Antonijevic I, Mousa SA, Schäfer M, Stein C. Perineural defect and peripheral opioid analgesia in inflammation. *J Neurosci* 1995; 15:165–172.

Attal N, Chen YL, Kayser V, Guilbaud G. Behavioural evidence that systemic morphine may modulate a phasic pain-related behaviour in a rat model of peripheral mononeuropathy. *Pain* 1991; 47:65–70.

Besse D, Weil-Fugazza, Lombard MC, Butler SH, Besson JM. Monoarthritis induces complex changes in endogenous μ-; δ-; and κ-opioid binding sites in the superficial dorsal horn of the rat spinal cord. *Eur J Pharmacol* 1992; 223:123–131.

Besson JM, Guilbaud G (Eds.) *The Arthritic Rat as a Model of Clinical Pain?* Amsterdam: Elsevier Science, 1988.

Bourgoin S, Benoliel JJ, Collin E, et al. Opioidergic control of the spinal release of neuropeptides. Possible significance for the analgesic effects of opioids. *Fundam Clin Pharmacol* 1994; 8:307–321.

Cesselin F. Endomorphines; récepteurs des opioïdes et nociception. In: Brasseur L, Chauvin M, Guilbaud G (Eds). *Douleurs, Bases fondamentales, Pharmacologie, Douleurs aigues, Douleurs chroniques, Thérapeutiques.* Paris: Maloine, 1997, pp 65–76.

Cesselin F, Montastruc JL, Gros C, Bourgoin S, Hammon M. Met-enkephalin levels and opiate receptors in the spinal cord of chronic suffering rats. *Brain Res* 1980; 191:289–293.

Cesselin F, Bourgoin S, Le Bars D, Hamon M. Central met-enkephalinergic systems in arthritic rats. In: Besson JM, Guilbaud G (Eds). *The Arthritic Rat as a Model of Clinical Pain?* Amsterdam: Elsevier Science, 1988, pp 185–202.

Chapman V, Besson JM. Pharmacological studies of nociceptive systems using the c-Fos immunohistochemical technique: an indicator of noxiously activated spinal neurones. In: Dickenson A, Besson JM (Eds). *The Pharmacology of Pain.* Handbook of Experimental Pharmacology, Vol. 130. Berlin: Springer-Verlag, 1997, pp 235–279.

Chapman V, Honoré P, Buritova J, Besson JM. Cholecystokinin B receptor antagonism enhances the ability of a low dose of morphine to reduce c-Fos expression in the spinal cord of the rat. *Neuroscience* 1995; 67:731–739.

Coggeshall RE, Zhou S, Carlton SM. Opioid receptors on peripheral sensory axons. *Brain Res* 1997; 764:126–132.

Collier HOJ, Francis DL, Schneider C. Modification of morphine withdrawal by drugs interacting with humoral mechanisms: some contradictions and their interpretation. *Nature* 1972; 237:220–223.

Colpaert FC. Can chronic pain be suppressed despite purported tolerance to narcotic analgesia. *Life Sci* 1979; 24:1201–1210.

Colpaert FC. Evidence that adjuvant arthritis in the rat is associated with chronic pain. *Pain* 1987; 28:201–222.

Colpaert FC, De Witte P, Maroli AN, et al. Self-administration of the analgesic suprofen in arthritic rats: evidence of mycobacterium butyricum-induced arthritis as an experimental model of chronic pain. *Life Sci* 1980; 27:921–928.

Czlonkowski A, Stein C, Herz A. Peripheral mechanisms of opioid antinociception in inflammation: involvement of cytokines. *Eur J Pharmacol* 1987; 142:183–184.

Dahl JB, Kehlet H. Non-steroidal anti-inflammatory drugs: rationale for use in severe postoperative pain. *Br J Anaesth* 1991; 66:703–712.

De Castro-Costa M, De Sutter P, Gybels J, Van Hees J. Adjuvant induced arthritis in rats; a possible model of chronic pain. *Pain* 1981; 10:173–186.

Delay-Goyet P, Kayser V, Zajac JM, et al. Lack of significant changes in μ; δ opioid binding sites and neutral endopeptidase EC 3.4.24.11 in the brain and spinal cord of arthritic rats. *Neuropharmacology* 1989; 28:1341–1346.

Desmeules JA, Kayser V, Gacel G, Guilbaud G, Roques BP. The highly selective δ agonist BUBU induces an analgesic effect in normal and arthritic rat and this action is not affected by repeated administration of low doses of morphine. *Brain Res* 1993; 611:243–248.

Dickenson A, Besson JM (Eds). *The Pharmacology of Pain.* Handbook of Experimental Pharmacology, Vol. 130. Berlin: Springer-Verlag, 1997.

Dourish CT, O'Neill MF, Coughlan J, et al. The selective CCK_B antagonist L-365,260 enhances morphine analgesia and prevents morphine tolerance in the rat: evidence for mediation of CCK/opioid interactions by CCK-B receptor. *Eur J Pharmacol* 1990; 176:35–44.

Draisci G, Kajander KC, Dubner R, Bennett G, Iadarola MJ. Up-regulation of opioid gene expression in spinal cord evoked by experimental nerve injuries and inflammation. *Brain Res* 1991; 560:186–192.

Dubner R, Ruda MA. Activity-dependent plasticity following tissue injury and inflammation. *Trends Neurosci* 1992; 15:96–103.

Faccini E, Uzumaki H, Govoni S, et al. Afferent fibers mediate the increase of Met-enkephalin elicited in rat spinal cord by localized pain. *Pain* 1984; 18:25–31.

Faris PL, Komisaruk BR, Watkins LR, Mayer DJ. Evidence for the neuropeptide cholecystokinin as an antagonist of opiate analgesia. *Science* 1983; 219:310–312.

Ferreira SH, Nakamura M. Prostaglandin hyperalgesia: the peripheral analgesic activity of morphine; meperidine; and brain stem stimulation in rats and cats. *Prostaglandins* 1979; 18:191–200.

Fields H, Emson PC, Leigh BK, Gilbert RFT, Iversen LL. Multiple opiate receptor sites on primary afferent fibers. *Nature* 1980; 284:351–353.

Fletcher D, Kayser V, Guilbaud G. Influence of timing of administration on the analgesic effect of bupivacaine infiltration in carrageenin-injected rats. *Anesthesiology* 1996; 84:1129–1137.

Fletcher D, Benoist JM, Gautron M, Guilbaud G. Isobolographic analysis of interactions between intravenous morphine; propacetamol; and diclofenac in carrageenin-injected rats. *Anesthesiology* 1997a; 87:318–326.

Fletcher D, Kayser V, Guilbaud G. The influence of the timing of bupivacaine infiltration induced by two carrageenin injections seven days apart. *Pain* 1997b; 69:303–309.

Fournié-Zaluski MC, Coric P, Turcaud S, et al. 'Mixed inhibitor prodrug' as a new approach toward systemically active inhibitors of enkephalin-degrading enzymes. *J Med Chem* 1992; 32:2473–2481.

Hamon M, Bourgoin S, Le Bars D, Cesselin F. In vivo and in vitro release of central neurotransmitters in relation to pain and analgesia. *Prog Brain Res* 1988; 77:433–446.

Hargreaves KM, Dubner R, Joris J. Peripheral actions of opiates in the blockade of carrageenin-induced inflammation. In: Dubner R, Gebhart GF, Bond MR (Eds). *Proceedings of the Vth World Congress on Pain.* Amsterdam, Elsevier Science, 1988, pp 55–60.

Hassan AHS, Ableitner A, Stein C, Herz A. Inflammation of the rat paw enhances axonal transport of opioid receptors in the sciatic nerve and increase their density in the inflamed tissue. *Neuroscience* 1993; 55:185–195.

Ho J, Mannes AJ, Dubner R, Caudle RM. Putative kappa-2 opioid agonists are antihyperalgesic in a rat model of inflammation. *J Pharmacol Exp Ther* 1997; 281:136–141.

Höllt V, Haarman I, Millan MJ, Herz A. Prodynorphin gene expression is enhanced in the spinal cord of chronic arthritic rats. *Neurosci Lett* 1987; 73:90–94.

Honoré MP, Buritova J, Besson JM. Intraplantar morphine depresses spinal c-Fos expression induced by carrageenin-inflammation but not by noxious heat. *Br J Pharmacol* 1996a; 118:671–680.

Honoré P, Chapman V, Buritova J, Besson JM. To what extent do spinal interactions between an alpha-2 adrenoceptor agonist and a mu opioid agonist influence noxiously evoked c-Fos expression in the rat? A pharmacological study. *J Pharmacol Exp Ther* 1996b; 278:393–403.

Honoré P, Chapman V, Buritova J, Besson JM. When is the maximal effect of pre-administered systemic morphine on carrageenin-evoked spinal c-Fos expression in the rat? *Brain Res* 1996c; 705:91–96.

Hylden JLK, Nahin RL, Traub RJ, Dubner R. Expansion of receptive fields of spinal lamina I projection neurons in rats with unilateral adjuvant-induced inflammation: the contribution of dorsal horn mechanisms. *Pain* 1989; 37:229–243.

Iadarola MJ, Brady LS, Draisci G, Dubner R. Enhancement of dynorphin gene expression in spinal cord following experimental inflammation: stimulus specificity; behavioural parameters and opioid receptor binding. *Pain* 1988; 35:313–326.

Idänpään-Heikkilä JJ, Perrot S, Guilbaud G, Kayser V. In mononeuropathic rats, the enhancement of morphine antinociception by L-365,260, a selective CCK$_B$ receptor antagonist, depends on the dose of systemic morphine and stimulus characteristics. *Eur J Pharmacol* 1997; 325:155–164.

Itoh S, Katsuura G, Maeda Y. Caerulein and cholecystokinin suppress beta-endorphin-induced analgesia in the rat *Eur J Pharmacol* 1982; 80:421–425

Jeanjean AP, Maloteaux JM, Laduron PM. IL-1β-like Freund's adjuvant enhances axonal transport of opiate receptors in sensory neurons. *Neurosci Lett* 1994; 177:75–78.

Ji RR, Zhang Q, Law PY, et al. Expression of μ-, δ-, and κ-opioid receptor like immunoreactivities in rat dorsal root ganglia after carrageenin-induced inflammation. *J Neurosci* 1995; 15:8136–8166.

Joris JL, Dubner R, Hargreaves KM. Opioid analgesia at peripheral sites: a target for opioids released during stress and inflammation? *Anesth Analg* 1987; 66:1277–1281.

Kalso E, Tramer MR, Carroll D, McQuay HJ, Moore RA. Pain relief from intra-articular morphine after knee surgery: a qualitative systematic review. *Pain* 1997; 71:127–134.

Kar S, Rees RG, Quirion R. Altered calcitonin gene-related peptide, substance P and enkephalin immunoreactivities and receptor binding sites in the dorsal spinal cord of the polyarthritic rat. *Eur J Neurosci* 1994; 6:345–354.

Kayser V. Endogenous opioid systems in the modulation of pain: behavioral studies in rat models of persistent hyperalgesia. In: Gebhart GF, Hammond DL, Jensen TS (Eds). *Proceedings of the 7th World Congress on Pain,* Progress in Pain Research and Management, Vol. 2. Seattle: IASP Press, 1994, pp 553–568.

Kayser V, Guilbaud G. Dose-dependent analgesic and hyperalgesic effects of systemic naloxone in arthritic rats. *Brain Res* 1981; 226:344–348.

Kayser V, Guilbaud G. The analgesic effects of morphine, but not those of the enkephalinase inhibitor Thiorphan, are enhanced in arthritic rats. *Brain Res* 1983; 267:131–138.

Kayser V, Guilbaud G. Local and remote modifications of nociceptive sensitivity during carrageenin-induced inflammation in the rat. *Pain* 1987; 28:99–107.

Kayser V, Guilbaud G. Differential effect of various doses of morphine and naloxone on two nociceptive test threshold in arthritic and normal rats. *Pain* 1990; 41:353–363.

Kayser V, Guilbaud G. Peripheral aspects of opioid activity: studies in animals. In: Besson JM, Guilbaud G, Ollat H (Eds). *Peripheral Neurons in Nociception: Physiopharmacological Aspects.* Paris: John Libbey Eurotext, 1994, pp 137–156.

Kayser V, Guilbaud G. Modèles animaux de douleur clinique. In: Brasseur L, Chauvin M, Guilbaud G (Eds.) *Douleurs, Bases fondamentales, Pharmacologie, Douleurs aigues, Douleurs chroniques, Thérapeutiques.* Paris: Maloine, 1997, pp 77–90.

Kayser V, Neil A, Guilbaud G. Repeated low doses of morphine induce a rapid tolerance in arthritic rats but a potentiation of opiate analgesia in normal animals. *Brain Res* 1986; 383:392–396.

Kayser V, Fournié-Zaluski MC, Guilbaud G, Roques BP. Potent antinociceptive effects of kelatorphan (a highly efficient inhibitor of multiple enkephalin-degrading enzymes) systemically administered in normal and arthritic rats. *Brain Res* 1989; 497:94–101.

Kayser V, Gobeaux D, Lombard MC, Guilbaud G, Besson JM. Potent and long lasting antinociceptive effects after injection of low doses of the mu-opioid receptor agonist, fentanyl, into the brachial plexus sheath of the rats. *Pain* 1990; 42:215–225.

Kayser V, Besson JM, Guilbaud G. Effects of the analgesic agent tramadol in normal and arthritic rats: comparison with the effects of different opioids, including tolerance and cross-tolerance to morphine. *Eur J Pharmacol* 1991a; 195:37–45.

Kayser V, Chen YL, Guilbaud G. Behavioural evidence for a peripheral component in the enhanced antinociceptive effect of a low dose of systemic morphine in carrageenin-induced hyperalgesic rats. *Brain Res* 1991b; 560:237–244.

Kayser V, Guilbaud G, Besson JM. Potent antinociceptive effects of clonidine systemically administered in an experimental model of clinical pain, the arthritic rat. *Brain Res* 1992; 593:7–13.

Kayser V, Lee S, Guilbaud G. Evidence for a peripheral component in the antinociceptive effect of systemic morphine in rats with peripheral neuropathy. *Neuroscience* 1995; 64:537–545.

Kayser V, Idänpään-Heikkilä J, Guilbaud G. Sensitization of the nervous system, induced by two successive hindpaw inflammations, is suppressed by a local anesthetic. *Brain Res* 1998; 794:19–27.

Kehlet H, Dahl JB. The value of 'multimodal' or 'balanced' analgesia in postoperative treatment. *Anesth Analg* 1993; 77:1048–1056.

Laduron P. Axonal transport of opiate receptors in the capsaicin sensitive neurones. *Brain Res* 1984; 294:157–160.

Loomis CW, Jhamandas K, Milne B, Cervenko F. Monoamine and opioid interactions in spinal analgesia and tolerance. *Pharmacol Biochem Behav* 1987; 26:445–451.

MacArthur L, Ren K, Pfaffenroth E, Franklin E, Ruda MA. Descending modulation of opioid-containing nociceptive neurons in rats with peripheral inflammation and hyperalgesia *Neuroscience* 1999; 88:499–506.

Maekawa K, Minami M, Masida T, Satoh M. Expression of μ- and κ-, but not δ-, opioid receptor mRNAs is enhanced in the spinal dorsal horn the arthritic rats. *Pain* 1996; 64:365–371.

Malberg AB, Yaksh TL. Pharmacology of the spinal action of ketorolac, morphine, ST-91, and L-PIA on the formalin test and an isobolographic analysis of NSAID interaction. *Anesthesiology* 1993; 79:270–281.

McQuay HJ. Is there a place for alpha2 adrenergic agonists in the control of pain? In: Besson JM, Guilbaud G (Eds). *Towards the Use of Noradrenergic Agonists for the Treatment of Pain.* Amsterdam: Elsevier Science, 1992, pp 219–232.

Meert TF, De Kock M, Janssen PA. Potentiation of the analgesic properties of fentanyl-like opioids with alpha 2-adrenoceptor agonists in rats. *Anesthesiology* 1994; 81:677–688.

Millan MJ. Multiple opioid systems and pain. *Pain* 1986; 27:303–347.

Millan MJ, Czlonkowski A, Pilcher CWT, et al. A model of chronic pain in the rat: functional correlates of alterations in the activity of opioid systems. *J Neurosci* 1987; 7:77–87.

Millan MJ, Czlonkowski A, Morris B, et al. Inflammation of the hind limb as a model of unilateral, localized pain: influence on multiple opioid systems in the spinal cord of the rat. *Pain* 1988; 35:299–312.

Monasky MS, Zinmeister AR, Stevens CW, Yaksh TL. Interaction of intrathecal morphine and ST91 on antinociception in the rat: dose-response analysis, antagonism and clearance. *J Pharmacol Exp Ther* 1990; 234:383–392.

Motsh J, Graber E, Ludwig K. Addition of clonidine enhances postoperative analgesia from epidural morphine: a double blind study. *Anesthesiology* 1990; 73:1067–1073.

Naguib M, Yaksh TL. Antinociceptive effects of spinal cholinesterase inhibition and isobolographic analysis of the interaction with mu and alpha2 receptor systems. *Anesthesiology* 1994; 80:1338–1348.

Neil A, Kayser V, Gacel G, Besson JM, Guilbaud G. Opioid receptor types and antinociceptive activity in chronic inflammation: both κ- and μ-opiate agonist effects are enhanced in arthritic rats. *Eur J Pharmacol* 1986; 130:203–208.

Neil A, Kayser V, Chen YL, Guilbaud G. Repeated low doses of morphine do not induce tolerance but increase the antinociceptive effect in rats with a peripheral neuropathy. *Brain Res* 1990; 522:140–143.

Nichols ML, Bian D, Ossipov MH, Lai J, Porreca F. Regulation of morphine antiallodynic efficacy by cholecystokinin in a model of neuropathic pain. *J Pharmacol Exp Ther* 1995; 275:1339–1345

Nichols ML, Bian D, Ossipov MH, Malan TP Jr, Porreca F. Antiallodynic effects of a CCKB antagonist in rats with nerve ligation injury: role of endogenous enkephalins *Neurosci Lett* 1996; 215:161–164

Ohta S, Niwa M, Nozaki M, et al. Changes in opioid receptor binding nature in rat brain and spinal cord following formalin or carrageenin-induced nociception. *Masui* 1997; 46:644–649.

Oliveras JL, Bruxelle J, Clot AM, Besson JM. Effects of morphine and naloxone on painful reaction in normal and chronic suffering rats *Neurosci Lett* 1979; (Suppl)3:S263.

O'Neil MF, Dourish CT, Ossipov MH, Malan TP Jr, Porreca F. Morphine induced analgesia in the rat paw pressure test is blocked by CCK and enhanced by the CCK antagonist MK-329. *Neuropharmacology* 1989; 28:243–249.

Ossipov MH, Suarez LJ, Spaulding TC. Antinociceptive interactions between alpha 2-adrenergic and opiate agonists at the spinal level in rodents. *Anesth Analg* 1989; 68:194–200.

Ossipov MH, Harris S, Lloyd P, Messineo E. An isobolographic analysis of the antinociceptive effect of systemically and intrathecally administered combination of clonidine and opiates *J Exp Pharmacol Ther* 1990; 255:1107–1116.

Pearson CM, Wood FD. Studies of polyarthritis and other lesions induced in rats by injection of mycobacterial adjuvant. I. General clinical and pathological characteristics and some modifying factors. *Arthritis Rheum* 1959; 2:440–459.

Pearson CM, Waksman BH, Sharp JJ. Studies of arthritis and other lesions induced in rats by injection of mycobacterial adjuvant. Changes affecting the skin and mucous membranes. Comparison of the experimental process with human disease. *J Exp Med* 1961; 113:485–509.

Perrot S, Kayser V, Fournié-Zaluski MC, Roques BP, Guilbaud G. Antinociceptive effect of systemic PC12, a prodrug mixed inhibitor of enkephalin-degrading enzymes, in normal and arthritic rats. *Eur J Pharmacol* 1993; 241:129–133.

Perrot S, Idänpään-Heikkilä JJ, Guilbaud G, Kayser V. The enhancement of morphine antinociception by a CCK_B receptor antagonist in the rat depends on the phase of inflammation and the intensity of carrageenin-induced hyperalgesia. *Pain* 1998; 269–274.

Pircio AW, Fedele CT, Bierwagen ME. A new method for the evaluation of analgesic activity using adjuvant induced arthritis in the rat. *Eur J Pharmacol* 1975; 31:207–215.

Pircio AW, Buyniski JP, Rocheel LE. Pharmacological effects of a combination of butorphanol and acetaminophen. *Arch Int Pharmacodyn* 1978; 235:116–123.

Przewloski R, Przewloska B, Lason W, et al. Opioid peptides, particularly dynorphin, and chronic pain. In: Besson JM, Lazorthes Y (Eds)*, Spinal Opioids and the Relief of Pain*. Paris: Editions INSERM, 1984, pp 159–170.

Quevauviller A, Chalchat MA, Brouilhet H, Delbarre F. Action des barbituriques chez le rat atteint de polyarthrite à adjuvant. *CR Soc Biol Paris* 1968; 162:618–621.

Reiber H, Suckling AJ, Rumsby MG. The effect of Freund's adjuvant on blood, cerebrospinal fluid barrier permeability. *J Neurol Sci* 1984; 63:55–61.

Rostaing S, Bonnet F, Levron JC, et al. Effect of epidural clonidine on analgesia and pharmacokinetics of epidural fentanyl in postoperative patients. *Anesthesiology* 1991; 75:420–425.

Ruda MA, Iadarola MJ, Cohen LV, Young WS. *In situ* hybridisation histochemistry and immunocytochemistry reveal an increase in spinal cord dynorphin biosynthesis in a rat model of peripheral inflammation and hyperalgesia. *Proc Nat Acad Sci USA* 1988; 85:622–626.

Schäfer M, Carter L, Stein C. Interleukin 1 beta and corticotropin-releasing factor inhibit pain by releasing opioids from immune cells in inflamed tissue. *Proc Natl Acad Sci USA* 1994; 91:4219–4223.

Schäfer M, Zhou L, Stein C. Cholecystokinin inhibits peripheral opioid analgesia in inflamed tissue. *Neuroscience* 1998; 82:603–611.

Schaible HG, Neugebauer B, Cervero F, Schmidt RF. Changes in tonic descending inhibition of spinal neurons with articular input during the development of acute arthritis in the cat. *J Neurophysiol* 1991; 66:1021–1032.

Selley DE, Breivogel CS, Childers SR. Modification of G protein-coupled functions by low-pH pretreatment of membranes from NG108-15 cells: increase in opioid efficacy by decreased inactivation of G-proteins. *Mol Pharmacol* 1993; 44:731–741.

Stanfa LC, Dickenson AH. Cholecystokinin as a factor in the enhanced potency of spinal morphine following carrageenin inflammation *Br J Pharmacol* 1993; 108:967–973.

Stein C, Yassouridis A. Peripheral morphine analgesia. *Pain* 1997; 71:119–121.

Stein C, Millan MJ, Shippenberg TS, Herz A. Peripheral effect of fentanyl upon nociception in inflamed tissue of the rat. *Neurosci Lett* 1988a; 84:225–228.

Stein C, Millan J, Yassouridis A, Herz A. Antinociceptive effects of μ- and κ-agonists in inflammation are enhanced due to a peripheral opioid receptor-specific mechanism. *Eur J Pharmacol* 1988b;155:255–264.

Stein C, Millan MJ, Shippenberg TS, Peter K, Herz A. Peripheral opioid receptors mediating antinociception in inflammation. Evidence for involvement of Mu, Delta and Kappa receptors. *J Pharmacol Exp Ther* 1989; 248:1269–1275.

Stein C, Hassan AHS, Przewlocki R, et al. Opioids from immunocytes interact with receptors on sensory nerves to inhibit nociception in inflammation. *Proc Natl Acad Sci USA* 1990; 87:5935–5939.

Sullivan AF, Dashwood MR, Dickenson AH. α-2-Adrenoreceptor modulation of nociception in rat spinal cord: location, effects and interactions with morphine. *Eur J Pharmacol* 1987; 138:169–177.

Tallarida RJ. Statistical analysis of drug combinations for synergism. *Pain* 1992; 49:93–97.

Valverde O, Maldonado, Fournie-Zaluski MC, Roques BP. Cholecystokinin B antagonists strongly potentiate antinociception mediated by endogenous enkephalins. *J Pharmacol Exp Ther* 1994; 270:77–88.

Van Veldhoven P, Carton H. Enkephalinase A activity in different regions of brain and spinal cord of normal and chronic arthritic rats. *FEBS Lett* 1982 138:76–78.

Van Essen EJ, Bovill JG, Ploeger EJ. Extradural clonidine does not potentiate analgesia produced by extradural morphine after meniscectomy. *Br J Anaesth* 1991; 66:237–241.

Vercauteren M, Lauwers E, Meert T, De Hert S, Adriensen H. Comparison of epidural sulfentanyl plus clonidine with sulfentanyl alone for postoperative pain relief. *Anaesthesiology* 1990; 45:531–534.

Wilson JL, Nayanar V, Walker JS. The site of anti-arthritic action of the kappa-opioid, U-50, 488H, in adjuvant arthritis: importance of local administration. *Br J Pharmacol* 1996; 118:1754–1760.

Yaksh TL. Pharmacology of spinal adrenergic systems which modulate spinal nociceptive processing. *Pharmacol Biochem Bhav* 1985; 22:845–858.

Yonehara N, Kudo T, Iwatsubo K, et al. possible involvement of the central endorphin system in the autoanalgesia induced by chronic administration of Freund's adjuvant solution in rats. *Pain* 1983; 17:91–98.

Young WS, Wamsley JK, Zarbin MA, Kuhar MJ. Opioid receptors undergo axonal flow. *Science* 1980; 210:76–78.

Zhou L, Zhang Q, Stein C, Schäfer M. Contribution of opioid receptors on primary afferent versus sympathetic neurons to peripheral opioid analgesia. *J Pharmacol Exp Ther* 1998; 286:1000–1006.

Correspondence to: Dr. Gisèle Guilbaud, MD, DSc, Unité de Recherches en Physiopharmacologie du Système Nerveux, U 161, INSERM, 2 rue d'Alésia, 75014, Paris, France. Tel: 33-1-458-93662; Fax: 33-1-458-81304; email: guilbaud@broca.inserm.fr.

Opioid Sensitivity of Chronic Noncancer Pain,
Progress in Pain Research and Management,
Vol. 14, edited by Eija Kalso, Henry J. McQuay,
and Zsuzsanna Wiesenfeld-Hallin, IASP Press,
Seattle, © 1999.

13

Opioid Modulation of Visceral Pain

G.F. Gebhart, Xin Su, Shailen Joshi, N. Ozaki, and J.N. Sengupta

*Department of Pharmacology, College of Medicine,
University of Iowa, Iowa City, Iowa, USA*

Opioids are widely and successfully used for management of visceral pain, especially when it arises from a malignancy. Morphine and other μ-opioid-receptor agonists are the standard for management of such pain, including palliative care at the end of life. There are several chronic, nonmalignant visceral pains, however, for which opioids are not generally given. Functional bowel disorders, in which pain and discomfort may be the principal complaint in up to 50% of patients, are notoriously difficult to manage. If a strategy were available that could significantly reduce the incidence of pain and discomfort, many such patients would enjoy an enhanced quality of life.

This brief review of some results from our own and other studies on the modulation of visceral nociception will discuss several key points: (1) κ-, but not either μ- or δ-opioid-receptor agonists, significantly attenuate visceral afferent input. (2) The peripheral actions of κ-opioid-receptor agonists are enhanced in the presence of chronic, but not acute inflammation of the viscera. (3) The peripheral receptor at which κ-opioid-receptor agonists act to attenuate visceral afferent input is different from the κ-opioid receptor cloned from the central nervous system (CNS).

OPIOID MODULATION OF RESPONSES TO VISCERAL STIMULATION

It has long been appreciated that pain arising from viscera differs in important ways from pain that arises from cutaneous structures (see Ness and Gebhart 1990 and Cervero 1994 for recent reviews). Until the 1980s most knowledge about pain mechanisms and pain modulation was derived from models of cutaneous pain. Because of our interest in visceral pain, we developed a model of visceral nociception in the rat that employed colorectal distension (CRD) as the adequate stimulus (Ness and Gebhart 1988). We used CRD because it reproduces a natural visceral stimulus, is noninvasive (a distending balloon is inserted via the anus), produces easily quantifiable responses, and most importantly, can be used in unanesthetized animals (see Gebhart and Sengupta 1995 for rationale and description of methods).

In early characterization of this model, we documented that morphine administered systemically or intrathecally produced dose-dependent, naloxone-reversible attenuation of responses to noxious CRD (Ness and Gebhart 1988; Danzebrink et al. 1995). Similar results on visceral nociception were reported by others (e.g., Jensen et al. 1988; Harada et al. 1995; Borgbjerg et al. 1996). Interestingly, Danzebrink et al. (1995) and Harada et al. (1995) noted that μ- and δ-opioid-receptor agonists given intrathecally (i.t.) attenuated responses to CRD in a dose-dependent manner, but that the κ-opioid-receptor agonist U50,488 given i.t. was ineffective (Fig. 1). In contrast, κ-opioid-receptor agonists dose-dependently attenuated responses to CRD in intact, unanesthetized rats when administered systemically (Diop et al. 1994; Langlois et al. 1994; Danzebrink et al. 1995; Harada et al. 1995; Burton and Gebhart 1998). We interpreted these results to mean that κ-opioid-receptor

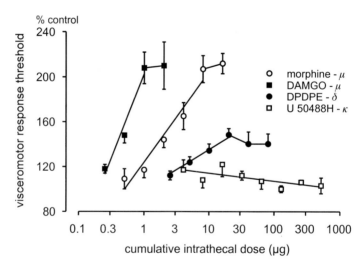

Fig. 1. Changes in the threshold for the visceromotor response to noxious colorectal distension produced by intrathecal administration of μ- (morphine and DAMGO), δ- (DPDPE), and κ- (U50,488) opioid-receptor agonists. The intracolonic distending pressure that produces a contraction of the peritoneal musculature (the visceromotor response) is 20–25 mm Hg. Intrathecal μ and δ agonists, but not the k agonist, significantly increase the visceromotor response threshold. Data derived from Danzebrink et al. (1995).

agonists may have a peripheral site of action and thus particular utility in the modulation of visceral nociception.

OPIOID MODULATION OF VISCERAL AFFERENT INPUT

Both nonpainful and painful sensations from the distal gut and urinary bladder are conveyed to the spinal cord via the pelvic nerve (see Ness and Gebhart 1990 for review). To examine peripheral effects of μ-, δ-, and κ-opioid-receptor agonists on responses to CRD, we conducted a series of experiments in rats on the responses of pelvic nerve afferent fibers to CRD before and after intravenous or intra-arterial opioid-receptor agonist administration. Because these experiments involve recording of pelvic nerve afferent fibers teased from the decentralized S1 dorsal rootlet, any drug effects must be restricted to the periphery (e.g., on colonic smooth muscle, at receptors located on nerve terminals in the colon or on nerve cell bodies in the S1 dorsal root ganglion, or on conduction of pelvic nerve axons). Many of the pelvic nerve afferent fibers that innervate the distal colon are mechanosensitive and encode distending pressure in their response (e.g., Sengupta and Gebhart 1994, 1995). We thus examined the dose-dependent effects of opioid-receptor agonists on responses of pelvic nerve afferent fibers to a noxious intensity of CRD (80 mm Hg). To our surprise, morphine was unable to attenuate responses of pelvic nerve afferent fibers to noxious CRD. Similarly, a δ-opioid-receptor agonist ([D-Pen^2,D-Pen^5]enkephalin, DPDPE) also failed to attenuate responses to CRD, but the κ-opioid-receptor agonist U50,488 dose-dependently attenuated such responses (Fig. 2). We went on to examine the effects of different μ- (morphine, fentanyl), δ- (DPDPE, SNC-80), and κ-opioid-receptor agonists (Sengupta et al. 1996; Su et al. 1997a) (Fig. 3) on responses to noxious CRD. The outcomes illustrated in Figs. 2 and 3 were not unique to pelvic nerve innervation of the colon because the same experimental outcomes were observed when we studied the effects of opioid-receptor agonists on responses of pelvic nerve afferent fibers to noxious urinary bladder distension (Su et al. 1997b) or on responses of vagal afferent fibers to gastric distension (Sengupta et al. 1997). Accordingly, the effects of κ-opioid-receptor agonists on pelvic nerve innervation were shown not to be unique to the colon.

Several features of these experimental outcomes suggest that the peripheral receptor at which these κ-opioid-receptor agonists acted to modulate visceral nociception was different from the κ-opioid receptor cloned from the CNS. Fig. 3 reveals an unusual clustering of dose-effect functions for the κ-opioid-receptor agonists tested, and this was true also for their

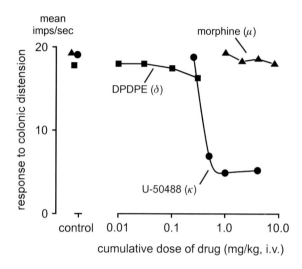

Fig. 2. Attenuation of responses of pelvic nerve afferent fibers (impulses per second) to noxious colorectal distension (80 mm Hg) by a κ (U50,488), but not μ (morphine) or δ (DPDPE) agonist.

effects on urinary bladder distension (see Su et al. 1997b). In other work (see Burton and Gebhart 1998, and references therein), the effective dose of systemic κ-opioid-receptor agonists ranges from low (micrograms per kilogram) to much higher doses (milligrams per kilogram), but the effective dose in our studies ranged only from about 2 to 12 mg/kg (see Fig. 3). Moreover, the κ-opioid-receptor agonists we tested have different selectivity for the receptor subtypes ($κ_1$, $κ_2$, and $κ_3$) and thus would be expected to exhibit different relative potencies if the receptor were a κ-opioid receptor. We consider the receptor to be an opioid-like receptor because naloxone, when given in a high, nonselective dose, partly antagonizes the effect of the κ-opioid-receptor agonists on responses to CRD. Doses of naloxone that are selective for the μ-opioid receptor are without effect. Unexpectedly, two κ-opioid-receptor-selective antagonists (nor-binaltorphimine [nor-BNI] and DIPPA) were unable to antagonize the effects of any of the κ-opioid-receptor agonists tested, regardless of the duration of pretreatment or dosage of the κ-opioid-receptor-selective antagonists (see Sengupta et al. 1996; Su et al. 1997a,b).

We also demonstrated that κ-, but not either μ- or δ-opioid-receptor agonists given intracolonically attenuate responses of pelvic nerve afferent fibers to CRD (Su et al. 1998) (Fig. 4). Accordingly, we are satisfied that these effects of κ-opioid-receptor agonists occur in the periphery and are not associated with effects either on smooth muscle contractility or on conduction in pelvic nerve afferent fibers (see Sengupta et al. 1996; Su et al. 1997a,b).

It has been well documented that peripheral antinociceptive effects of opioids can be enhanced in the presence of tissue inflammation (see Stein 1993 for review and Chapters 3 and 12 of this volume), and so we reexamined the effects of μ-, δ-, and κ-opioid-receptor agonists on pelvic nerve fiber responses to CRD in rats following both acute (intracolonic acetic acid) and chronic (4 days after intracolonic trinitrobenzene sulfonic acid,

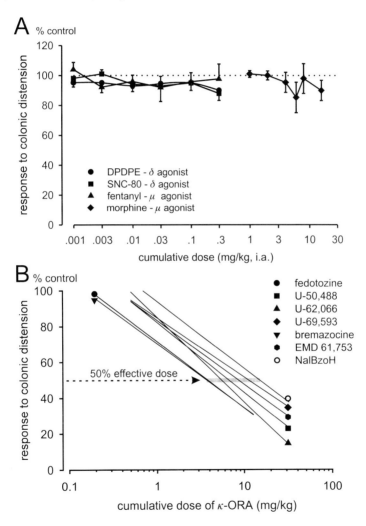

Fig. 3. Summary of effects of opioid-receptor agonists on pelvic nerve afferent fiber responses to noxious colorectal distension (CRD) (80 mm Hg). (A) Summary of failure of μ- and δ-opioid-receptor agonists to attenuate responses of pelvic nerve afferent fibers to noxious CRD. (B) Summary of dose-dependent effects of κ-opioid-receptor agonists (ORA) on responses of pelvic nerve afferent fibers to noxious CRD. Data are summarized from Sengupta et al. (1996) and Su et al. (1997a).

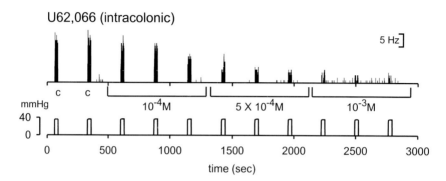

Fig. 4. Example of the effect of intracolonic instillation of a κ-opioid receptor agonist (U62,066) on responses of a pelvic nerve afferent fiber to CRD. Responses are presented as peristimulus-time histograms to 40 mm Hg colonic distension (illustrated bottom-most). Control (c) responses to distension are illustrated, as are reduced responses to the same stimulus as the intracolonic concentration of U62,066 is serially increased. From X. Su and G.F. Gebhart (unpublished data).

TNBS) colonic inflammation. Neither morphine nor the δ-opioid-receptor agonist SNC-80 were effective in attenuating responses of pelvic nerve afferent fibers to CRD in either the acetic acid- or TNBS-inflamed colon. The dose-effect function for the κ-opioid-receptor agonists EMD61,753, however, was shifted leftward in the presence of chronic colonic inflammation (Sengupta et al. 1999) (Fig. 5). Thus, as in other peripheral tissues when

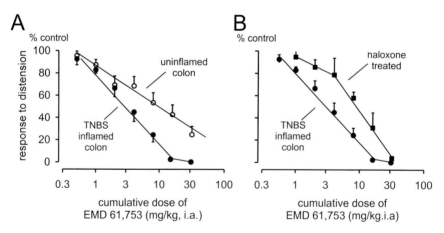

Fig. 5. (A) Summary of dose-effect functions of the κ-opioid receptor agonist EMD 61,753 on pelvic nerve fiber responses to CRD in uninflamed and trinitrobenzene sulfonic acid (TNBS)-inflamed rat colon. The dose-effect function is shifted significantly leftward in the presence of chronic inflammation. (B) Illustration of the rightward shift in the dose-effect function for EMD 61,753 in TNBS-inflamed rats pretreated with naloxone (2 mg/kg). Data modified from Sengupta et al. (1999).

inflamed, the antinociceptive effects of exogenous opioids were enhanced. Interestingly, even in the presence of chronic inflammation, neither μ- nor δ-opioid-receptor agonists were effective in attenuating responses to CRD. As noted above, a nonopioid-receptor-selective dose of naloxone, but not the κ-opioid-receptor-selective antagonist nor-BNI, was able to antagonize the enhanced effects of the κ-opioid-receptor agonist EMD 61,753 in TNBS-inflamed colon (Fig. 5).

KAPPA-OPIOID-RECEPTOR KNOCK-DOWN

We believe that the effects of κ-opioid-receptor agonists summarized above occur at a opioid-like receptor in the periphery that is different from the κ-opioid receptor cloned from the CNS. This conclusion was derived principally on the basis of the clustered dose-effect functions and the ability of naloxone (and failure of nor-BNI) to antagonize the effects of κ-opioid-receptor agonists. In subsequent experiments we used an antisense strategy to specifically knock down the cloned κ-opioid receptor. We administered antisense oligodeoxynucleotides (ODNs) targeting the cloned κ-opioid receptor i.t. twice daily for 4 days. To assess the efficacy of the antisense ODN treatment, we evaluated the antinociception produced by μ-, δ-, and κ-opioid-receptor agonists given into a hindpaw on formalin-produced hindpaw flinching. The experimental strategy is shown in Fig. 6. The same rats were deeply anesthetized after the formalin test and prepared for electrophysiological study of pelvic nerve afferent fiber responses to colonic distension. As

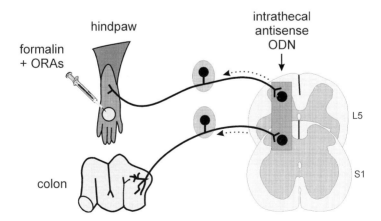

Fig. 6. Illustration of the experimental design for the study of κ-opioid-receptor knockdown using antisense oligodeoxynucleotides (ODN) and peripherally administered opioid-receptor agonists (ORAs) (see text for details).

anticipated, antisense, but not mismatch ODN treatment given i.t. for 4 days blocked the antinociceptive actions of κ-opioid-receptor agonists administered into the paw without affecting the antinociception produced by either the μ-opioid-receptor agonist DAMGO ([D-Ala-N-Me-Phe⁴,Gly⁵-OL]enkephalin) or the δ-opioid-receptor agonist deltorphin given into the paw (Joshi et al. 1998) (Fig. 7). In the same rats, the ability of κ-opioid-receptor agonists to dose-dependently attenuate responses of pelvic nerve afferent fibers to noxious CRD was unaffected. These results support the view that the opioid-like receptor in the colon at which κ-opioid-receptor agonists act to attenuate responses to noxious distension is different from the κ-opioid receptor cloned in the CNS.

SUMMARY AND CONCLUSIONS

Regardless of the receptor at which κ-opioid-receptor agonists produce their effect in the viscera, it is clear from this work that such compounds could be useful in the management of chronic visceral pain. Kappa-opioid-receptor agonists are undeniably analgesic when given systemically, but their utility has been limited by undesirable psychotomimetic, dysphoric,

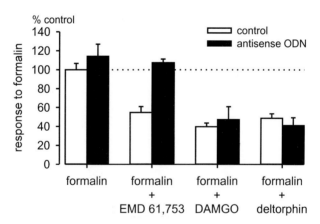

Fig. 7. Summary of the efficacy of intrathecal antisense oligodeoxynucleotide (ODN) administration against the target receptor (κ-opioid receptor). Formalin (50 μL, 2.5%) was used as the peripheral noxious stimulus. Either vehicle (control) or μ-, δ-, or κ-opioid-receptor agonists were injected into the hindpaw before intraplantar injection of formalin, and the number of paw flinches was counted over the subsequent 60 min. Different groups received antisense or mismatch ODNs intrathecally. Only the antinociceptive effects of the κ-opioid receptor agonist EMD 61,753 was affected by prior antisense treatment; neither the μ (DAMGO) nor δ (deltorphin) agonists injected into the hind paw were affected by κ-opioid-receptor antisense ODN treatment. From S. Joshi and G.F. Gebhart (unpublished data).

and sedating CNS effects (Pfeiffer et al. 1986; Peters and Gaylor 1989). Accordingly, a new therapeutic approach could arise from the development of a κ-opioid-receptor agonist with actions restricted to the periphery.

While these findings promise an attractive therapeutic approach to the treatment of visceral pain, much remains to be learned about the site and mechanism of action of such a compound. The results summarized above point to a novel opioid-like receptor in the viscera. There is, however, no published evidence that such a receptor exists. We have considered previously that this novel receptor may be an orphan receptor similar to opioid-receptor-like 1 (ORL1), at which the endogenous orphanin FQ/nociceptin peptide acts (Meunier et al. 1995; Reinscheid et al. 1995). The ORL1 receptor most closely resembles the κ-opioid receptor, although it is distinct from the κ- and other opioid receptors (Meunier 1997). We tested nociceptin on responses of pelvic nerve afferent fibers to CRD and observed no effect (V. Julia and G.F. Gebhart, unpublished observations). While our conclusions are not definitive, it appears that the opioid-like receptor at which κ-opioid-receptor agonists act in modulating visceral pain is distinct from any opioid or orphan receptor cloned to date.

Not only the nature of the receptor, but also its location is still unresolved. Pharmacological and electrophysiological investigations provided early evidence for opioid effects localized to the gut. Binding studies localized opioid receptors to nerves and smooth muscle in the gastrointestinal (GI) tract (Pert and Snyder 1973; Miller and Kirning 1989; Daniel and Fox-Threlkeld 1992). Opioid receptors associated with sensory innervation of the GI tract are derived from their cell bodies in spinal dorsal root ganglia (e.g., Ji et al. 1995; Minami et al. 1995). Bagnol and colleagues (1997) used antibodies to epitopes of the cloned receptors to study the cellular localization and distribution of μ- and κ-opioid receptors in the rat GI tract. Neurons expressing the μ-opioid receptor were more prevalent in the submucosal plexus, whereas neurons expressing the κ-opioid receptor were found in greater number in the myenteric plexus. Interestingly, smooth muscle cells in the colon did not exhibit immunoreactivity for either μ- or κ-opioid receptors. Although distributed almost exclusively on nerve fibers and neurons in the GI tract, κ-opioid receptors were not definitively associated with terminals of pelvic nerve afferent fibers innervating the colon. Bagnol et al.'s report thus may not be particularly relevant to our results unless the antibody they used is shown to label the receptor that is the site of the drug effects summarized above.

In our examination of pelvic nerve afferent fiber responses to colonic distension, we concluded that the principal effects of the κ-opioid-receptor agonists studied are produced at or near the terminals of pelvic nerve afferent fibers in the GI tract. These sites of action need not be on the pelvic nerve terminals themselves, but could be associated with neurons of the enteric or intrinsic nervous system of the gut, which interacts with sensory afferent nerve terminals in the pelvic nerve. Further data are needed to resolve the issue of site of action of κ-opioid-receptor agonists.

ACKNOWLEDGMENTS

Work described here was supported by National Institutes of Health awards NS 19912, DA 02879, and NS 35790. The authors gratefully acknowledge the excellent secretarial support of Susan Birely and assistance by Michael Burcham with production of graphics.

REFERENCES

Bagnol D, Mansour A, Akil H, Watson SJ. Cellular localization and distribution of the cloned mu and kappa opioid receptors in rat gastrointestinal tract. *Neuroscience* 1997; 81:579–591.

Borgbjerg FM, Frigast C, Madsen JB, Mikkelsen LF. The effect of intrathecal opioid receptor agonists on visceral noxious stimulation in rabbits. *Gastroenterol* 1996; 110:139–146.

Burton MB, Gebhart GF. Effects of *kappa*-opioid receptor agonists on responses to colorectal distension in rats with and without acute colonic inflammation. *J Pharmacol Exp Ther* 1998; 285:707–715.

Cervero F. Sensory innervation of the viscera: peripheral basis of visceral pain. *Physiol Rev* 1994; 74:95–138.

Daniel EE, Fox-Threlkeld JET. Role of opioid receptor subtypes in control of the gastrointestinal tract. In: Holle GH, Wood JD (Eds). *Advances in the Innervation of the Gastrointestinal Tract*. Amsterdam: Elsevier, 1992, pp 329–340.

Danzebrink RM, Green SA, Gebhart GF. Spinal mu and delta, but not kappa, opioid receptor agonists attenuate responses to noxious colorectal distension in the rat. *Pain* 1995; 63:39–47.

Diop L, Riviere PJ, Pascaud X, Dassaud M, Junien J-L. Role of vagal afferents in the antinociception produced by morphine and U-50,488H in the colonic pain reflex in rats. *Eur J Pharmacol* 1994; 257:181–187.

Gebhart GF, Sengupta JN. Evaluation of visceral pain. In: Gaginella TS (Ed). *Handbook of Methods in Gastrointestinal Pharmacology*. Boca Raton, FL: CRC Press, 1995, pp 359–373.

Harada Y, Nishioka K, Kitahata LM, Nakatani K, Collins JG. Contrasting actions of intrathecal U50,488H, morphine or [D-Pen2, D-Pen5] enkephalin, or intravenous U50,488H on the visceromotor response to colorectal distension in the rat. *Anesthesiology* 1995; 83:336–343.

Jensen FM, Madsen JB, Ringsted CV, Christensen A. Intestinal distension test, a method for evaluating intermittent visceral pain in the rabbit. *Life Sci* 1988; 43:747–753.

Ji R-R, Zhang Q, Law P-Y, Low HH, Elde R, Hökfelt T. Expression of μ-, δ-, and κ-opioid receptor-like immunoreactivities in rat dorsal root ganglia after carrageenan-induced inflammation. *J Neurosci* 1995; 15:8156–8166.

Joshi SK, Su X, Sengupta JN, Gebhart GF. Investigation of a peripheral, κ-opioid-like receptor using antisense-mediated knock-down. *Neurosci Abs* 1998; 24:890.

Langlois A, Diop L, Reviere PJN, Pascaud X, Junien J-L. Effect of fedotozine on the cardiovascular pain reflex induced by distension of the irritated rat colon in the anesthetized rat. *Eur J Pharmacol* 1994; 271:245–251.

Meunier J-C. Nociceptin/orphanin FQ and the opioid receptor-like ORL1 receptor. *Eur J Pharmacol* 1997; 340:1–15.

Meunier J-C, Mollereau C, Toll L, et al. Isolation and structure of the endogenous agonist of opioid receptor-like ORL1 receptor. *Nature* 1995; 337:532–535.

Miller RJ, Kirning LD. Opioid peptides of the gut. In: Shultz ST, Makhlouf GN, Rauner BB (Eds). *Handbook of Physiology, The Gastrointestinal Tract*, Vol. II. Bethesda: American Physiological Society, 1989, pp 631–660.

Minami M, Maekawa K, Yabuuchi K, Sato HM. Double *in situ* hybridization study on coexistence of the μ-, δ-, and κ-opioid receptor mRNAs with preprotachykinin A mRNA in the rat dorsal root ganglia. *Mol Brain Res* 1995; 30:203–210.

Ness TJ, Gebhart GF. Colorectal distension as a noxious visceral stimulus: physiologic and pharmacologic characterization of pseudaffective reflexes in the rat. *Brain Res* 1988; 450:153–169.

Ness TJ, Gebhart GF. Visceral pain: a review of experimental studies. *Pain* 1990; 41:167–234.

Pert CB, Snyder SH. Opioid receptor: demonstration in nervous tissue. *Science* 1973; 179:1011–1014.

Peters GR, Gaylor S. Human central nervous system effects of a selective kappa opioid agonist. *Clin Pharmacol Ther* 1989; 51:1–5.

Pfeiffer A, Brantl V, Herz A, Emrich HM. Psychotomimesis mediated by the κ-opiate receptors. *Science* 1986; 233:774–776.

Reinscheid RK, Nothacker HP, Bourson A, et al. Orphanin FQ: a neuropeptide that activates an opioid like G protein-coupled receptor. *Science* 1995; 270:792–794.

Sengupta JN, Gebhart GF. Characterization of mechanosensitive pelvic nerve afferent fibers innervating the colon of the rat. *J Neurophysiol* 1994; 71:2046–2060.

Sengupta JN, Gebhart GF. Mechanosensitive afferent fibers in the gastrointestinal and lower urinary tracts. In: Gebhart GF (Ed). *Visceral Pain,* Progress in Pain Research and Management, Vol. 5. Seattle: IASP Press, 1995, pp 75–98.

Sengupta JN, Su X, Gebhart GF. κ, but not μ or δ, opioids attenuate responses to distension of afferent fibers innervating the rat colon. *Gastroenterology* 1996; 111:968–980.

Sengupta JN, Ozaki N, Gebhart GF. Differential effects of the μ- and κ-opioid receptor agonists on responses of gastric vagal afferent fibers in the rat. *Neurosci Abs* 1997; 23:1002.

Sengupta JN, Snider A, Su X, Gebhart GF. Effects of kappa opioids in the inflamed rat colon. *Pain* 1999; 79:175–185.

Stein C. Peripheral mechanisms of opioid analgesia. *Anesth Analg* 1993; 76:182–191.

Su X, Sengupta JN, Gebhart GF. Effects of kappa opioid receptor agonists on mechanosensitive pelvic nerve afferent fibers innervating the colon of the rat. *J Neurophysiol* 1997a; 78:1003–1012.

Su X, Sengupta JN, Gebhart GF. Effects of opioids on mechanosensitive pelvic nerve afferent fibers innervating the urinary bladder of the rat. *J Neurophysiol* 1997b; 77:1566–1580.

Su X, Julia V, Gebhart GF. Modulation of mechanosensitive pelvic nerve afferents by intracolonic κ-opioid agonists. *Neurosci Abs* 1998; 24:890.

Correspondence to: G.F. Gebhart, PhD, Department of Pharmacology, College of Medicine, 2-471 Bowen Science Building, University of Iowa, Iowa City, IA 52242-1109, USA. Tel: 319-335-7946; Fax: 319-335-8930; email: gf-gebhart@uiowa.edu.

Opioid Sensitivity of Chronic Noncancer Pain,
Progress in Pain Research and Management,
Vol. 14, edited by Eija Kalso, Henry J. McQuay,
and Zsuzsanna Wiesenfeld-Hallin, IASP Press,
Seattle, © 1999.

14

Opioid Sensitivity in Antinociception: Role of Anti-Opioid Systems with Emphasis on Cholecystokinin and NMDA Receptors

Zsuzsanna Wiesenfeld-Hallin, Pawel Alster, Stefan Grass, Orsolya Hoffmann, Guilherme de Araújo Lucas, Aida Plesan, and Xiao-Jun Xu

Department of Medical Laboratory Sciences and Technology, Division of Clinical Neurophysiology, Karolinska Institute, Huddinge University Hospital, Huddinge, Sweden

It is well established that the antinociceptive or analgesic effect of opioids can be physiologically antagonized by a range of nonopioid peptides (Cesselin 1995; Xu and Wiesenfeld-Hallin 1999). Recent evidence also suggests that activation of opioid receptors leads to subsequent activation of the N-methyl-D-aspartate (NMDA) receptors for glutamate, which may also counteract the effects of opioids (Mao et al. 1995a; Wiesenfeld-Hallin 1998). This chapter reviews recent progress in defining the role of one of the anti-opioid peptides, cholecystokinin, and of NMDA receptors in delineating opioid sensitivity under pathological states and in opioid tolerance and dependence.

THE ANTI-OPIOID EFFECT OF CHOLECYSTOKININ

The concept of endogenous anti-opioid peptides has been discussed for some time (see Cesselin 1995 for review). These peptides include cholecystokinin (CCK), FMRFamide-related peptides, angiotensin II, and melanocyte-inhibiting factor (MIF)-related peptides (Faris et al. 1983; Kastin et al. 1984; Yang et al. 1985). Among these, the anti-opioid effect of CCK has been most extensively studied, and the development of specific nonpeptide antagonists of CCK receptors has helped to characterize the role of endogenous CCK in mediating opioid analgesia.

CCK belongs to the gastrin family of peptides. In the nervous system it is mainly present in the form of the C-terminal octapeptide CCK-8 (Rehfeld 1978). CCK-like immunoreactivity (CCK-LI) and CCK mRNA are widely distributed in the central nervous system (CNS) (Williams et al. 1987; Schiffmann and Vanderhaeghen 1991; Lindefors et al. 1993). In general, there is an overlap in the anatomical distribution of CCK and endogenous opioids and their receptors in the spinal cord and brain, which may underlie the documented interaction between the opioid and CCK systems.

CCK receptors are heterogeneous; receptors predominantly located in the periphery (CCK$_A$ or CCK-1) differ from those in the CNS (CCK$_B$ or CCK-2) (Moran et al. 1986). However, it is now known that even the "peripheral" CCK$_A$ receptor is present to some extent in the CNS, particularly in primates (Hill et al. 1990). Receptor-binding sites for CCK have been visualized throughout the spinal dorsal horn, with the highest density in the superficial laminae. In the rat these receptors are predominantly the B-type, whereas in primates most receptors are of the A-type (Hill et al. 1990; Ghilardi et al. 1992). Only a few rat dorsal root ganglion (DRG) neurons express CCK-receptor mRNA under normal conditions (Zhang et al. 1993).

Itoh et al. (1982) and Faris et al. (1983) were the first to demonstrate that CCK attenuated antinociception induced by β-endorphin or morphine. A large body of literature has since accumulated to show that CCK reduces the effect of exogenous opioids upon local, systemic, intrathecal (i.t.), or intracerebral (i.c.) injection as tested in behavioral and electrophysiological studies (see Cesselin 1995 and Wiesenfeld-Hallin and Xu 1996 for review). CCK also blocks the antinociceptive effect of endogenous opioids produced by electroacupuncture or electric shocks (Watkins et al. 1985; Han et al. 1986). The inhibition by CCK of opioid antinociception appears to be tonic because blockade of endogenous CCK by receptor antagonists results in enhanced opioid-induced antinociception (see Wiesenfeld-Hallin and Xu 1996 for review). Comparison of the potency of CCK-receptor antagonists in studies using receptor antisense oligonucleotides has indicated that the CCK$_B$ receptor is responsible for the interaction between the CCK and opioid systems in rodents (Dourish et al. 1990; Wiesenfeld-Hallin et al. 1990; Vanderah et al. 1994). The antinociceptive effect of endogenously released opioids following the administration of endopeptidases and electroacupuncture is also potentiated by CCK-receptor antagonists (Han et al. 1986; Valverde et al. 1994). Interestingly, clinical placebo analgesia, which may be opioid mediated, is also potentiated by a CCK-receptor antagonist (Benedetti 1996).

The mechanism by which CCK antagonizes opioid analgesia is not fully understood. It is clear that the blockade of morphine analgesia by CCK is not due to a direct hyperalgesic effect, because CCK does not alter baseline pain threshold. Most studies of receptor binding fail to show an affinity of CCK for opioid receptors (cf. Wang et al. 1992). However, one study indicates that binding of CCK-8 to the CCK receptor reduces the binding affinity of μ-receptor ligands (Wang and Han 1989). There is also evidence that CCK may counteract intracellular events subsequent to opioid receptor activation (Wang et al. 1992).

CCK AND OPIOID SENSITIVITY IN RATS WITH NERVE INJURY OR INFLAMMATION

The analgesic effect of morphine varies in different clinical pain states. Neuropathic pain, involving injury to the nervous system, usually responds poorly to opioids (Arnér and Meyerson 1993), an observation supported by studies in rats showing that morphine causes less spinal antinociception after peripheral nerve injury (Xu and Wiesenfeld-Hallin 1991; Xu et al. 1994; Lee et al. 1995; Mao et al. 1995b; Ossipov et al. 1995). Peripheral axotomy induces an upregulation of CCK and CCK_B-receptor mRNA in rat DRG cells (Verge et al. 1993; Xu et al. 1993; Zhang et al. 1993). Electrophysiological and behavioral experiments have verified the role of CCK in morphine-induced antinociception (or the lack of it) in nerve-injured rats. Systemic morphine reduced antinociceptive potency in axotomized rats compared to normal controls, and addition of the CCK_B-receptor antagonist CI-988 strongly potentiated the effect of morphine (Xu et al. 1994). Furthermore, CCK_B-receptor antagonists reversed the ineffectiveness of i.t. morphine in alleviating neuropathic pain-like behaviors after complete or partial peripheral nerve injury in rats (Xu et al. 1993; Nichols et al. 1995). In one study, a CCK_B-receptor antagonist produced analgesia after constriction injury of the sciatic nerve in rats (Yamamoto and Nozakitaguchi 1995). Thus, it appears that, at least in rats, opioid insensitivity after nerve injury may be related to enhanced activity of the endogenous CCK system (Fig. 1).

Modulation by CCK of the degree of sensitivity to opioids may also be observed in animal models of inflammation, although the response is the opposite of that observed following nerve injury. It has been clearly established that the antinociceptive effect of opioids is enhanced in animals during acute inflammation (Stanfa and Dickenson 1993). While exogenous CCK is still able to attenuate the antinociceptive effect of morphine, CCK-receptor antagonists no longer enhance the effect of morphine (Stanfa and Dickenson 1993).

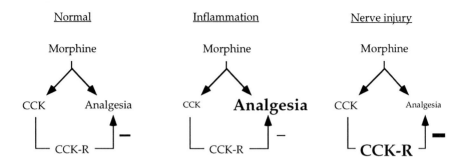

Fig. 1. Schematic illustration of the dynamic interaction between CCK and morphine. In normal rats, morphine administration induces analgesia and release of CCK, which may reduce (–) the effect of morphine through activation of CCK receptors (CCK-R). In rats with acute inflammation, the reduced release of CCK by morphine results in diminished antagonism by the peptide of morphine analgesia and enhances the effect of morphine. In rats with nerve injury, morphine releases CCK similarly as in normal rats. However, more CCK receptors are available, leading to the stronger inhibition of morphine analgesia that underlies morphine insensitivity in neuropathic pain. Type size indicates the magnitude of the effect.

Thus, although the mechanism by which CCK reduces the action of morphine is still intact, the availability of CCK within the spinal cord may decrease following inflammation, due to either decreased release of CCK or reduced concentration of this peptide within the dorsal horn (Fig. 1).

MORPHINE-INDUCED RELEASE OF CCK IN THE SPINAL CORD UNDER NORMAL AND PATHOLOGICAL CONDITIONS

One mechanism through which CCK modulates opioid-induced antinociception is that such drugs may evoke the release of CCK. Studies using in vitro and in vivo perfusion techniques have shown that spinal or systemic morphine increased the release of CCK-LI materials from the spinal cord (Tang et al. 1984; Benoliel et al. 1991; Zhou et al. 1993). We recently developed a spinal microdialysis technique to monitor the in vivo release of CCK-LI from dorsal spinal cord in anesthetized, intact rats (Lucas et al. 1998). With this technique, we have been able to show that systemic or i.t. administration of physiological doses of morphine that elicit antinociception cause significant spinal release of CCK-LI in normal rats (Lucas et al. 1998; Fig. 2).

As described above, nerve injury or inflammation may change the tone of endogenous CCK activity and modulate sensitivity to opioids. We used the microdialysis technique to explore the underlying mechanisms of this phenomenon (Lucas et al. 1998). In rats in which the sciatic nerve was

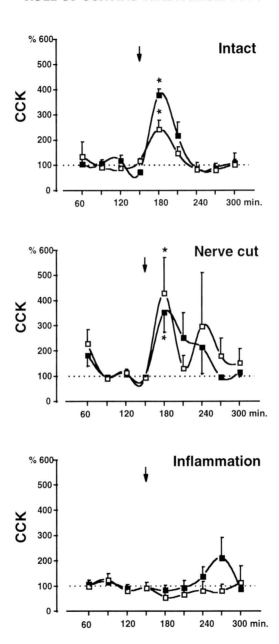

Fig. 2. Time course of the release of CCK in the spinal cord dorsal horn during basal conditions and following i.v. (solid squares) or i.t. (open squares) morphine administration (arrows) in halothane-anesthetized rats with normal peripheral nerves, 2–3 weeks after unilateral section of the sciatic nerve, or 1 day after carrageenan-induced inflammation. Changes in CCK levels are expressed as percentage (mean ± 1 SE) of basal values (average concentration from the three samples obtained before drug administration, defined as 100%). *$P < 0.05$ compared to basal values with the Wilcoxon signed-ranks test. Modified from Lucas et al. (1998), with permission.

unilaterally transected 2–3 weeks prior to the microdialysis experiment, systemic or i.t. morphine induced spinal release of CCK-LI, similar to the response in normal rats (Fig. 2). However, morphine failed to induce any measurable CCK release in rats 16–18 hours after peripheral inflammation induced by subcutaneous injection of carrageenan in the plantar skin of the hindpaw (Fig. 2).

The lack of CCK release by morphine during acute inflammation is unlikely to be due to a reduced level of CCK-LI in the spinal cord, as we have shown that the density of CCK-LI terminals in the dorsal spinal cord was not different on the control side than on the side of carrageenan-induced inflammation (G. Lucas et al., unpublished observations). Thus, acute inflammation may alter the release mechanisms for CCK or change the coupling between opioid receptor activation and terminals releasing CCK. Another interesting finding from the release experiments is that nerve section did not significantly increase CCK release (Lucas et al. 1998). Peripheral nerve injury induces upregulation of CCK mRNA in sensory neurons (Verge et al. 1993; Xu et al. 1993). However, an increase in CCK-LI in sensory neurons and the spinal cord cannot be demonstrated in axotomized animals (Verge et al. 1993). Our results indicate low translation of increased CCK mRNA into peptide in axotomized sensory neurons. Thus, increased CCK activity in nerve-injured rats is probably not due to increased release of CCK. Instead, the released CCK may act on increased numbers of CCK_B receptors in the spinal cord (Zhang et al. 1993), leading to increased efficacy.

CCK AND OPIOID TOLERANCE

Repeated administration of opioids induces a gradual reduction in their ability to induce analgesia, a condition known as tolerance. As CCK antagonizes opioid analgesia, it was suspected that widely distributed endogenous CCK may be involved in tolerance development. Studies with CCK-receptor antagonists have show this to be the case. Both the weak, nonspecific antagonists proglumide and lorglumide and the more recently developed potent CCK_B-receptor antagonists L-365,260 and CI-988 prevented (when applied chronically together with morphine) (Dourish et al. 1990; Xu et al. 1992) and reversed tolerance (when applied acutely in already tolerant animals) (Hoffmann and Wiesenfeld-Hallin 1994). However, the symptoms of physical dependence induced by chronic morphine were not prevented by CCK_B-receptor antagonists, and CCK did not precipitate withdrawal symptoms, indicating that opioid dependence does not involve CCK mechanisms (Dourish et al. 1990; Xu et al. 1992).

The mechanism for the prevention and reversal of morphine tolerance by CCK antagonists has been studied, but the results have been inconsistent. Two studies observed that repeated administration of morphine induced upregulation of CCK mRNA in the spinal cord and in discrete brain areas, a response accompanied by increased CCK content in the brain and spinal cord (Ding and Bayer 1993; Zhou et al. 1994). Other studies reported that the level of preproCCK mRNA (Pohl et al. 1992) and release of CCK (Lucas et al. 1999) were unaffected by acute or chronic morphine treatment. Thus, it is unclear whether opioid tolerance may be related to an upregulation of endogenous CCK levels that induces greater blockade of opioid analgesia. Alternatively, opioid tolerance may be associated with increased levels of CCK-receptor protein (Munro et al. 1998). Blockade of the action of the upregulated CCK system by receptor antagonists may thus restore some of the analgesic effect of the opioid, resulting in the reversal of morphine tolerance (Hoffmann and Wiesenfeld-Hallin 1994). Upregulation of the CCK system may require chronic stimulation of CCK receptors by repeated opioid administration, as CCK antagonists also prevent morphine tolerance.

ACTIVATION OF THE NMDA RECEPTORS BY ACUTE ADMINISTRATION OF OPIOIDS

Opioid antagonists are able to elicit withdrawal symptoms after administration of a single dose of agonist under certain conditions (Eisenberg 1982; Ramabadran 1985). When antagonists are used to reverse the depressive effect of opioids on neuronal activity, the response level often exceeds the original level of activity (Zieglgänsberger and Tölle 1993). This phenomenon has been termed acute opioid dependence or tolerance (Grilly and Gowans 1986; Zieglgänsberger and Tölle 1993). It has been hypothesized that even a single administration of an opioid elicits adaptive changes in the nervous system that attenuate the effect of the ligand. These adaptive changes persist when the depressive effects of opioids are reversed, resulting in hyperexcitability and withdrawal (Zieglgänsberger and Tölle 1993).

Activation of NMDA receptors constitutes an important step in these adaptive changes (Zieglgänsberger and Tölle 1993; Mao et al. 1995a). Iontophoretically applied opioids, in addition to blockade of glutamate-induced responses in dorsal horn neurons, enhanced the response to glutamate upon wash-out (Zieglgänsberger and Tulloch 1979). The enhancement of NMDA-receptor-mediated neuronal responses by opioids has been also reported in other CNS areas (see Zieglgänsberger and Tölle 1993 for review). In particular, intracellular recordings from dorsal horn neurons in vitro indicated that μ agonists enhanced neuronal responsiveness to NMDA (Rusin and Randic 1991; Chen and Huang 1991). Activation of protein kinase C (PKC) by opioids may play an important role in this process (see Mao et al. 1995a for review).

A form of acute opioid dependence or tolerance has been demonstrated in some rat strains, in which a single dose of morphine may induce a delayed hyperalgesic response upon recovery from its antinociceptive effect (Hoffmann et al. 1998). A recent study reported that a single injection of heroin may also induce prolonged hyperalgesia in rats (Laulin et al. 1998). Furthermore, the delayed hyperalgesic effect of morphine or heroin can be abolished by NMDA-receptor antagonists (Laulin et al. 1998; O. Hoffmann et al., unpublished observations), which again suggests the involvement of NMDA receptors in acute opioid dependence or tolerance.

ENHANCEMENT OF ACUTE MORPHINE ANTINOCICEPTION BY NMDA-RECEPTOR ANTAGONISTS

Acute opioid tolerance involving activation of NMDA receptors may reduce the magnitude and duration of opioid-induced antinociception. Thus, blockade of NMDA receptors would be expected to enhance opioid-induced antinociception during acute drug administration. Surprisingly, however, no such enhancement was observed in most earlier studies examining the acute interaction between morphine and NMDA-receptor antagonists (Trujillo and Akil 1991; Tiseo and Inturrisi 1993; Elliott et al. 1994a,b; but see Ben-Eliyahu et al. 1992), perhaps because the design of these studies was not optimal to detect an increase in the magnitude and duration of morphine-induced antinociception. More recently, several studies using various techniques have demonstrated an enhancement of morphine-induced antinociception by several NMDA-receptor antagonists acting at various sites on the receptor complex (Chapman and Dickenson 1992; Advokat and Rhein 1995; Feng and Kendig 1996; Mao et al. 1996; Bhargava 1997).

We systematically examined the interaction between morphine and NMDA-receptor antagonists in behavioral studies in rats, and were able to show a significant potentiation and prolongation of morphine-induced antinociception by NMDA antagonists. We observed potentiation with both the noncompetitive antagonists dextromethorphan, ketamine, and MK-801, and the competitive antagonist CGS-19755 (Hoffmann and Wiesenfeld-Hallin 1996; Grass et al. 1996; Plesan et al. 1998) (Fig. 3). The association of the NMDA-receptor antagonists with morphine did not increase morphine-induced sedation. Moreover, these NMDA antagonists at the doses employed

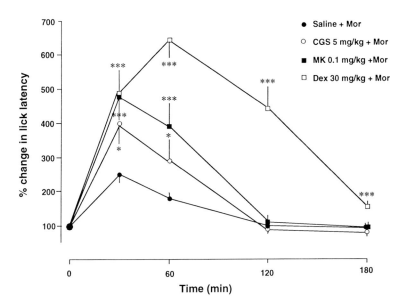

Fig. 3. Effects of 5 mg/kg i.p. morphine on the hindpaw lick latency of rats in the hot-plate test after pretreatment with saline, 5 mg/kg CGS-19755, 0.1 mg/kg MK-801, or 30 mg/kg dextromethorphan. There was a significant overall difference among the four groups as measured by repeated-measures analysis of variance (ANOVA). Data are expressed as mean ± SEM. Individual comparisons were made with factorial ANOVA followed by Fisher's protected least significant difference (PLSD) test. Asterisks indicate statistical significance compared with saline plus morphine: *$P < 0.05$, **$P < 0.01$. Reprinted from Grass et al. (1996), with permission.

did not produce motor impairment or antinociception on their own. Thus, the effects observed after the combined administration of morphine and NMDA antagonists reflect a potentiation of antinociception. Furthermore, as the potentiation was observed with antagonists that had different mechanisms of action, it is likely that the observed effect principally reflected a blockade of the NMDA channel.

The potentiation of morphine-induced antinociception was most profound with dextromethorphan, a noncompetitive blocker of the NMDA channel (Grass et al. 1996; Hoffmann and Wiesenfeld-Hallin 1996; Plesan et al. 1998). In contrast, ketamine (another noncompetitive NMDA-channel blocker) produced the least potentiation, which may be due to its short duration of action (Plesan et al. 1998) (Fig. 4). Dextromethorphan and its metabolite dextrorphan are centrally acting antitussives with no or very weak opioid activity (Tortella et al. 1989). Although dextromethorphan is less potent in blocking the NMDA channel than are MK-801 and CGS-19755, it has a rapid kinetic interaction with the channel (Lipton 1993) and pro-

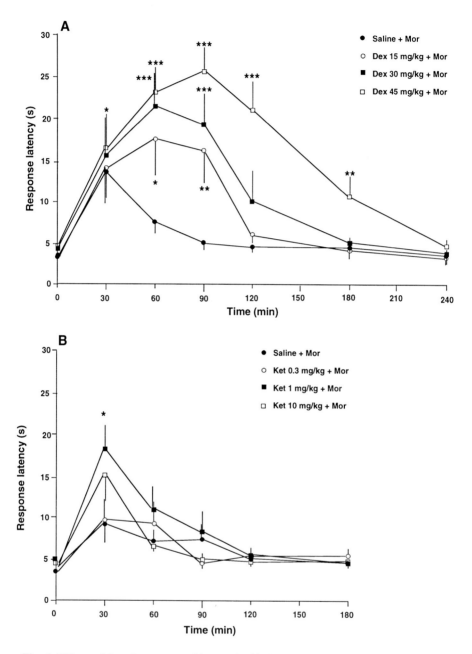

Fig. 4. Effects of 5 mg/kg s.c. morphine on the hindpaw lick latency in the hot-plate test after pretreatment with saline and various doses of (A) dextromethorphan or (B) ketamine. The data are analyzed with ANOVA followed by Fisher's PLSD test and are expressed as mean ± SEM. Asterisks indicate significance compared to saline plus morphine: *$P < 0.05$, **$P < 0.01$, ***$P < 0.001$. Note that ketamine potentiated morphine antinociception at 1 mg/kg at only one time point. Reprinted from Plesan et al. (1998), with permission.

duces fewer side effects than do the other two compounds. It is therefore possible to use a higher dose of dextromethorphan, which may more effectively block the NMDA receptor, rather than MK-801 and CGS-19755 in the relatively low doses necessary to avoid disturbance in motor function. Thus, the observed difference in the morphine-potentiating effect of the various NMDA antagonists may be due to a different level of receptor blockade at the doses used. However, we cannot rule out the possibility that dextromethorphan has other effects unrelated to NMDA-receptor antagonism (Carpenter et al. 1988; Tortella et al. 1989), which may also contribute to its pronounced potentiating effect on morphine-induced antinociception.

NMDA-RECEPTOR ACTIVATION AND OPIOID SENSITIVITY

The role of NMDA-receptor activation in opioid insensitivity in neuropathic pain has been studied recently. Mao et al. (1995b) showed that in rats with chronic sciatic nerve constriction injury, i.t. MK-801 alleviated thermal hyperalgesia but did not reverse the reduced effect of morphine. In contrast, Yamamoto and Yaksh (1992) reported that i.t. MK-801 enhanced the reduced effect of morphine on thermal hyperalgesia after nerve constriction injury. Similarly, Nichols et al. (1997) observed that in the neuropathic pain model of spinal nerve ligation, coadministration of MK-801 with morphine totally reversed the ineffectiveness of morphine in producing anti-allodynia and antinociception in the tail-flick test.

We recently studied this issue using a photochemically induced sciatic nerve ischemia model of neuropathic pain (Kupers et al. 1998). In this model, rats developed mechanical and cold allodynia-like behavior that was not alleviated by systemic morphine at doses that did not cause sedation (Kauppila et al. 1998). However, combining dextromethorphan (which by itself had no effect) with morphine produced strong anti-allodynia (Kauppila et al. 1998). The opioid-receptor antagonist naloxone totally reversed the anti-allodynic effect of the coadministration of morphine and dextromethorphan. Thus, this drug combination mediates its anti-allodynic effect primarily via opioid receptors.

THE NMDA RECEPTOR AND OPIOID TOLERANCE

Coadministration of different classes of NMDA antagonists prevents or reduces morphine tolerance (Marek et al. 1991; Trujillo and Akil 1991; Ben-Eliyahu et al. 1992; Tiseo and Inturrisi 1993; Elliot et al. 1994a,b; Lutfy et al. 1995; Mao et al. 1996). It has been proposed that acute enhancement of

NMDA-receptor activity by opioids may lead to persistent changes in the state of these receptors following chronic opioid administration, possibly involving the production of nitric oxide or activation of PKC (Mao et al. 1995a). Such changes in NMDA receptors increase excitatory transmission in the nervous system and may partially contribute to opioid tolerance (see Mao et al. 1995a for review). After tolerance has developed, the administration of NMDA antagonists could reestablish the antinociceptive effect of opioids (Tiseo and Inturrisi 1993; Elliot et al. 1994a,b). The interpretation of the results of these studies is based on the assumption that there is no acute potentiation of opioid-induced antinociception by NMDA antagonists. This notion, however, is not supported by other data. Therefore, it is possible that the apparent reversal of tolerance may result from the potentiation of the residual effect of the opioid by the NMDA antagonists, rather than representing a genuine reversal of tolerance (Hoffmann and Wiesenfeld-Hallin 1996).

CONCLUSIONS

CCK and glutamate acting on NMDA receptors may have a role in mediating the magnitude of opioid analgesia and in the development of tolerance and opioid insensitivity that is observed in some pain states. Thus, blockade of CCK and NMDA receptors may have potential clinical applications in pain management. This effect may reduce the required analgesic dose of the opioid, leading to fewer and weaker side effects. It may also delay the development of tolerance because of low-level stimulation of opioid receptors. Furthermore, in opioid-insensitive pain states or in patients tolerant to opioids, antagonists of the CCK and NMDA receptors may be analgesic or may reinstate the analgesic effect of opioids. These concepts should be vigorously tested in clinical studies, primarily with clinically available drugs with NMDA-receptor-blocking properties.

ACKNOWLEDGMENTS

The studies in the authors' laboratory were conducted with the support of the Swedish Medical Research Council (projects 07913 to ZWH and 12168 to XJX), the Biomed II program of the European Commission (project BMH4 CT95 0172), Astra Pain Control AB, and the Clinical Research Center at Huddinge University Hospital.

REFERENCES

Advokat C, Rhein FQ. Potentiation of morphine-induced antinociception in acute spinal rats by the NMDA antagonist dextrophan. *Brain Res* 1995; 699:157–160.

Arnér S, Meyerson B. Opioids in neuropathic pain. *Pain Digest* 1993; 3:15–22.

Benedetti F. The opposite effects of the opiate antagonist naloxone an+d the cholecystokinin antagonist proglumide on placebo analgesia. *Pain* 1996; 64:535–543.

Benoliel JJ, Bourgoin S, Mauborgne A, et al. Differential inhibitory/stimulatory modulation of spinal CCK release by mu and delta opioid agonists, and selective blockade of mu-dependent inhibition by kappa receptor stimulation. *Neurosci Lett* 1991; 124:204–207.

Ben-Eliyahu S, Marek P, Vaccarino AL, et al. The NMDA receptor antagonist MK-801 prevents long-lasting non-associative morphine tolerance in the rat. *Brain Res* 1992; 575:304–308.

Bhargava HN. Enhancement of morphine actions in morphine-naive and morphine-tolerant mice by LY 235959, a competitive antagonist of the NMDA receptor. *Gen Pharmacol* 1997; 28:61–64.

Carpenter CL, Marks SS, Watson DL, Greenberg DA. Dextromethorphan and dextrorphan as calcium channel antagonists. *Brain Res* 1988; 439:372–375.

Cesselin F. Opioid and anti-opioid peptides. *Fundam Clin Pharmacol* 1995; 9:409–433.

Chapman V, Dickenson AH. The combination of NMDA antagonism and morphine produces profound antinociception in the rat dorsal horn. *Brain Res* 1992; 573:321–323.

Chen L, Huang LY. Sustained potentiation of NMDA receptor-mediated glutamate responses through activation of protein-kinase C by μ-opioids. *Neuron* 1991; 7:319–326.

Ding XZ, Bayer BM. Increases of CCK mRNA and peptide in different brain areas following acute and chronic administration of morphine. *Brain Res* 1993; 625:139–144.

Dourish CT, O'Neill MF, Coughlan J, et al. The selective CCK-B receptor antagonist L-365,260 enhances morphine analgesia and prevents morphine tolerance in the rat. *Eur J Pharmacol* 1990; 176:35–44.

Eisenberg RM. Further studies on the acute dependence produced by morphine in opiate naive rats. *Life Sci* 1982; 31:1531–1540.

Elliott K, Hynansky A, Inturrisi CE. Dextromethorphan attenuates and reverses analgesic tolerance to morphine. *Pain* 1994a; 59:361–368.

Elliott K, Minami N, Kolesnikov YA, Pasternak GW, Inturrisi CE. The NMDA receptor antagonists, LY274614 and MK-801, and the nitric oxide synthase inhibitor, NG-nitro-L-arginine, attenuate analgesic tolerance to the mu-opioid morphine but not to kappa opioids. *Pain* 1994b; 56:69–75.

Faris PL, Komisaruk BR, Watkins LR, Mayer DJ. Evidence for the neuropeptide cholecystokinin as an antagonist of opiate analgesia. *Science* 1983; 219:310–312.

Feng J, Kendig JJ. The NMDA receptor antagonist MK-801 differentially modulates μ and κ opioid actions in spinal cord in vitro. *Pain* 1996; 66:342–349.

Ghilardi JR, Allen CJ, Vigna SR, McVey DC, Mantyh PW. Trigeminal and dorsal root ganglion neurons express CCK receptor binding sites in the rat, rabbit and monkey: possible site of opiate-CCK analgesic interactions. *J Neurosci* 1992; 12:4854–4866.

Grass S, Hoffmann O, Xu X-J, Wiesenfeld-Hallin Z. N-methyl-D-aspartate receptor antagonists potentiate morphine's antinociceptive effect in the rat. *Acta Physiol Scand* 1996; 158:269–273.

Grilly DM, Gowans GC. Acute morphine dependence: effects observed in shock and light discrimination tasks. *Psychopharmacology* 1986; 88:500–504.

Han JS, Ding XZ, Fan SG. Cholecystokinin octapeptide (CCK-8): antagonism to electroacupuncture analgesia and a possible role in electroacupuncture tolerance. *Pain* 1986; 27:101–115.

Hill DR, Shaw TM, Graham W, Woodruff GN. Autoradiographical detection of cholecystokinin-A receptors in primate brain using 125I-bolton hunter CCK-8 and 3H-MK-329. *J Neurosci* 1990; 10:1070–1081.

Hoffmann O, Wiesenfeld-Hallin Z. The CCK-B receptor antagonist Cl 988 reverses tolerance to morphine in rats. *Neuroreport* 1994; 5:2565–2568.

Hoffmann O, Wiesenfeld-Hallin Z. Dextromethorphan potentiates morphine antinociception, but does not reverse tolerance in rats. *Neuroreport* 1996; 7:838–840.

Hoffmann O, Plesan A, Wiesenfeld-Hallin Z. Genetic differences in morphine sensitivity, tolerance and withdrawal in rats. *Brain Res* 1998; 806:232–237.

Itoh S, Katsuura G, Maeda Y. Caerulein and cholecystokinin suppress b-endorphin-induced analgesia in rats. *Eur J Pharmacol* 1982; 80:421–425.

Kastin AJ, Stephens E, Ehrensing RH, Fischman AJ. Tyr-MIF-I acts as an opiate antagonists in the tail flick test. *Pharmacol Biochem Behav* 1984; 21:937–941.

Kupers R, Yu W, Persson J, Xu X-J, Wiesenfeld-Hallin Z. Photochemically-induced ischemia of the rat sciatic nerve produces a dose-dependent and highly reproducible mechanical, heat and cold allodynia and signs of spontaneous pain. *Pain* 1998; 76:45–60.

Kauppila T, Xu X-J, Yu W, Wiesenfeld-Hallin Z. Dextromethorphan potentiates the anti-allodynic effect of morphine in rats with peripheral neuropathy. *Neuroreport* 1998; 9:1071–1074.

Laulin J-P, Larcher A, Célèrier E, Le Moal M, Simonnet G. Long-lasting increased pain sensitivity in rat following exposure to heroin for the first time. *Eur J Neurosci* 1998; 10:782–785.

Lee Y-W, Chaplan SR, Yaksh TL. Systemic and supraspinal, but not spinal, opiates suppress allodynia in a rat neuropathic pain model. *Neurosci Lett* 1995; 186:111–1114.

Lindefors N, Linden A, Brene S, Sedvall G, Persson H. CCK peptides and mRNA in the human brain. *Prog Neurobiol* 1993; 40:671–690.

Lipton SA. Prospects for clinically tolerated NMDA antagonists: open-channel blockers and alternative redox states of nitric oxide. *Trends Neurosci* 1993; 16:527–532.

Lucas GA, Alster P, Brodin E, Wiesenfeld-Hallin Z. Differential release of cholecystokinin by morphine in rat spinal cord. *Neurosci Lett* 1998; 245:13–16.

Lucas G, Hoffmann O, Alster P, Wiesenfeld-Hallin Z. Extracellular cholecystokinin levels in the rat spinal cord following chronic morphine exposure: an *in vivo* microdialysis study. *Brain Res* 1999; 821:79–86.

Lutfy K, Shen KZ, Kwon IS, et al. Blockade of morphine tolerance by ACEA-1328, a novel NMDA receptor/glycine site antagonist. *Eur J Pharmacol* 1995; 273:187–189.

Mao J, Price DD, Mayer DJ. Mechanisms of hyperalgesia and morphine tolerance: a current view of their possible interactions. *Pain* 1995a; 62:259–274.

Mao J, Price DD, Mayer DJ. Experimental mononeuropathy reduces the antinociceptive effects of morphine: implications for common intracellular mechanisms involved in morphine tolerance and neuropathic pain. *Pain* 1995b; 61:353–364.

Mao J, Price DD, Caruso FS, Mayer DJ. Oral administration of dextromethorphan prevents the development of morphine tolerance and dependence in rats. *Pain* 1996; 67:361–368.

Marek P, Ben-Eliyahu S, Gold M, Liebeskind JC. Excitatory amino acid antagonists (kynurenic acid and MK-801) attenuate the development of morphine tolerance in the rat. *Brain Res* 1991; 547:77–81.

Moran T, Robinson P, Goldrich MS, McHugh P. Two brain cholecystokinin receptors: implications for behavioural actions. *Brain Res* 1986; 362:175–179.

Munro G, Pumford KM, Russell JA. Altered cholecystokinin binding site density in the supraoptic nucelus of morphine-tolerant and -dependent rats. *Brain Res* 1998; 780:190–198.

Nichols ML, Bian D, Ossipov MH, Lai J, Porreca F. Regulation of morphine antiallodynic efficacy by cholecystokinin in a model of neuropathic pain in rats. *J Pharmacol Exp Ther* 1995; 275:1399–1345.

Nichols ML, Lopez Y, Ossipov MH, Bian D, Porreca F. Enhancement of the antiallodynic and antinociceptive efficacy of spinal morphine by antisera to dynorphin A (1–13) or MK-801 in a nerve-ligation model of peripheral neuropathy. *Pain* 1997; 69:317–322.

Ossipov MH, Lopez Y, Nichols ML, Bian D, Porreca F. Inhibition by spinal morphine of the tail-flick response is attenuated in rats with nerve ligation injury. *Neurosci Lett* 1995; 199:83–86.

Plesan A, Hedman U, Xu X-J, Wiesenfeld-Hallin Z. Comparison of ketamine and dextromethorphan in potentiating the antinociceptive effect of morphine in rats. *Anesth Analg* 1998; 86:825–829.

Pohl M, Collin E, Benoliel JJ, et al. Cholecystokinin (CCK)-like material and CCK mRNA levels in the rat brain and spinal cord after acute or repeated morphine treatment. *Neuropeptides* 1992; 21:193–200.

Ramabadran K. An analysis of precipitated withdrawal in rats acutely dependent on morphine. *Jap J Pharmacol* 1985; 37:307–316.

Rehfeld JF. Immunochemical studies of cholecystokinin: distribution and molecular heterogeneity of cholecystokinin in the central nervous system and small intestine of man and hog. *J Biol Chem* 1978; 253:4022–4030.

Rusin KI, Randic M. Modulation of NMDA-induced currents by mu-opioid receptor agonist DAGO in acutely isolated rat spinal dorsal horn neurons. *Neurosci Lett* 1991; 124:208–212.

Schiffmann SN, Vanderhaeghen J-J. Distribution of cells containing mRNA encoding cholecystokinin in the rat central nervous system. *J Comp Neurol* 1991; 304:219–233.

Stanfa LC, Dickenson AH. Cholecystokinin as a factor in the enhanced potency of spinal morphine following carrageenan inflammation. *Br J Pharmacol* 1993; 108:967–973.

Tang J, Chou J, Iadarola M, Yang HY, Costa E. Proglumide prevents and curtails acute tolerance to morphine in rats. *Neuropharmacology* 1984; 23:715–718.

Tiseo PJ, Inturrisi CE. Attenuation and reversal of morphine tolerance by the competitive N-methyl-D-aspartate receptor antagonist LY274614. *J Pharmacol Exp Ther* 1993; 264:1090–1096.

Tortella FC, Pellicano M, Bowery NG. Dextromethorphan and neuromodulation: old drug coughs up new activities. *Trends Pharmacol Sci* 1989; 10:501–507.

Trujillo KA, Akil H. Inhibition of morphine tolerance and dependence by the NMDA receptor antagonist MK-801. *Science* 1991; 251:85–87.

Valverde O, Maldonado R, Fournie-Zaluski MC, Roques BP. Cholecystokinin B antagonists strongly potentiate antinociception mediated by endogenous enkephalins. *J Pharmacol Exp Ther* 1994; 270:77–88.

Vanderah TW, Lai J, Yamamura HI, Porreca F. Antisense oligodeoxynucleotide to the CCKB receptor produces naltrindole and [Leu5]enkephalin antiserum-sensitive enhancement of morphine antinociception. *Neuroreport* 1994; 5:1–5.

Verge VMK, Wiesenfeld-Hallin Z, Hökfelt T. Cholecystokinin in mammalian primary sensory neurons and spinal cord: in situ hybridization studies in rat and monkey. *Eur J Neurosci* 1993; 5:240–250.

Wang XJ, Han JS. Modification by cholecystokinin octapeptide of the binding of μ-, δ- and k-opioid receptors. *J Neurochem* 1989; 55:1379–1382.

Wang JF, Ren MF, Han JS. Mobilization of calcium from intracellular stores is one of the mechanisms underlying the antiopioid effect of cholecystokinin octapeptide. *Peptides* 1992; 13:947–951.

Watkins LR., Kinscheck IB, Kaufman EF, et al. Cholecystokinin antagonists selectively potentiate analgesia induced by endogenous opiates. *Brain Res* 1985; 327:181–190.

Wiesenfeld-Hallin Z. Combined opioid–NMDA antagonist therapies. What advantage do they offer for the control of pain syndromes? *Drugs* 1998; 55:1–4.

Wiesenfeld-Hallin Z, Xu X-J. The role of cholecystokinin in nociception, neuropathic pain and opiate tolerance. *Regul Pept* 1996; 65:23–28.

Wiesenfeld-Hallin Z, Xu X-J, Hughes J, Horwell DC, Hökfelt T. PD134308, a selective antagonist of cholecystokinin type B receptor, enhances the analgesic effect of morphine and synergistically interacts with intrathecal galanin to depress spinal nociceptive reflexes. *Proc Natl Acad Sci USA* 1990; 87:7105–7109.

Williams RG, Dimaline R, Varro A, et al. Cholecystokinin octapeptide in rat central nervous system: immunocytochemical studies using a monoclonal antibody that does not react with CGRP. *Neurochem Int* 1987; 11:433–442.

Xu X-J, Wiesenfeld-Hallin Z. The threshold for the depressive effect of intrathecal morphine on the spinal nociceptive flexor reflex is increased during autotomy after sciatic nerve section in rats. *Pain* 1991; 46:223–229.

Xu X-J, Wiesenfeld-Hallin Z. Opioid-antiopioid interaction in Analgesia. In: Stein C (Ed). *Opioids and Pain Control.* New York: Cambridge University Press, 1999, pp 131–142.

Xu X-J, Wiesenfeld-Hallin Z, Hughes J, Horwell DC, Hökfelt T. CI988, a selective antagonist of cholecystokinin type-B receptor, prevents morphine tolerance in the rat. *Br J Pharmacol* 1992; 105:591–596.

Xu X-J, Puke MJC, Verge VMK, et al. Up-regulation of cholecystokinin in primary sensory neurons is associated with morphine insensitivity in experimental neuropathic pain. *Neurosci Lett* 1993; 152:129–132.

Xu X-J, Hökfelt T, Hughes J, Wiesenfeld-Hallin Z. The CCK-B antagonist CI988 enhances the reflex-depressive effect of morphine in axotomized rats. *Neuroreport* 1994; 5:718–720.

Yamamoto T, Nozakitaguchi N. Role of cholecystokinin-B receptor in the maintenance of thermal hyperalgesia induced by unilateral constriction injury to the sciatic nerve in the rat. *Neurosci Lett* 1995; 202:89–92.

Yamamoto T, Yaksh TL. Studies on the spinal interaction of morphine and the NMDA antagonist MK-801 on the hyperesthesia observed in a rat model of sciatic mononeuropathy. *Neurosci Lett* 1992; 135:67–70.

Yang HYT, Fratta W, Majabe EA, Costa E. Isolation, sequencing, synthesis and pharmacological characterization of two brain neuropeptides that modulate the action of morphine. *Proc Natl Acad Sci USA* 1985; 82:7757–7761.

Zhang X, Dagerlind Å, Elde RP, et al. Marked increase in cholecystokinin B receptor messenger RNA levels in rat dorsal root ganglia after peripheral axotomy. *Neuroscience* 1993; 57:227–233.

Zhou Y, Sun YH, Zhang ZW, Han JS. Increased release of immunoreactive cholecystokinin octapeptide by morphine and potentiation of ∝-opioid analgesia by CCKB receptor antagonist L365,260 in rat spinal cord. *Eur J Pharmacol* 1993; 234:147–154.

Zhou Y, Sun YH, Zhang ZW, Han JS. Accelerated expression of cholecystokinin gene in the brain of rats rendered tolerant to morphine. *Neuroreport* 1994; 3:1121–1123.

Zieglgänsberger W, Tölle TR. The pharmacology of pain signalling. *Curr Opin Neurobiol* 1993; 3:611–618.

Zieglgänsberger W, Tulloch IF. The effects of methionine- and leucine-enkephalin on spinal neurones of the cat. *Brain Res* 1979; 167:53–64.

Correspondence to: Professor Zsuzsanna Wiesenfeld-Hallin, PhD, Division of Clinical Neurophysiology, Karolinska Institute, Huddinge University Hospital, S-141 86 Huddinge, Sweden. Tel: 46-8-585 87085; Fax: 46-8-585 87050; email: zsuzsanna.wiesenfeld-hallin@neurophys.hs.sll.se.

Opioid Sensitivity of Chronic Noncancer Pain,
Progress in Pain Research and Management,
Vol. 14, edited by Eija Kalso, Henry J. McQuay,
and Zsuzsanna Wiesenfeld-Hallin, IASP Press,
Seattle, © 1999.

15

Alpha, Omega, and In Between

Sandra R. Chaplan

*Anesthesiology Research Laboratory, University of California, San Diego,
La Jolla, California, USA*

NONOPIOID-RESPONSIVE NEUROPATHIC PAIN

More than 10 years ago, Arnér and Meyerson suggested that opioids may be ineffective in the treatment of pain due to worsening of the underlying condition, the development of opioid tolerance, or the prior existence or development of a nonopioid-responsive condition (Arnér and Meyerson 1988). While therapeutic improvements may follow opioid dose increases in the first two cases, it has been recognized for some time that certain forms of pain are simply not effectively treated with opioids, whatever the useful effects of such drugs may be on mood or level of consciousness.

Many nonopioid-responsive pain conditions are neuropathic in nature. These conditions are the result of some form of injury to neural tissue, whether to the peripheral nerve, spinal cord, or brain. Many mechanisms of nerve injury result in neuropathic syndromes with strikingly similar manifestations; etiologies include (but are not limited to) trauma (accidental or surgical), infection (as in herpetic or HIV-related neuritides), ischemia, metabolic derangement (as in diabetes), solid tumor invasion, and cancer treatment (surgery, radiation, and chemotherapy). These numerous forms of nerve injury result in neuropathic states that typically exhibit spontaneous burning and intermittent lancinating pain, paresthesias/dysesthesias, hyperalgesia, and allodynia (pain evoked by light touch). Although allodynia is also displayed in other pain syndromes, it is a hallmark of neuropathic pain (Wahren and Torebjörk 1992; Koltzenburg et al. 1994).

Allodynia most likely results from several different mechanisms, and displays varying degrees of response to morphine depending on its etiology. We chose to focus on the L5/L6 spinal nerve ligation (SNL) model of Kim and Chung (1992). This model has readily apparent clinical correlations, is

highly reproducible, represents an anatomically well-delineated injury, and
does not respond to lumbar intrathecal (i.t.) morphine administration up to
highly sedative doses (Bian et al. 1995; Lee et al. 1995). As such, it is a
useful model of nonopioid-responsive pain due to focal, traumatic nerve injury.

    A working explanation for the ineffectiveness of lumbar i.t. morphine is
suggested by the observation that capsaicin, administered to neonatal rats at
doses high enough to destroy virtually all C fibers (Nagy et al. 1983), has no
effect on the development of allodynia after subsequent nerve ligation at 5
weeks of age (Fig. 1) (Okuse et al. 1997). This observation strongly suggests
that C fibers are not required during either the initiation process or the
maintenance phase of allodynia, and concurs with previous findings that
established allodynia is transduced by Aβ fibers (Price et al. 1989; Shir and
Seltzer 1990). The lack of effect of lumbar i.t. morphine administration on
the Aβ fibers that transduce allodynia is reasonable in that μ-opioid receptors are associated with small nociceptive neurons, or with the central terminals of thinly myelinated/unmyelinated fibers in lamina II, and not with Aβ
fibers or their cell bodies (Honda and Arvidsson 1995; Taddese et al. 1995).

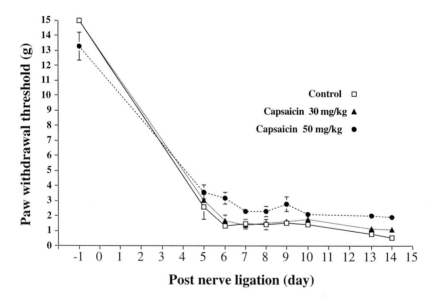

Fig. 1. Development of allodynia in the spinal nerve ligation (SNL) model after
neonatal capsaicin treatment. Male Harlan Sprague-Dawley rats were treated i.p. with
capsaicin 50 mg/kg, capsaicin 30 mg/kg, or vehicle alone, within 48 hours of birth. At
5 weeks of age, all underwent left L5/L6 tight SNL under halothane/oxygen anesthesia.
Tactile allodynia was measured in awake rats by touching the left hindpaw with von
Frey filaments and using responses to calculate the 50% threshold for paw withdrawal
in grams ($n = 6$ rats per group). No difference was seen between control and treated
groups; all developed robust allodynia (threshold below 4 g) of the same magnitude
and time course. Error bars denote SEM.

ALTERNATIVE DRUGS

Several alternative therapeutic agents have proven to be useful in the pain clinic, and more are in preclinical phases of development; others are still on the drawing board. This chapter discusses the following drug classes: α_2-adrenoceptor agonists, N-type voltage-dependent calcium channel (VDCC) blockers, $\alpha_2\delta$ VDCC subunit blockers, nitric oxide synthase (NOS) inhibitors, and sodium channel (NaC) blockers.

ALPHA-2 ADRENOCEPTOR AGONISTS

Ample research has shown that α_2 adrenoceptor agonists have analgesic as well as antiallodynic properties, in both clinical and preclinical models (Kauppila et al. 1991; Rauck et al. 1993; Puke et al. 1994). Activation of the α_2 adrenoceptor appears to suppress VDCC activation and thereby prohibit neurotransmitter release (Adamson et al. 1989; Xiang et al. 1990). In our own laboratory, the i.t. administration of a panel of α_2 agonists has shown efficacy for all agents tested, with potency ranking: dexmedetomidine > clonidine > UK14304 > ST-91 > oxymetazoline > guanfacine (Yaksh et al. 1995). Fig. 2 shows dose-response curves for these agents in the SNL model, with morphine and methoxamine (an α_1-adrenoceptor agonist), both lacking in antiallodynic effects, for comparison. Clear evidence for a direct spinal site of action for α_2-agonist analgesia includes not only the large antiallodynic/analgesic dose ratio of systemic to spinal α_2-agonist administration, but also work utilizing knockout mice with inoperative α_2-receptor subtypes, which has delineated the α_{2A} receptor as responsible for spinal analgesia (Stone et al. 1997). Previous attempts to explain α_2-agonist analgesia on the basis of inhibition of sympathetic outflow and decreased catecholaminergic interaction with afferent fibers appear less powerful in the context of observations that these agents are analgesic in models that have not shown analgesic responses to sympathectomy (Ahlgren and Levine 1993; Calcutt and Chaplan 1997). The SNL model has shown varying responses to sympathectomy in different laboratories (Kim and Chung 1991), and there appear to be important strain influences on the contribution of the sympathetic nervous system to hyperalgesia, lacking in Sprague-Dawley rats; this is an active area of research (Lee et al. 1997). Curious findings are that the distribution of the α_{2A} adrenoceptor subtype mainly includes smaller, capsaicin-sensitive neurons that co-express substance P (Stone et al. 1998), and that α_{2A} expression is dramatically *diminished* by rhizotomy and nerve ligation. These observations are difficult to reconcile with the clear antihyperalgesic effects of α_2 agonists after nerve injury, despite reduced receptor presence, and so further studies are required.

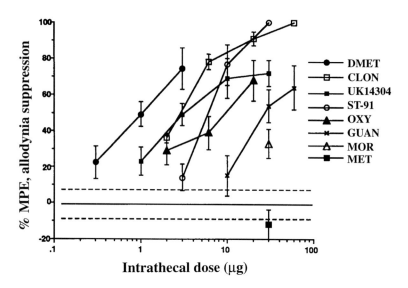

Fig. 2. Responses to α_2 adrenoceptor agonists (percentage of maximal possible effect [MPE] in suppressing allodynia, up to the maximum tolerated dose) in male Harlan Sprague-Dawley rats that underwent left L5/L6 SNL at approximately 5 weeks of age, followed by lumbar i.t. drug dosing (n = 4–6 rats per dose). Tactile allodynia was assessed in the left hindpaw as described for Fig. 1. DMET = dexmedetomidine, α_2 agonist; CLON = clonidine, α_2 agonist; UK14304 = α_2 agonist; ST-91 = α_2 agonist; OXY = oxymetazoline, α_2 agonist; GUAN = guanfacine, α_2 agonist; MOR = morphine, μ agonist; MET = methoxamine, α_1 agonist. The α_2 agonists as a group provide antiallodynic effects, with differing potencies and efficacies in the range of 70–100%. In comparison, morphine has an insignificant effect at maximum dose, and methoxamine has no effect or may possibly augment allodynia.

Clinical use of α_2-adrenoceptor agonists may be limited by cross-tolerance with morphine, despite a strong unidirectional tolerance bias. While rats made tolerant to α_2 agonists are also tolerant to morphine, rats made tolerant to morphine do not exhibit immediate α_2-agonist tolerance (Stevens et al. 1988). Clinical α_2-agonist side effects of hypotension, sedation, and mouth dryness require specific attention in management. Since tolerance does develop to α_2-agonist administration, dose escalation may be necessary, and the risk of abstinence syndrome (with profound hypertension) is present if the drug is abruptly withheld.

VOLTAGE-DEPENDENT CALCIUM CHANNEL BLOCKERS

For some time, it has been recognized that control of neurotransmitter release in pain states could be beneficial. Since Ca^{2+} channels play an intimate role in neurotransmitter release, a therapeutic role for calcium channel antagonists was postulated several years ago, but clinical studies with cardioactive calcium channel blockers available at that time proved disappointing. The VDCC family is now better understood and includes increasingly numerous cloned subtypes. These channels consist of an α_1 pore-forming subunit associated with a β subunit and an $\alpha_2\delta$ subunit consisting of two peptide moieties encoded by the same gene (De Jongh et al. 1990). All clinically available Ca^{2+} channel blocking agents interact with the L-type VDCC, prominent in cardiac tissue. The P-type VDCC is widely found in the brain, and the N-type in neural tissue. Our studies of Ca^{2+} channel subtype antagonists in the SNL model (Chaplan et al. 1994) demonstrate the specificity of the role of these receptor subtypes in allodynia. L-type VDCC blockers are completely ineffective against allodynia in the SNL model by both the intravenous (i.v.) and the lumbar i.t. routes. Omega conotoxins (conopeptides), derived from the venom of the fish-hunting sea snail, provide a powerful research tool as highly selective N-type VDCC blockers. Fig. 3 shows the significant efficacy with which these extremely potent compounds inhibit allodynia. These compounds are highly effective, but only by the i.t. route: they cross the blood–brain barrier only in the most

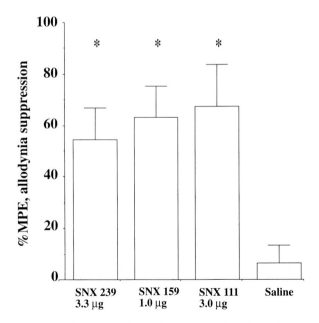

Fig. 3. Responses to voltage-dependent calcium channel (VDCC) blockers (percentage of maximal possible effect [MPE] in suppressing allodynia, up to the maximum tolerated dose). Male Harlan Sprague-Dawley rats with SNL and indwelling lumbar i.t. catheters were treated with SNX 239, SNX 159, or SNX 111, all N-type selective VDCC-blocking conotoxins ($n = 6$ rats per dose). Efficacy ranges from 55% to 65%. * $P < 0.05$, one-way ANOVA, Fisher's protected least significant differences (PSLD); error bars denote SEM.

limited amounts, and so the site of action appears to be in the spinal cord. Motor side effects are limiting; tremor and ataxia become problematic at doses above those illustrated. These agents have recently entered clinical trials for terminal cancer pain as well as refractory neuropathic pain of benign origin. Their clinical efficacy appears to be comparable to preclinical observations (Presley et al. 1998), and it remains to be seen whether they will be accepted into the clinical repertoire. The necessity of intraspinal administration limits their use to situations where lumbar puncture/cannulation is appropriate. We have also examined the effects of P-type channel blockade; P-type channels appear to be so ubiquitous in the nervous system and brain, and their function so fundamentally important, that their blockade is lethal; in preclinical studies, it was not possible to show analgesic effects below a dose that was immediately fatal.

GABAPENTINOIDS

It is appropriate to consider the gabapentinoids in the context of agents that act upon VDCC. This drug class, presently consisting of gabapentin and S-isobutyl-GABA, has marked antiallodynic actions (Mellick et al. 1995; Xiao and Bennett 1997; Partridge et al. 1998). Gabapentin has been in clinical use for neuropathic pain since its first introduction to the market as an anticonvulsant. Its preclinical evaluation in this context was prompted by clinicians' reports of favorable effects in pain patients. Gabapentin exerts marked dose-responsive antiallodynic effects in the SNL model (Hwang and Yaksh 1997). S-isobutyl-GABA shows the same profile as gabapentin in preclinical trials, with increased potency (Partridge et al. 1998).

The mechanism of action of these drugs is unknown. They do not interact with any known receptor or channel that has been associated with pain; despite their name, they do not have any effect on γ-aminobutyric acid (GABA) receptors (Taylor 1995). However, gabapentin has recently been shown to bind to the $\alpha_2\delta$ VDCC subunit in homogenized porcine brain (Gee et al. 1996). The relevance of this finding to pain states remains to be elucidated. The $\alpha_2\delta$ Ca^{2+} channel subunit exists in several tissue-specific splice variants (Angelotti and Hofmann 1996). The role of this subunit is incompletely understood (Wiser et al. 1996): it modulates the binding affinity of ω-conotoxins to the N-type VDCC (Brust et al. 1993), and augments the inward current amplitude of the α_{1C} subunit (Singer et al. 1991).

Recent data from our laboratory show marked upregulation of the $\alpha_2\delta$ VDCC subunit in the dorsal root ganglia (DRG) and spinal cord of SNL rats. In semiquantitative studies using ribonuclease (RNase) protection assays, we used an antisense probe designed to protect a specific, unique base sequence of the mRNA encoding the $\alpha_2\delta$ protein. Fig. 4 shows electrophoretic migration of protected mRNA bands of the expected size for the $\alpha_2\delta$ subunit (Luo et al. 1999). Six- to seven-fold upregulation of $\alpha_2\delta$ mRNA is seen by day 2, and 14-fold upregulation by 1 week postligation in the ipsilateral L5/L6 DRG. Western blotting shows that $\alpha_2\delta$ protein follows suit and is similarly upregulated. These results would suggest that $\alpha_2\delta$ subunits may play a role in allodynia, and that they may be in fact a target of drug action for gabapentin and congeners. However, we cannot afford to be complacent, and must await more stringent confirmation of a causal role of $\alpha_2\delta$.

NITRIC OXIDE SYNTHASE INHIBITORS

We have recently explored the role of neuronal nitric oxide synthase (nNOS) in tactile allodynia. NOS clearly appears to play a role in thermal hyperalgesia (Yonehara et al. 1977; Meller et al. 1992; Lam et al. 1996; Wu et al. 1998; Yoon et al. 1998). nNOS mRNA is upregulated, along with NOS protein, in the DRG of ligated spinal nerves in SNL rats (Fig. 5). However, specific pharmacological inhibition does not decrease pain behavior (Fig. 6), either prospectively or as treatment after injury. Furthermore, upregulation

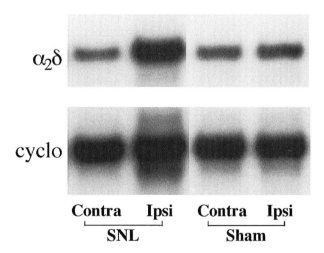

Fig. 4. Upregulation of $\alpha_2\delta$ VDCC subunit mRNA in the L5/L6 dorsal root ganglia (DRG) in the SNL model. Total RNA was extracted from tissues of male Harlan Sprague-Dawley rats 1 week after SNL, and RNase protection assays were performed using probes designed to protect a 413-base sequence of the $\alpha_2\delta$ subunit. Normalization of the protected $\alpha_2\delta$ band densities against a 300-base cyclophilin (cyclo) internal control sequence reveals an approximately 400% increase in $\alpha_2\delta$ mRNA in the L5/L6 DRG of the ligated (ipsi) side compared to the contralateral (contra) side in the second lane. A correspondingly large increase in $\alpha_2\delta$ protein was also observed (data not shown).

outlasts the pain behavior. Also, a strain of rats that does not display allodynia after nerve injury still shows nNOS upregulation (Luo et al. 1998). Work with knockout mice substantiates this finding (Traub et al. 1994; Crosby et al. 1995). In summary, nNOS regulation does not correlate with allodynia behavior. We interpret these results to mean that whatever other role nNOS may play, it is not directly involved in allodynia. This does not mean that nNOS may not have a vitally important role in controlling events that are important in the pathogenesis of allodynia; it merely indicates that it is not a useful drug target either for the prevention or the reversal of allodynia. Other forms of NOS may be more important; however, we have not seen increases in inducible NOS (iNOS) mRNA.

SODIUM CHANNEL BLOCKERS

Anecdotal data on the usefulness of sodium channel blockers in neuropathic pain states date back to the 1960s (Morton et al. 1949; Keats et al. 1951; Shanbrom 1961). More recently, double-blinded and placebo-controlled studies have yielded firm support for the clinical antiallodynic, antihyperalgesic effects of lidocaine and mexiletine, an orally bioavailable lidocaine analogue (Kastrup et al. 1986; Dejgård et al. 1988; Chabal et al. 1992). These compounds have come to be useful in the pain clinic for their

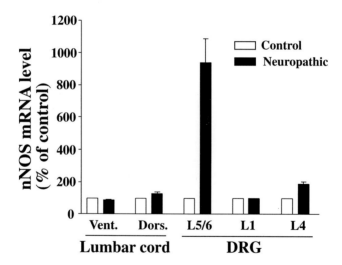

Fig. 5. Neuronal nitric oxide synthase (NOS) mRNA upregulation in the SNL model. Total RNA was extracted from tissues of Harlan Sprague-Dawley rats with SNL and control rats, and RNase protection assays were performed using probes designed to protect a partial sequence of NOS mRNA. Relative quantification was performed by normalizing the resulting band densities against a cyclophilin internal control sequence. Vent = ventral; dors = dorsal. Error bars denote SEM.

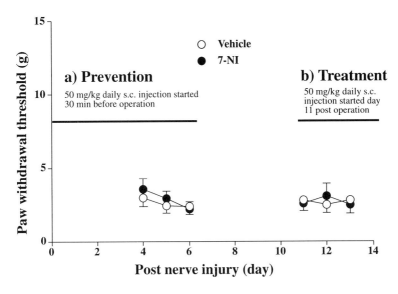

Fig. 6. Responses to systemic 7-nitroindazole, a specific nNOS inhibitor. Male Harlan Sprague-Dawley rats with SNL were treated with (a) preventive dosing of 50 mg/kg daily subcutaneous injection of 7-nitroindazole, beginning 30 minutes before nerve ligation, or vehicle alone; (b) the same drug regimen, begun 11 days post nerve ligation, or vehicle alone ($n = 6$ rats per data point). Neither preventive nor postligation regimen had any effect on the appearance of allodynia, measured as paw withdrawal threshold to von Frey filaments. Error bars denote SEM.

sensory-modality-specific ability to suppress allodynia without disrupting touch or other noxious stimulus perception. Delivered systemically, the plasma levels required for effect are within the cardiac antiarrhythmic range and well below any concentration associated with neuronal conduction blockade (Chaplan et al. 1995). The site of action has not clearly been demonstrated, although there is evidence that it may be at the injured nerve terminal (Tanelian and MacIver 1991), the neuroma (Devor et al. 1992), the DRG (Devor et al. 1992; Sotgiu et al. 1994), and the spinal cord dorsal horn (Sotgiu et al. 1991, 1992). Substantial evidence points to a central site of action, postsynaptic to the primary afferent. Woolf and Wiesenfeld-Hallin (1985) described the suppression by systemic lidocaine and tocainide, at nontoxic doses, of C-fiber-evoked polysynaptic reflexes generated by sural nerve stimulation in the rat. Bach and colleagues (1990) found an increase in nociceptive flexion reflex thresholds by i.v. lidocaine infusion in normal subjects and in diabetic pain patients, with no effect on the Hoffman reflex, indicating a spinal cord site of drug action. Other investigators have reported similar results for in vitro electrophysiological studies (Nagy and Woolf 1996).

Sodium channels consist of a pore-forming α channel and a β subunit whose role is incompletely understood (Nuss et al. 1995). To date, at least 10 subtypes of sodium channels have been identified and cloned. No subtype-specific pharmacological reagents have yet been developed. However, sodium channels can be divided into two pharmacological classes based on their response to tetrodotoxin (TTX), with over 1000-fold differences in susceptibility to TTX blockade (Taylor and Meldrum 1995). A special role has been described for TTX-resistant currents in lidocaine-suppressed nociception (Nagy and Woolf 1996). It is widely believed, although not proven, that use-dependent sodium channel blockade underlies the ability of lidocaine (and congeners) to provide exquisitely specific blockade only to "hyperactive" channels, sparing routine sensory modalities. Sodium channels susceptible to use-dependent blockade are TTX resistant (Roy and Narahashi 1992). Thus, there is some basis for the speculation that the sodium channels responsible for allodynia and susceptible to i.v. lidocaine/mexiletine may be TTX-resistant. We have infused TTX i.v. in SNL rats and have seen no antiallodynic effects up to a dose that is lethal in approximately 20% of subjects (Chaplan et al. 1996).

The structure–activity relationship of sodium channel blockade in allodynia is not clear. We infused sodium channel blockers in SNL rats at a dose just below that required to elicit central nervous system toxicity (demonstrated by sedation and ataxia). Fig. 7 illustrates the varying efficacies of a panel of sodium channel blockers in this model. Lidocaine, mexiletine, and tocainide were highly effective. Other agents were not at all effective; while mepivacaine was effective, it caused significant ataxia at the minimum effective dose. The property of allodynia blockade fails to correlate with major structural qualities such as ester/amine backbone, or presence or absence of an aromatic subgroup. Interestingly, allodynia suppression showed stereoselectivity. In a separate group of experiments, we compared the effects of the S(+) and R(–) isomers of mexiletine on allodynia in the SNL model. A marked antiallodynic effect was seen for the S(+) isomer, but no effect whatsoever for the R(–) isomer. These isomers had equal potency and efficacy in blocking the compound action potential when applied directly to the rat sciatic nerve in vivo (S.R. Chaplan and N.A. Calcutt, unpublished observations).

Sodium channels appear to cluster at neuromas (England et al. 1996). Upregulation of at least one type of sodium channel message apparently occurs in the DRG after nerve damage, namely type III, normally seen in the embryonic and not in the adult peripheral nerve (Waxman et al. 1994). Type III is a TTX-sensitive channel. Two types of TTX-resistant channel have been described so far: SNS/PN3 (Akopian et al. 1996; Sangameswaran et al.

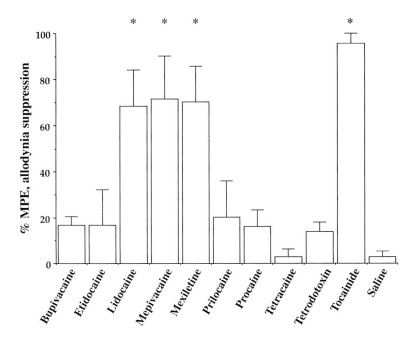

Fig. 7. Responses to sodium channel blockers (percentage of maximal possible effect [MPE] in suppressing allodynia, up to the maximum tolerated dose). Male Harlan Sprague-Dawley rats with allodynia after SNL underwent i.v. infusion of drugs for 60 minutes; allodynia was measured during the infusion and for 60 minutes after completion of infusion (n = 6 rats per group). Drug doses were: bupivacaine 7.5 mg/kg, etidocaine 7.5 mg/kg, lidocaine 20 mg/kg, mepivacaine 30 mg/kg, mexiletine 30 mg/kg, prilocaine 30 mg/kg, procaine 60 mg/kg, tetracaine 7.5 mg/kg, tetrodotoxin 30 µg/kg, tocainide 100 mg/kg. * P < 0.05, one-way ANOVA, Fisher's PLSD; error bars denote SEM.

1996) and the cardiac channel (Rogart et al. 1989) (cf. the denervated skeletal muscle channel, SkM2; White et al. 1991). We hypothesized that SNS/PN3 might be upregulated in nerve injury models. We therefore measured levels of SNS mRNA in the DRG of SNL rats with allodynia, SNL rats from a strain that does not display allodynia after nerve injury, diabetic rats with painful neuropathy, nondiabetic control rats, rats that had been neonatally treated with capsaicin to destroy C fibers and subsequently nerve ligated at the age of 5 weeks (with resulting allodynia), and controls (capsaicin treatment and sham ligation; and vehicle treatment plus real or sham ligation). In all instances of nerve injury, SNS message was decreased, from mildly in diabetic neuropathy (20%) to severely (80%) after combined capsaicin treatment and nerve ligation (Okuse et al. 1997). Site-specific upregulation of SNS may in fact occur in A cells (cell bodies giving rise to Aβ fibers), particularly in the L4 DRG (Porreca et al. 1998); this work was conducted using a polyclonal antibody raised against the SNS/PN3 protein. We compared mRNA levels of SNS/PN3, using RNase protection assays, from L4 DRG from nerve-ligated/contralateral and sham-operated SNL rats, and see no evidence to support upregulation in L4 (S.R. Chaplan and B.P. Scott, unpublished observations). However, this technique does not permit us to assess cellular localization, and if upregulation in A cells is counterbalanced by downregulation in B cells, it would not be detectable using this whole-tissue assay.

The relative contributions of the L4 and L5/L6 DRG to neuropathic pain are a subject of controversy and speculation. Spontaneous activity in the neuroma and DRG has been documented at the L5/L6 levels, but has not been reported in uninjured DRG. Section of the L5/L6 dorsal roots in SNL rats abolishes neuropathic behavior, and section of the L4 dorsal root abolishes evoked, but not spontaneous pain (Yoon et al. 1996). It remains unknown whether abnormal sensation is the result of changes in L4 (following injury to L5/L6), or whether abnormal sensation (necessarily transduced through L4, the only remaining sensory innervation of the paw) results from spinal cord alterations evoked and maintained by pathology in L5/L6. Since evidence suggests that the site of action of lidocaine and congeners is within the spinal cord, the relevance of upregulation of elements in the DRG remains to be clarified.

REFERENCES

Adamson P, Xiang JZ, Mantzourides T, Brammer MJ, Campbell IC. Presynaptic alpha 2-adrenoceptor and kappa-opiate receptor occupancy promotes closure of neuronal (N-type) calcium channels. *Eur J Pharmacol* 1989; 174:63–70.

Ahlgren SC, Levine JD. Mechanical hyperalgesia in streptozotocin-diabetic rats is not sympathetically maintained. *Brain Res* 1993; 616:171–175.

Akopian AN, Sivilotti L, Wood JN. A tetrodotoxin-resistant voltage-gated sodium channel expressed by sensory neurons. *Nature* 1996; 379:257–262.

Angelotti T, Hofmann F. Tissue-specific expression of splice variants of the mouse voltage-gated calcium channel alpha2/delta subunit. *FEBS Lett* 1996; 397:331–337.

Arnér S, Meyerson BA. Lack of analgesic effect of opioids on neuropathic and idiopathic forms of pain. *Pain* 1988; 33:11–23.

Bach FW, Jensen TS, Kastrup J, Stigsby B, Dejgård A. The effect of intravenous lidocaine on nociceptive processing in diabetic neuropathy. *Pain* 1990; 40:29–34.

Bian D, Nichols ML, Ossipov MH, Lai J, Porreca F. Characterization of the antiallodynic efficacy of morphine in a model of neuropathic pain in rats. *Neuroreport* 1995; 6:1981–1984.

Brust PF, Simerson S, McCue AF, et al. Human neuronal voltage-dependent calcium channels: studies on subunit structure and role in channel assembly. *Neuropharmacology* 1993; 32:1089–1102.

Calcutt NA, Chaplan SR. Spinal pharmacology of tactile allodynia in diabetic rats. *Br J Pharmacol* 1997; 122:1478–1482.

Chabal C, Jacobson L, Mariano A, Chaney E, Britell CW. The use of oral mexiletine for the treatment of pain after peripheral nerve injury. *Anesthesiology* 1992; 76:513–517.

Chaplan SR, Pogrel JW, Yaksh TL. Role of voltage-dependent calcium channel subtypes in experimental tactile allodynia. *J Pharmacol Exp Ther* 1994; 269:1117–1123.

Chaplan SR, Bach FW, Shafer SL, Yaksh TL. Prolonged alleviation of tactile allodynia by intravenous lidocaine in neuropathic rats. *Anesthesiology* 1995; 83:775–785.

Chaplan SR, Scott BP, Hua X-Y, Yaksh TL. Effect of tetrodotoxin on experimental tactile allodynia in the rat: alteration by neonatal capsaicin treatment. *Soc Neurosci Abstr* 1996; 22:876.

Crosby G, Marota JJ, Huang PL. Intact nociception-induced neuroplasticity in transgenic mice deficient in neuronal nitric oxide synthase. *Neuroscience* 1995; 69:1013–1017.

Dejgård A, Petersen P, Kastrup J. Mexiletine for treatment of chronic painful diabetic neuropathy. *Lancet* 1988; 1:9–11.

De Jongh KS, Warner C, Catterall WA. Subunits of purified calcium channels. Alpha 2 and delta are encoded by the same gene. *J Biol Chem* 1990; 265:14738–14741.

Devor M, Wall PD, Catalan N. Systemic lidocaine silences ectopic neuroma and DRG discharge without blocking nerve conduction. *Pain* 1992; 48:261–268.

England JD, Happel LT, Kline DG, et al. Sodium channel accumulation in humans with painful neuromas. *Neurology* 1996; 47:272–276.

Gee NS, Brown JP, Dissanayake VU, et al. The novel anticonvulsant drug, gabapentin (Neurontin), binds to the alpha2delta subunit of a calcium channel. *J Biol Chem* 1996; 271:5768–5776.

Honda CN, Arvidsson U. Immunohistochemical localization of delta- and mu-opioid receptors in primate spinal cord. *Neuroreport* 1995; 6:1025–1028.

Hwang JH, Yaksh TL. Effect of subarachnoid gabapentin on tactile-evoked allodynia in a surgically induced neuropathic pain model in the rat. *Reg Anesth* 1997; 22:249–256.

Kastrup J, Angelo HR, Petersen P, Dejgård A, Hilsted J. Treatment of chronic painful diabetic neuropathy with intravenous lidocaine infusion. *BMJ* 1986; 292:173.

Kauppila T, Kemppainen P, Tanila H, Pertovaara A. Effect of systemic medetomidine, an alpha 2 adrenoceptor agonist, on experimental pain in humans. *Anesthesiology* 1991; 74:3–8.

Keats AS, D'Alessandro GL, Beecher HK. A controlled study of pain relief by intravenous procaine. *JAMA* 1951; 147:1761–1763.

Kim SH, Chung JM. Sympathectomy alleviates mechanical allodynia in an experimental animal model for neuropathy in the rat. *Neurosci Lett* 1991; 134:131–134.

Kim SH, Chung JM. An experimental model for peripheral neuropathy produced by segmental spinal nerve ligation in the rat. *Pain* 1992; 50:355–363.

Koltzenburg M, Torebjörk HE, Wahren LK. Nociceptor modulated central sensitization causes mechanical hyperalgesia in acute chemogenic and chronic neuropathic pain. *Brain* 1994; 117:579–591.

Lam HH, Hanley DF, Trapp BD, et al. Induction of spinal cord neuronal nitric oxide synthase (NOS) after formalin injection in the rat hind paw. *Neurosci Lett* 1996; 210:201–204.

Lee DH, Chung K, Chung JM. Strain differences in adrenergic sensitivity of neuropathic pain behaviors in an experimental rat model. *Neuroreport* 1997; 8:3453–3456.

Lee YW, Chaplan SR, Yaksh TL. Systemic and supraspinal, but not spinal, opiates suppress allodynia in a rat neuropathic pain model. *Neurosci Lett* 1995; 199:111–114.

Luo ZD, Scott BP, Calcutt NA, Yaksh TL, Chaplan SR. Up-regulation of neuronal nitric oxide synthase mRNA in dorsal root ganglion of rats with neuropathic pain. *Soc Neurosci Abstr* 1998; 24:363.

Luo ZD, Higuera E, Chaplan SR. Up-regulation of $\alpha 2\delta$ calcium channel subunit in dorsal root ganglia and spinal cord of rats with tactile allodynia. *IASP Abstracts*. Seattle: IASP Press, 1999, in press.

Meller ST, Pechman PS, Gebhart GF, Maves TJ. Nitric oxide mediates the thermal hyperalgesia produced in a model of neuropathic pain in the rat. *Neuroscience* 1992; 50:7–10.

Mellick GA, Mellicy LB, Mellick LB. Gabapentin in the management of reflex sympathetic dystrophy [Letter]. *J Pain Symptom Manage* 1995; 10:265–266.

Morton R, Spitzer K, Steinbrocker O. Intravenous procaine as an analgesic and therapeutic procedure in painful, chronic neuromusculoskeletal disorders. *Anesthesiology* 1949; 10:629–633.

Nagy I, Woolf CJ. Lignocaine selectively reduces C fibre-evoked neuronal activity in rat spinal cord in vitro by decreasing N-methyl-D-aspartate and neurokinin receptor-mediated post-synaptic depolarizations; implications for the development of novel centrally acting analgesics. *Pain* 1996; 64:59–70.

Nagy JI, Iversen LL, Goedert M, Chapman D, Hunt SP. Dose-dependent effects of capsaicin on primary sensory neurons in the neonatal rat. *J Neurosci* 1983; 3:399–406.

Nuss HB, Chiamvimonvat N, Perez-Garcia MT, Tomaselli GF, Marban E. Functional association of the beta 1 subunit with human cardiac (hH1) and rat skeletal muscle (mu 1) sodium channel alpha subunits expressed in Xenopus oocytes. *J Gen Physiol* 1995; 106:1171–1191.

Okuse K, Chaplan SR, McMahon SB, et al. Regulation of expression of the sensory neuron-specific sodium channel SNS in inflammatory and neuropathic pain. *Mol Cell Neurosci* 1997; 10:196–207.

Partridge B, Chaplan SR, Sakamoto E, Yaksh TL. Characterization of the effects of gabapentin and 3-isobutyl GABA on substance-P induced thermal hyperalgesia. *Anesthesiology* 1998; 88:196–205.

Porreca F, Bian D, Kassotakis L, et al. An antisense oligodoxynucleotide to the novel, TTX-resistant sodium channel PN3 prevents and reverses hyperalgesia after peripheral nerve injury. *Soc Neurosci Abstr* 1998; 24:640–647.

Presley R, Charapata S, Ferrar-Brechner T, et al. Chronic, opioid resistant, neuropathic pain: marked analgesic efficacy of intrathecal ziconitide. *Am Pain Soc Abstr* 1998:122.

Price DD, Bennett GJ, Rafii A. Psychophysical observations on patients with neuropathic pain relieved by a sympathetic block. *Pain* 1989; 36:273–288.

Puke MJ, Luo L, Xu XJ. The spinal analgesic role of alpha 2-adrenoceptor subtypes in rats after peripheral nerve section. *Eur J Pharmacol* 1994; 260:227–232.

Rauck RL, Eisenach JC, Jackson K, Young LD, Southern J. Epidural clonidine treatment for refractory reflex sympathetic dystrophy. *Anesthesiology* 1993; 79:1163–1169; 1127A.

Rogart RB, Cribbs LL, Muglia LK, Kephart DD, Kaiser MW. Molecular cloning of a putative tetrodotoxin-resistant rat heart Na+ channel isoform. *Proc Natl Acad Sci USA* 1989; 86:8170–8174.

Roy ML, Narahashi T. Differential properties of tetrodotoxin-sensitive and tetrodotoxin-resistant sodium channels in rat dorsal root ganglion neurons. *J Neurosci* 1992; 12:2104–2111.

Sangameswaran L, Delgado SG, Fish LM, et al. Structure and function of a novel voltage-gated, tetrodotoxin-resistant sodium channel specific to sensory neurons. *J Biol Chem* 1996; 271:5953–5956.

Shanbrom E. Treatment of herpetic pain and postherpetic neuralgia with intravenous procaine. *JAMA* 1961; 176:1041–1043.

Shir Y, Seltzer Z. A-fibers mediate mechanical hyperesthesia and allodynia and C-fibers mediate thermal hyperalgesia in a new model of causalgiform pain disorders in rats. *Neurosci Lett* 1990; 115:62–67.

Singer D, Biel M, Lotan I, et al. The roles of the subunits in the function of the calcium channel. *Science* 1991; 253:1553–1557.

Sotgiu ML, Lacerenza M, Marchettini P. Selective inhibition by systemic lidocaine of noxious evoked activity in rat dorsal horn neurons. *Neuroreport* 1991; 2:425–428.

Sotgiu ML, Lacerenza M, Marchettini P. Effect of systemic lidocaine on dorsal horn neuron hyperactivity following chronic peripheral nerve injury in rats. *Somatosens Mot Res* 1992; 9:227–233.

Sotgiu ML, Biella G, Castagna A, Lacerenza M, Marchettini P. Different time-courses of i.v. lidocaine effect on ganglionic and spinal units in neuropathic rats. *Neuroreport* 1994; 5:873–876.

Stevens CW, Monasky MS, Yaksh TL. Spinal infusion of opiate and alpha-2 agonists in rats: tolerance and cross-tolerance studies. *J Pharmacol Exp Ther* 1988; 244:63–70.

Stone LS, MacMillan LB, Kitto KF, Limbird LE, Wilcox GL. The alpha2a adrenergic receptor subtype mediates spinal analgesia evoked by alpha2 agonists and is necessary for spinal adrenergic-opioid synergy. *J Neurosci* 1997; 17:7157–7165.

Stone LS, Broberger C, Vulchanova L, et al. Differential distribution of alpha2A and alpha2C adrenergic receptor immunoreactivity in the rat spinal cord. *J Neurosci* 1998; 18:5928–5937.

Taddese A, Nah SY, McCleskey EW. Selective opioid inhibition of small nociceptive neurons. *Science* 1995; 270:1366–1369.

Tanelian DL, MacIver MB. Analgesic concentrations of lidocaine suppress tonic A-delta and C-fiber discharges produced by acute injury. *Anesthesiology* 1991; 74:934–936.

Taylor CP. Gabapentin: mechanisms of action. In: Levy RH, Mattson RH, Meldrum BS (Eds). *Antiepileptic Drugs,* 4th ed. Raven Press: New York, 1995, pp 829–841.

Taylor CP, Meldrum BS. Na$^+$ channels as targets for neuroprotective drugs. *Trends Pharmacol Sci* 1995; 16:309–316.

Traub RJ, Solodkin A, Meller ST, Gebhart GF. Spinal cord NADPH-diaphorase histochemical staining but not nitric oxide synthase immunoreactivity increases following carrageenan-produced hindpaw inflammation in the rat. *Brain Res* 1994; 668:204–210.

Wahren LK, Torebjörk E. Quantitative sensory tests in patients with neuralgia 11 to 25 years after injury. *Pain* 1992; 48:237–244.

Waxman SG, Kocsis JD, Black JA. Type III sodium channel mRNA is expressed in embryonic but not adult spinal sensory neurons, and is reexpressed following axotomy. *J Neurophysiol* 1994; 72:466–470.

White MM, Chen LQ, Kleinfield R, Kallen RG, Barchi RL. SkM2, a Na$^+$ channel cDNA clone from denervated skeletal muscle, encodes a tetrodotoxin-insensitive Na$^+$ channel. *Mol Pharmacol* 1991; 39:604–608.

Wiser O, Trus M, Tobi D, et al. The alpha 2/delta subunit of voltage sensitive Ca^{2+} channels is a single transmembrane extracellular protein which is involved in regulated secretion. *FEBS Lett* 1996; 379:15–20.

Woolf CJ, Wiesenfeld-Hallin Z. The systemic administration of local anesthetics produces a selective depression of C-afferent fibre evoked activity in the spinal cord. *Pain* 1985; 23:361–374.

Wu J, Lin Q, Lu Y, Willis WD, Westlund KN. Changes in nitric oxide synthase isoforms in the spinal cord of rat following induction of chronic arthritis. *Exp Brain Res* 1998; 118:457–465.

Xiang JZ, Morton J, Brammer MJ, Campbell IC. Regulation of calcium concentrations in synaptosomes: alpha 2-adrenoceptors reduce free Ca^{2+} by closure of N-type Ca^{2+} channels. *J Neurochem* 1990; 55:303–310.

Xiao W-H, Bennett GJ. Gabapentin has an antinociceptive effect mediated via a spinal site of action in a rat model of painful peripheral neuropathy. *Analgesia* 1997; 2:267–273.

Xie Y, Zhang J, Petersen M, LaMotte RH. Functional changes in dorsal root ganglion cells after chronic nerve constriction in the rat. *J Neurophysiol* 1995; 73:1811–1820.

Yaksh TL, Pogrel JW, Lee YW, Chaplan SR. Reversal of nerve ligation-induced allodynia by spinal alpha-2 adrenoceptor agonists. *J Pharmacol Exp Ther* 1995; 272:207–214.

Yonehara N, Takemura M, Yoshimura M, et al. Nitric oxide in the rat spinal cord in Freund's adjuvant-induced hyperalgesia. *Jpn J Pharmacol* 1997; 75:327–335.

Yoon YW, Na HS, Chung JM. Contributions of injured and intact afferents to neuropathic pain in an experimental rat model. *Pain* 1996; 64:27–36.

Yoon YW, Sung B, Chung JM. Nitric oxide mediates behavioral signs of neuropathic pain in an experimental rat model. *Neuroreport* 1998; 9:367–372.

Correspondence to: Sandra R. Chaplan, MD, Anesthesiology Research Laboratory, University of California, San Diego, 9500 Gilman Drive, La Jolla, CA 92093-0818, USA. Tel: 619-543-3962; Fax: 619-543-6070; email: schaplan@ucsd.edu.

Opioid Sensitivity of Chronic Noncancer Pain,
Progress in Pain Research and Management,
Vol. 14, edited by Eija Kalso, Henry J. McQuay,
and Zsuzsanna Wiesenfeld-Hallin, IASP Press,
Seattle, © 1999.

16

Alternatives to Mu-Opioid Analgesics: Delta-Opioid- and Galanin-Receptor-Selective Compounds

Andy Dray

*Department of Pharmacology, AstraZeneca R&D Montreal,
St.-Laurent, Quebec, Canada*

Pain therapy with opioids is limited by several long-recognized problems, including adverse side effects at therapeutic doses and lack of efficacy in certain pain conditions, particularly neuropathic pain. Several approaches would lead to obvious improvements in therapy: side effects could be reduced by selecting alternatives to μ-selective types of opioid analgesics, and analgesic efficacy improved through nonopioid mechanistic strategies. This chapter describes the potential advantages in developing other classes of nonpeptidic compounds with selectivity for the δ-opioid receptor and highlights the role of galanin in nociception and the potential use of specific galanin-receptor ligands as novel analgesics.

DELTA OPIOIDS

Opioids inhibit nociception by attenuating transmission in the spinal cord (Yaksh and Rudy 1978) by acting on μ, δ, and κ subtypes of opioid receptors located in the spinal dorsal horn and on central terminals of fine primary afferent fibers (Arvidsson et al. 1995a,b; Zaki et al. 1996). Several studies have shown that opioid receptors are also expressed in the periphery. Thus, all three opioid-receptor subtypes are expressed in primary sensory neurons (Mansour et al. 1995; Zhang et al. 1998) and can be visualized in fine cutaneous nerves (Stein et al. 1990; Hassan et al. 1993; Coggeshall et al. 1997).

Activity at μ-opioid receptors causes analgesia but is also responsible for most of the adverse side effects such as sedation, respiratory depression, and dependence (Matthes et al. 1996; Sora et al. 1997). Activation of κ-opioid receptors also produces analgesia, with dysphoria and diuresis as common side effects (Pfeiffer et al. 1986; Peters et al. 1987). However, molecular and functional studies have suggested that δ receptors are also important in nociception and that selective ligands are analgesic with a lower propensity for causing adverse effects. Until recently, functional studies of δ-opioid receptors in pain have been restricted to the use of peptidic agonists such as [D-Pen^2,D-Pen^5]enkephalin (DPDPE) and deltorphin II. The relative affinity and selectivity of several peptidic and nonpeptidic opioid agonists and antagonists at human opioid receptors are shown in Table I.

Direct administrations of δ-selective peptides at supraspinal and spinal sites have produced antinociception in various rodent pain models (Yaksh et al. 1980; Tung and Yaksh 1982; Galligan et al. 1984; Heyman et al. 1987; Malmberg and Yaksh 1992). Typical δ-peptidergic agonists, when injected spinally into rats, are potent in reducing thermal, chemical, and mechanical nociception, despite their weakness as analgesics upon supraspinal administration (Miaskowski et al. 1991, 1993; Stewart et al. 1994).

Genetic studies have shown that inhibition of δ-opioid-receptor expression with antisense oligonucleotides (Standifer et al. 1994; Zaki et al. 1996) prevented the analgesic effects of several centrally administered δ-selective agonists. Moreover, deletion of the μ-opioid-receptor gene in transgenic mice prevented the effects of morphine but did not alter the analgesic activity of centrally administered δ-opioid-receptor ligands (Matthes et al. 1996,

Table I
Opioid receptor ligands: activity at human delta receptors
and receptor subtype selectivity

Compound	δ Activity, K_i (nmol/L)	δ Efficacy, EC_{50} (nmol/L)	δ/μ	δ/κ
Fentanyl	158	—	0.001	1.6
DAMGO	429	709	0.001	1.0
Naloxone	18	Antagonist	0.03	0.1
CTOP	5202	Antagonist	9×10^{-5}	1.0
DPDPE	0.8	13	112	>3300
Deltorphin II	1.2	5.0	163	>2200
SNC80	1.1	2.1	295	1586
Naltrindole	0.17	Antagonist	23	38

Note: EC_{50} = median effective concentration. δ/μ and δ/κ are ratios of δ to μ and κ receptor selectivity; higher numbers indicate greater δ selectivity.

1998; Sora et al. 1997). Additionally, in μ-deficient (CXBK) mice, the potency of morphine and DAMGO were greatly reduced, whereas the potency of a δ-selective peptide was virtually unaffected (Vaught et al. 1998). However, others have observed an additional loss of δ-ligand efficacy in μ-knockout mice (Sora et al. 1999).

Further antisense oligonucleotide studies have blocked spinal antinociception induced by both DPDPE and deltorphin II, and have blocked supraspinal antinociception induced by deltorphin II but not that produced by DPDPE (Bilsky et al. 1994). This finding supports the hypothesis proposing subtypes of δ-opioid receptors. Thus, spinal analgesia may involve a deltorphin II-selective site (δ_2 receptors), whereas both δ_1 (DPDPE-selective) and δ_2 receptors mediate supraspinal analgesia. Attempts to clone the putative δ_1-receptor subtype by homology have been unsuccessful (Zaki et al. 1996).

For δ-opioid-receptor agonists, potential clinical advantages include analgesia without respiratory depression (Cheng et al. 1993), constipation, or other adverse gastrointestinal effects (Sheldon et al. 1990), and with minimal development of physical dependence (Cowan et al. 1988). Additionally, the specific mechanism of the gastrointestinal action of δ agonists (an increase in net basal intestinal fluid absorption) may be particularly significant for clinical management of disorders such as diarrhea and the pain of cholecystitis (Sheldon et al. 1990).

DEVELOPMENT OF HIGHLY SELECTIVE PEPTIDE AND NONPEPTIDE DELTA-OPIOID-RECEPTOR LIGANDS

In general, peptidic drugs have several disadvantages: their bioavailability and central penetration are poor, they are unstable by oral administration, and they can be metabolically labile and thus are unsuitable for administration by systemic routes. However, pseudopeptides such as TIPP[psi] are highly selective δ antagonists (Schiller et al. 1993). Although few studies have been reported, these compounds are likely to supplant less selective nonpeptidic δ-receptor ligands such as naltrindole (Table I) (Takemori and Portoghese 1992).

Several poorly selective agonists such as BW373U86 (Chang et al. 1993; Wild et al. 1993) have been developed, but SNC80, the optically pure methyl ether of BW373U86 (Calderon et al. 1994) showed considerably improved activity and was highly selective for δ- over μ-opioid receptors (Calderon et al. 1994) (Table I). This drug produced naloxone- and naltrindole-reversible analgesia following either systemic administration or direct administration into the brain or spinal cord (Bilsky et al. 1995). High δ-receptor selectivity was also accompanied by a reduced incidence of convulsive side effects noted with BW373U86 (Bilsky et al. 1995). More recent studies with intramuscular SNC80 in rhesus monkeys produced analgesia to mild noxious heating of the tail, with no evidence of convulsions or other untoward behaviors. The efficacy of SNC80 was less than that of fentanyl or U5488, and its analgesic effect was reversed by naltrindole but not by the μ-receptor-selective antagonist quidozacine or by the κ-receptor antagonist nor-BNI. These findings suggest a predominantly δ-receptor-mediated mechanism of action (Negus et al. 1998). Of equal significance, perhaps, were the observations that SNC80 produced a cocaine-like discriminative response, although the response was mechanistically dissimilar from that of cocaine and did not produce drug self-administration, which suggests low potential for abuse.

GALANIN RECEPTORS AND SELECTIVE LIGANDS AS ANALGESICS

Compelling data indicate the involvement of galanin in pain transmission. Normally, modest amounts of galanin-like immunoreactivity occur in spinal cord interneurons and in small dorsal root ganglion (DRG) neurons (Ch'ng et al. 1985; Skofitsch and Jacobowitz 1985). However, following peripheral (sciatic) nerve section a dramatic increase in galanin-like immunoreactivity and galanin mRNA occurs in small and large sensory neurons (Hökfelt et al. 1987, 1994; Villar et al. 1989) and in the spinal dorsal horn, together with an enhanced galanin release from the spinal dorsal horn (Hope et al. 1994; Colvin et al. 1997).

Functional studies have shown that direct spinal administration of galanin produces a biphasic excitation followed by inhibition of spinal nociceptive reflexes (Yanagisawa et al. 1986; Wiesenfeld-Hallin et al. 1989, 1994; Xu et al. 1990; Nussbaumer and Yanagisawa 1998). The more prominent depressive effect was much enhanced after peripheral nerve section (Wiesenfeld-Hallin et al. 1989; Xu et al. 1990), and following painful injury, galanin decreased the allodynia induced by various sensory stimuli (Yu et al. 1999). In addition, galanin significantly decreased abnormal pain behaviors after painful ischemic lesions of the sciatic nerve (Hao et al. 1999), even though the increase of galanin in sensory neurons was modest compared with that seen after peripheral nerve injury. Also, spinal intrathecal administrations of galanin induced behavioral antinociception and potentiated the analgesic effect of morphine (Wiesenfeld-Hallin et al. 1990). In accordance with these behavioral measures, galanin reduced C-fiber-evoked flexor-reflex activity and diminished the increase in spinal excitability after repetitive C-fiber activation (wind-up) (Yanagisawa et al. 1986; Xu et al. 1990; Nussbaumer and Yanagisawa 1998). This effect may be due to depression of excitability in spinal afferent nerve terminals or in spinal dorsal and ventral horn neurons. The effects of galanin in the spinal cord are probably due to neural hyperpolarization, which has been demonstrated in the spinal dorsal horn (Randic et al. 1987). Interestingly the effect of galanin on DRG excitability is markedly enhanced after axotomy (Xu et al. 1997), and indication that this may also be an important site of action for galanin.

The description of chimeric peptidic antagonists (galantide, M32, M40, C7) has further characterized galanin functions (Bartfai et al. 1991) (Table II). Their actions demonstrated in vivo have supported the view of a predominantly inhibitory role for galanin (Verge et al. 1993; Wiesenfeld-Hallin et al. 1994). Thus, spinal infusion of the antagonist alone produced an

Table II
Receptor affinity and agonist activity of galanin$_{(1-16)}$-NH$_2$ analogues

Compound	Stability†	Binding, EC$_{50}$ (nmol/L)		Activation, EC$_{50}$ (nmol/L)	
		Gal-R1	Gal-R2	Gal-R1	Gal-R2
Gal$_{(1-16)}$-NH$_2$	0	0.174	1.39	14.5	8.80
[1-Nal^2]gal		3.63	80.5	256	
[2-Nal^2]gal		2.71	43.6	1560	90.2
[Bta^2]gal	9	3.92	555	3630	263
[αMeTrp^2,D-Ala^{12}]gal	83	143	26.8	>10,000	64.5
[Aib^{12}]gal	25	1.66	12.0	1660	53.8
[D-Ala^{12}]gal-OH	38	0.590	5.97	186	
[Sar^1,D-Ala^{12}]gal	83	0.403	1.74	118	7.12
c[Asp^4,Lys^8]gal		0.601	1.75	1690	9.97
c[Glu^4,Lys^8]gal		2.66	1.72	4980	13.3
c[Asp^4,Orn^8]gal		300		>10,000	857
Galantide (M15)		17.9	102		5.4
M32		0.65	5.35	166	115
M40		0.3	1.9	7.4	98.1
C7		0.4	11.7	76.1	90.5

Source: Schmidt et al. (1999).

Note: EC$_{50}$ = median effective concentration.

†Determined as percentage remaining following 30-min incubations in rat brain homogenates. Note that [αMeTrp^2,D-Ala^{12}]gal$_{(1-16)}$-NH$_2$ was stable and Gal-R2-selective. Several dimeric peptide antagonists, galantide, M32, M40, and C7, had greater affinity for Gal-R1, but also acted as agonists.

increase in spinal excitability following peripheral nerve inflammation or injury, and points to an endogenous inhibitory action of galanin in the spinal cord (Xu et al. 1998a). Further support for an inhibitory role in the spinal cord comes from treatment with a galanin antisense oligonucleotide, which produced markedly increased autotomy in rats following sciatic nerve axotomy. This finding suggests an increase in excitability in the absence of endogenous galanin (Bartfai et al. 1992; Ji et al. 1995).

However, other research has suggested that galanin can also produce hyperalgesia and hyper-responsiveness to sensory stimuli (Kuraishi et al. 1991; Cridland and Henry 1998). Also, changes in spinal excitability during neuropathic pain may be better correlated with changes in substance P content rather than galanin, since the latter appears to be a predominantly inhibitory neuropeptide but is significantly elevated in the spinal cord in chronic pain (Ramer et al. 1998). However, during painful peripheral inflammation, galanin-like immunoreactivity increased in the spinal dorsal horn but was reduced in the DRG (Togunaga et al. 1992; Ji et al. 1995). In this condition, spinal sensitization and wind-up were decreased (Xu et al. 1998a) and C-fiber-evoked reflex activity was depressed. Galanin was a less potent depressant of spinal excitability under these circumstances. The increased galanin expression in the spinal cord was also accompanied by an increase in basal release, but this was suppressed with peripheral nerve stimulation (Hope et al. 1994). However, other changes that occur in galanin receptors after peripheral injury or inflammation make it difficult to ascribe a general role for galanin in pain modulation. For example, during inflammation Gal-R1 mRNA was downregulated whereas Gal-R2 mRNA was upregulated, but both receptor subtypes were downregulated in the DRG after axotomy (Shi et al. 1997; Xu et al. 1998b).

In addition to modulating neuronal excitability, galanin may also be a trophic peptide and appears to be involved in the processes of nerve maturation and regeneration. Thus, galanin expression in the DRG is high in gestation and falls to low levels in adults (Xu et al. 1996), but can be strikingly upregulated after peripheral nerve injury (Hökfelt et al. 1987). In accordance with this hypothesis, deletion of the galanin gene delayed functional regeneration following painful peripheral nerve lesions in the mouse (Wynick et al. 1998). Little is known about the molecular events involved in this function, but as with effects on nerve excitability, there is a strong likelihood of galanin receptor involvement.

GALANIN RECEPTORS

While several functional roles have been identified for galanin in the aftermath of peripheral injury, it is unclear through which receptors these are mediated, since various receptor subtypes have been cloned: Gal-R1, Gal-R2, and Gal-R3 (Branchek et al. 1998). To date, limited characterization of Gal-R1 and Gal-R2 have been achieved in pain modulation. In situ hybridization studies of the distribution of the human (h) and rat (r) Gal-R1 receptor (Ahamad et al. 1998; O'Donnell et al. 1999) show high levels of Gal-R1 mRNA in various structures that have been related to pain transmission and modulation. Prominent among these are the spinal cord dorsal horn, trigeminal ganglia, and thalamus (Ahamad et al. 1998; O'Donnell et al. 1999).

There is an overall molecular identity of 35% of rGal-R2 compared with Gal-R1. There is a relatively low abundance of Gal-R2 mRNA in the spinal cord and in discrete brain areas associated with pain signaling. In contrast, there is high abundance of Gal-R2 in rat dorsal root ganglia. Gal-R3 has 35% homology with R1 and 52% with R2. It has been found in spinal cord but not in the DRG (Branchek et al. 1998).

Galanin-receptor expression undergoes several changes in sensory ganglia in persistent pain conditions Gal-R1 mRNA is downregulated in sensory ganglia after peripheral inflammation, but Gal-R2 mRNA is upregulated. Both receptor subtypes are downregulated in the DRG after axotomy (Shi et al. 1997; Xu et al. 1998b), but specific upregulation of Gal-R2 mRNA occurred in the spinal ventral horn after a sciatic nerve lesion (Ahamad et al. 1998). Interestingly, an enhanced inward current in the DRG was induced by galanin after axotomy (Xu et al. 1997), which raises the possibility that the functional expression of another receptor subtype, perhaps Gal-R3, was increased.

DEVELOPMENT AND CHARACTERIZATION OF GAL-R1 AND GAL-R2 LIGANDS

The characterization of galanin receptors and their function has been impeded by the lack of subtype-selective agonists and antagonists. Thus, it is presently unclear which receptor is a more desirable target for the development of a novel analgesic. To address this question, receptor-selective compounds have been developed using ^{125}I-galanin binding to membranes expressing rGal-R2 (Table II). The activation of rGal-R2 resulted in increased intracellular calcium through a G_q-mediated signaling pathway. This assay was used to distinguish compounds with agonist or antagonistic activity

(Smith et al. 1997; Schmidt et al. 1999). Evaluation of hGal-R1 activity was also made using Ca^{2+} release in human Bowes melanoma cells, which endogenously express the receptor.

Several earlier studies have demonstrated a structure–activity relationship in galanin ligands. We synthesized several peptidic analogues to enhance Gal-R1 versus Gal-R2 receptor selectivity (Table II). Other modifications were made to improve metabolic stability. Such compounds provided stable but selective tools for the in vivo functional evaluation of antinociceptive properties. Stability was assayed in homogenates of whole rat brain. Some compounds were also administered directly into the lumbar spinal intrathecal space in rats with mechanical allodynia 7 days after a sciatic nerve injury. Of particular note was the compound [D/L-αMeTrp^2,D-Ala^{12}]gal$_{(1-16)}$-NH$_2$, which showed Gal-R2 selectivity (Table II) and antiallodynic activity, which suggests that Gal-R2 selective ligands may have analgesic potential. Clearly, further characterization with antagonists will be required to consolidate these preliminary data.

SUMMARY

Several alternative approaches to μ-opioid-receptor-mediated analgesia are possible. Delta-receptor-selective peptides exert analgesic activity without the range of untoward effects exhibited by μ-receptor-selective compounds. This also seems to be the case with the first generation of nonpeptidic δ-receptor-selective compounds such as SNC80, which are also active systemically.

These recent findings hold great promise for future improvements in therapy. Nonopioid mechanisms may also be used to advantage with the characterization of the role of galanin in inflammatory and neuropathic pain and in neural regeneration. With the development of selective tools, we may discover several galanin-receptor subtypes through which these effects are mediated.

REFERENCES

Ahamad S, O'Donnell D, Payza K, et al. Cloning and evaluation of the role of rat GALR-2, a novel subtype of galanin receptor, in the control of pain perception. In: Hökfelt T, Bartfai T, Crawley J (Eds). *Galanin: Basic Research Discoveries and Therapeutic Implications.* New York: New York Academy of Sciences, 1998, 108–119.

Arvidsson U, Dado RJ, Riedl M, et al. Opioid receptor immunoreactivity; distribution in brainstem and spinal cord, and relationship to biogenic amines and enkephalin. *J Neurosci* 1995a; 15:1215–1235.

Arvidsson U, Riedl M, Chakabarti S, et al. Distribution and targeting of μ-opioid receptor (MOR-1) in brain and spinal cord. *J Neurosci* 1995b; 15:3328–3341.

Bartfai T, Bedecs K, Land T, et al. M-15: high affinity chimeric peptide that blocks the neuronal action of galanin in the hippocampus, locus coeruleus and spinal cord. *Proc Natl Acad Sci USA* 1991; 88:10961–10965.

Bartfai T, Fisone G, Langel U. Galanin and galanin antagonists: molecular and biochemical perspectives. *Trends Pharmacol Sci* 1992; 13:312–316.

Bilsky EJ, Bernstein RN, Pasternak GW, et al. Selective inhibition of [D-Ala^2, Glu^4] deltorphin antinociception by supraspinal, but not spinal, administration of an antisense oligodeoxy-nucleotide to an opioid delta receptor. *Life Sci* 1994; 55:L37–L43.

Bilsky EJ, Calderon SN, Wang T, et al. SNC 80, a selective, non-peptidic and systemically-active opioid delta agonist. *J Pharmacol* 1995; 273:359–366.

Branchek TA, Smith KE, Walker MW. Molecular biology and pharmacology of galanin receptors. In: Hökfelt T, Bartfai T, Crawley J (Eds). *Galanin: Basic Research Discoveries and Therapeutic Implications.* New York: New York Academy of Science, 1998, 94–107.

Calderon SN, Izenwasser S, Heller B, et al. Novel 1-phenylcyloalkanecarboxylic acid derivatives are potent and selective sigma 1 ligands. *J Med Chem* 1994; 37:2285–2291.

Ch'ng JL, Christofides ND, Anand P, et al. Distribution of galanin immunoreactivity in the central nervous system and the responses of galanin-containing neuronal pathways to injury. *Neuroscience* 1985; 16:343–354.

Chang KJ, Rigdon GC, Howard JL, McNutt RW. A novel, potent and selective non-peptide delta receptor agonist BW 373U86. *Pharmacology* 1993; 267:852–857.

Cheng PY, Wu D, Decena J, et al. Opioid induced stimulation of fetal respiratory activity [D-Ala^2] deltorphin I. *J Pharmacol* 1993; 230:85–88.

Coggeshall RE, Zhou S, Carlton SM. Opioid receptors on peripheral sensory axons. *Brain Res* 1997; 764:126–132.

Colvin LA, Mark MA, Duggan AW. The effect of peripheral mononeuropathy on immunoreactive (ir)-galanin release in the spinal cord of the rat. *Brain Res* 1997; 766:259–261.

Cowan A, Zhu XZ, Mosberg HI, Porreca F. Direct dependence studies in rats with agents selective for different subtypes of opioid receptor. *J Pharmacol* 1988; 246:950–955.

Cridland RA, Henry J. Effects of intrathecal administration of neuropeptides on a spinal nociceptive reflex in the rat; VIP, galanin, CGRP, TRH, somatostatin and angiotensin II. *Neuropeptides* 1998; 11:23–32.

Galligan JJ, Mosberg HI, Hurst R, Hruby VJ, Burks TF. Cerebral delta opioid receptors mediate analgesia but not the intestinal motility effects of intracerebroventricularly administered opioids. *J Pharmacol* 1984; 229:641–648.

Hao J-X, Shi T-J, Xu IS, et al. Intrathecal galanin alleviates allodynia-like behaviour in rats after partial peripheral nerve injury. *Eur J Neurosci* 1999; 11:427–432.

Hassan AHS, Ableiter A, Stein C, Herz A. Inflammation of the rat paw enhances axonal transport of opioid receptors in the sciatic nerve and increases their density in the inflamed tissue. *Neuroscience* 1993; 55:185–195.

Heyman JS, Mulvaney SA, Mosberg HI, Porreca F. Opioid delta receptor involvement in supraspinal and spinal antinociception in mice. *Brain Res* 1987; 420:100–108.

Hope PJ, Lang CW, Grubb BD, Duggan AW. Release of immunoreactive galanin in the spinal cord of rats with ankle inflammation: studies with antibody microprobes. *Neuroscience* 1994; 60:810–807.

Hökfelt T, Wiesenfeld-Hallin Z, Villar M, Milander T. Increase of galanin-like immunoreactivity in rat dorsal root ganglion cells after peripheral axotomy. *Neurosci Lett* 1987; 83:217–220.

Hökfelt T, Zhang X, Wiesenfeld-Hallin Z. Messenger plasticity in primary sensory neurons following axotomy and its functional implications. *Trends Neurosci* 1994; 17:22–30.

Ji RR, Zhang Q, Dagerlind A, et al. Central and peripheral expression of galanin in response to inflammation. *Neuroscience* 1995; 68:563–576.

Kuraishi Y, Kawamura M, Yamaguchi T, et al. Intrathecal injection of galanin and its antiserum affect nociceptive response of rat to mechanical but not thermal stimuli. *Pain* 1991; 44:321–324.

Malmberg AB, Yaksh TL. Isobolographic and dose-response analyses of the interaction between intrathecal mu and delta agonist: effects of naltrindole and its benzofuran analog (NTB). *J Pharm Exp Ther* 1992; 263:264–275.

Mansour A, Fox CA, Burke S, Akil H, Watson SJ. Immunohistochemical localization of the cloned mu opioid receptor in the rat CNS. *J Chem Neuroanat* 1995; 8:283–305.

Matthes HW, Maldonado R, Simonin F, et al. Loss of morphine-induced analgesia, reward effects and withdrawal symptoms in mice lacking the mu-opioid receptor gene. *Nature* 1996; 383:819–823.

Matthes HW, Smadja C, Valverde O, et al. Activity of the delta-opioid receptor is partially reduced, whereas activity of the kappa-receptor is maintained in mice lacking the mu-receptor. *J Neurosci* 1998; 18:7285–7295.

Miaskowski C, Sutters KA, Taiwo YO, Levine JD. Comparison of the antinociceptive and motor effects of intrathecal opioid agonists in the rat. *Brain Res* 1991; 553:105–109.

Miaskowski C, Taiwo YO, Levine JD. Antinociception produced by receptor selective opioids. Modulation of supraspinal antinociceptive effects by spinal opioids. *Brain Res* 1993; 608:87–94.

Negus SS, Gatch MB, Zhang X, Rice K. Behavioral effects of the delta-selective opioid agonist SNC80 and related compounds in rhesus monkey. *J Pharm Exp Ther* 1998; 286:362–375.

Nussbaumer JC, Yanagisawa M. Pharmacological properties of a C-fibre response evoked by saphenous nerve stimulation in an isolated spinal cord—nerve preparation of the newborn rat. *Br J Pharmacol* 1998; 98:373–382.

O'Donnell D, Ahmad S, Wahlestedt C, Walker P. Expression of the novel galanin receptor subtype GalR2 in the adult rat CNS: distinct distribution from GalR1. *J Comp Neurol* 1999; in press.

Peters GR, Antal EG, Lai PY, deMaar EW. Diuretic actions in man of a selective kappa opioid agonist: U-62,066E. *J Pharm Exp Ther* 1987; 240:128–131.

Pfeiffer A, Brantl V, Herz A, Emrich HM. Psychotomimesis mediated by kappa-opiate receptors. *Science* 1986; 233:774–775.

Ramer MS, Ma W, Murphy PG, Richardson PM, Bisby MA. Galanin expression in neuropathic pain: friend or foe. In: Hökfelt T, Bartfai T, Crawley J (Eds). *Galanin: Basic Research Discoveries and Therapeutic Implications*. New York: New York Academy of Science 1998; 390–401.

Randic M, Gerber G, Ryu PD, Kangra I. Inhibitory action of galanin and somatostatin 28 on rat spinal dorsal horn neurons. *Soc Neurosci Abstracts* 1987; 17:1308–1308.

Schiller P, Weltrowska, G, Nguyen TM, et al. TIPP[psi]: a highly potent and stable pseudopeptide delta opioid receptor antagonist with extraordinary delta selectivity. *J Med Chem* 1993; 36:3182–3187.

Schmidt R, Carpenter K, Yue S, et al. Linear and cyclic galanin (1–16)-NH$_2$ analogues: structure activity relationships, metabolic stability and conformational analysis. In: Bajusz S, Hudecz F (Eds). *Peptides 1998*. Budapest: Akademia Kiado, 1999, in press.

Sheldon RJ, Riviere PJM, Malarchik ME, et al. Opioid regulation of mucosal ion transport in mouse isolated jejunum. *J Pharmacol Exp Ther* 1990; 253:144–151.

Shi TJ, Zhang X, Holmberg K, Xu ZQD, Hökfelt T. Expression and regulation of gal R2 receptors in rat primary sensory neurons. Effects of axotomy and inflammation. *Neurosci Lett* 1997; 237:57–60.

Skofitsch G, Jacobowitz G. Galanin like immunoreactivity in capsaicin sensitive sensory neurons and ganglia. *Brain Res Bull* 1985; 15:191–195.

Smith KE, Forray C, Walker MW, et al. Expression cloning of a rat hypothalmic galanin receptor coupled to phosphoinositide turnover. *J Biol Chem* 1997; 272:24612–24616.

Sora I, Takahashi N, Funada M, et al. Opiate receptor knockout mice define μ receptor role in endogenous nociceptive responses and morphine-induced analgesia. *Proc Natl Acad Sci USA* 1997; 94:1544–1549.

Sora I, Li X-F, Funada M, Kinsey S, Uhl GR. Visceral chemical nociception in mice lacking μ-opioid receptors: effects of morphine, SNC80 and U-50,488. *Eur J Pharmacol* 1999; 366:R3–R5.

Standifer KM, Chien CC, Wahlestedt C, Brown GP, Pasternak GW. Selective loss of delta opioid analgesia and binding by antisense oligodeoxynucleotides to a delta opioid receptor. *Neuron* 1994; 12:805–810.

Stein C, Hassan AHS, Przewlocki R, Gramsch C, Peter KHA. Opioids from immunocytes react with receptors on sensory nerves to inhibit nociception in inflammation. *Proc Natl Acad Sci USA* 1990; 87:5935–5939ss.

Stewart PE, Holper EM, Hammond DL. Delta antagonist and kappa agonist activity of naltriben: evidence for differential kappa interaction with the delta1 and delta2 opioid receptor subtypes. *Life Sci* 1994(Suppl); 55:PL79–PL84.

Takemori AE, Portoghese PS. Selective naltrexone-derived opioid receptor antagonists. *Ann Rev Pharmacol Toxicol* 1992; 32:239–269.

Togunaga A, Senba E, Manabe Y, et al. Orofacial pain increase mRNA level for galanin in the trigeminal nucleus caudalis of the rat. *Peptides* 1992; 13:1067–1072.

Tung AS, Yaksh TL. In vivo evidence for multiple opiate receptors mediating analgesia in the rat spinal cord. *Brain Res* 1982; 247:75–83.

Vaught JL, Mathiasen JR, Raffa RB. Examination of the involvement of supraspinal and spinal mu delta opioid receptors in analgesia using the mu receptor deficient CXBK mouse. *J Pharmacol Exp Ther* 1998; 245:13–16.

Verge VMK, Xu X-J, Langel U, Hökfelt T. Evidence for an endogenous inhibition of autotomy, a behavioral sign of neuropathic pain, by galanin in rat after sciatic nerve section: demonstration by chronic intrathecal infusion of a high affinity galanin receptor antagonist. *Neurosci Lett* 1993; 149:193–197.

Villar MJ, Cortes R, Theodorsson E, et al. Neuropeptide expression in rat dorsal root ganglion cells and spinal cord after peripheral nerve injury with special reference to galanin. *Neuroscience* 1989; 33:587–604.

Wiesenfeld-Hallin Z, Xu X-J, Villar MJ, Hökfelt T. The effect of intrathecal galanin on the flexor reflex of the rat: increased depression after sciatic nerve section. *Neurosci Lett* 1989; 105:149–154.

Wiesenfeld-Hallin Z, Xu X-J, Villar MJ, Hökfelt T. Intrathecal galanin potentiates the spinal analgesic effect of morphine: electrophysiological and behavioural studies. *Neurosci Lett* 1990; 109:217–221.

Wiesenfeld-Hallin Z, Xu X, Langel U, et al. Galanin-mediated control of pain: enhanced role after nerve injury. *Proc Natl Acad Sci* 1994; 89:3334–3337.

Wild KD, Horan PJ, Jiang Q, et al. Antinociceptive pharmacology of BW 373U86: a novel nonpeptidic and selective opioid delta receptor agonist with an atypical profile. *J Pharmacol Exp Ther* 1993; 267:858–865.

Wynick D, Small CJ, Bloom SR. Targeted disruption of the murine galanin gene. In: Hökfelt T, Bartfai T, Crawley J (Eds). *Galanin: Basic Research Discoveries and Therapeutic Implications.* New York: New York Academy of Science, 1998, pp 22–47.

Xu LS, Grass S, Xu XJ, Wiesenfeld-Hallin Z. On the role of galanin in mediating spinal reflex excitability in inflammation. *Neuroscience* 1998a; 85:827–835.

Xu X-J, Wiesenfeld-Hallin Z, Villar MJ, Hökfelt T. On the role of galanin substance and other neuropeptides in primary sensory neurons of the rat: studies on spinal reflex excitability and peripheral axotomy. *Eur J Pharmacol* 1990; 2:733–743.

Xu Z, Xu ZQ, Shi T-J, et al. Regulation of expression of galanin and galanin receptors in dorsal root ganglia and spinal cord after axotomy and inflammation. In: Hökfelt T, Bartfei T, Crawley J (Eds). *Galanin: Basic Research Discoveries and Therapeutic Implications.* New York: New York Academy of Science, 1998b, pp 402–413.

Xu ZQ, Shi TJ, Landry M, Hökfelt T. Evidence for galanin receptors in primary sensory neurones and effects of axotomy and inflammation. *Neuroreport* 1996; 8:237–242.

Xu ZQ, Zhang X, Grillner S, Hökfelt T. Electrophysiological studies on rat dorsal root ganglion neurons after peripheral axotomy: changes in responses to neuropeptides. *Proc Natl Acad Sci* 1997; 94:13262–13266.

Yaksh TL, Rudy TA. Narcotic analgesics: CNS sites and mechanisms of action as revealed by intracerebral injection techniques. *Pain* 1978; 4:299–359.

Yaksh TL, Jessell TM, Leeman SE. Intrathecal morphine inhibits substance P release from mammalian spinal cord in vivo. *Nature* 1980; 286:155–157.

Yanagisawa M, Yagi N, Otsuka M, Yanaihara C,Yanaihara N. Inhibitory effects of galanin on the isolated spinal cord of the newborn rat. *Neurosci Lett* 1986; 70:278–282.

Yu LC, Lundenberg S, An H, Wang FX, Lundenberg T. Effects of intrathecal galanin on nociceptive responses in rats with mononeuropathy. *Life Sci* 1999; 64:1145–1153.

Zaki, PA, Bilsky EJ, Vanderah TW, et al. Opioid receptor types and subtypes: the δ receptor as a model. *Ann Rev Pharmacol Toxicol* 1996; 36:379–410.

Zhang Q, Schäfer M, Elde R, Stein C. Effects of neurotoxins and hindpaw inflammation on opioid receptor immunoreactivities in dorsal root ganglia. *Neuroscience* 1998; 85:281–291.

Correspondence to: Andy Dray, PhD, Department of Pharmacology, AstraZeneca R&D Montreal, 7171 Frederick Banting Building, St.-Laurent, Quebec, Canada H4S 1Z9. Fax: 514-832-3229; email: andy.dray@ arcm.ca.astra.com.

Opioid Sensitivity of Chronic Noncancer Pain,
Progress in Pain Research and Management,
Vol. 14, edited by Eija Kalso, Henry J. McQuay,
and Zsuzsanna Wiesenfeld-Hallin, IASP Press,
Seattle, © 1999.

17

Opioid Gene Knockouts: New Answers to Old Questions?

Ian Kitchen

Pharmacology Research Group, School of Biological Sciences, University of Surrey, Guildford, Surrey, United Kingdom

OPIOID PEPTIDES AND RECEPTORS

More than a decade after reports of the cloning of the opioid peptide precursors in the late 1970s and early 1980s, groups in Europe and the USA cloned the first opioid receptor subtype (Evans et al. 1992; Kieffer et al. 1992). It is now clear that at least three, and possibly four, families of opioid peptides exert their effects on at least three opioid receptor subtypes. The three precursors that have been cloned are pro-opiomelanocortin (POMC), proenkephalin, and prodynorphin (see Rossier 1982). Proteolytic cleavage of these peptides by processing enzymes gives rise to a number of structurally related opioid peptides, generically known as the endorphins. The main opioid peptide product of POMC is β-endorphin, those of proenkephalin are met- and leu-enkephalin, and that of prodynorphin is dynorphin A (Table I). Two novel opioid peptides, termed endomorphins, have recently been isolated (Zadina et al. 1997), and the cloning of their precursor is awaited to confirm a new family of endogenous opioids. Only three opioid receptors have been cloned (μ, δ, and κ) (see Kieffer 1995), and although the opioid peptide families have some selectivity for these subtypes, it is doubtful whether there is a correlation between a specific peptide precursor and a particular receptor subtype throughout the brain (Mansour et al. 1988). Binding studies show that the dynorphins are κ-opioid-receptor-preferring ligands, that the enkephalins prefer δ-opioid receptors, and that β-endorphin is equiactive at μ- and δ-opioid receptors (Paterson et al. 1983). Perhaps surprisingly, the newly discovered endomorphins are the only highly selective opioid ligands, with more than 4000-fold selectivity for the μ-opioid receptor (Zadina et al. 1997). An orphan clone isolated during the cloning of the

Table I
Structural homology of the major opioid peptides

Met-enkephalin	Tyr-Gly-Gly-Phe-Met
Leu-enkephalin	Tyr-Gly-Gly-Phe-Leu
Dynorphin A	Tyr-Gly-Gly-Phe-Leu-Arg-Arg-Ile-Arg-Pro-Lys-Leu-Lys-Trp-Asp-Asn-Gln
β-Endorphin	Tyr-Gly-Gly-Phe-Met-Thr-Ser-Glu-Lys-Ser-Gln-Thr-Pro-Leu-Val-Thr-Leu ...*
Endomorphin 1	Tyr-Pro-Trp-Phe-NH₂
Nociceptin/ orphanin FQ	Phe-Gly-Gly-Phe-Thr-Gly-Ala-Arg-Lys-Ser-Ala-Arg-Lys-Leu-Ala-Asn-Gln

Note: Amino acid homology in all the major products of the opioid peptide precursors are underlined. The common N-Tyr is crucial in conferring opioid receptor affinity. Note the common C-terminal sequences between the κ-preferring ligand dynorphin and the ORL1 ligand nociceptin.
*β-Endorphin (31 amino acids) is truncated at amino acid 17 for brevity and to allow sequence comparison with other peptides.

opioid receptors had nearly 70% sequence homology with the opioid receptors and is now commonly termed the ORL1 (opioid-receptor-like) receptor (see Henderson and McKnight 1997; Meunier 1997). The endogenous ligand for this receptor was isolated by two groups and named nociceptin (Meunier et al. 1995) and orphanin FQ (Reinscheid et al. 1995) (OFQ); both names are commonly used (Meunier 1997). The pharmacology of this system shows some level of association with opioid peptide systems, and both anti-opioid and analgesic actions have been reported for nociceptin/OFQ (see Henderson and McKnight 1997; Meunier 1997).

OPIOID KNOCKOUT MICE

The first reports of the generation of transgenic mice deficient in endogenous genes (known as knockout mice) appeared at the end of the 1980s. These knockouts are produced primarily by inactivating the genes by homologous recombination techniques in embryonic stem cells and transferring this mutation into a developing mouse (Capecchi 1989). Attempts to generate mice deficient in the genes encoding for opioid peptides and receptors have led to the successful deletion of genes encoding for all three opioid peptide families and the three opioid receptors and also knockout of nociceptin/OFQ and its receptor, ORL1. This progress has occurred in just a few years, rather shorter than the time we had to wait for the successful cloning of the opioid receptors.

The first opioid peptide to be disrupted was β-endorphin (Rubinstein 1993); the characterization of mice deficient in this opioid peptide was reported in early 1996 (Rubenstein et al. 1996). The gene mutation produced a truncated POMC by insertion of a premature translational stop codon by site-directed mutagenesis. Although the resulting knockout mice were deficient in β-endorphin, they were still able to produce adrenocorticotropic hormone (ACTH) and melanocyte-stimulating hormone (MSH), the other major hormones generated from this precursor. Mice deficient in pro-enkephalin were generated later in 1996 by replacement of part of exon 3, which contains all the enkephalin coding sequences (Konig et al. 1996). Most recently, an abstract report of mice deficient in prodynorphin has appeared with initial characterization of the behavioral phenotype of these knockout mice (Benoliel et al. 1998).

The first opioid receptor to be disrupted was the μ receptor, and the behavioral phenotype of μ-opioid-knockout animals was reported at the end of 1996 (Matthes et al. 1996). The knockout strategy involved disruption of exon 2 by homologous recombination. The generation of δ-receptor knockouts was reported in abstract form in 1997 (Zhu et al. 1997), and the characterization of κ-receptor knockouts followed in 1998 (Simonin et al. 1998). Work on deleting the μ receptor has been the most successful, and five different molecular genetics teams have now generated μ-knockout mice. These groups have used different gene disruption processes including insertion in exon 2 (Matthes et al. 1996), exon 1 disruption (Sora et al. 1997b; Tian et al. 1997; Schuller et al. 1999), and complete replacement of exon 2 and 3 (Loh et al. 1998), the major coding region of the μ-receptor gene. Table II presents the cited literature grouped by the lead investigator from each molecular genetics team.

Although not an opioid peptide (as defined by an action at a naloxone-sensitive opioid receptor), nociceptin/OFQ and its receptor ORL1 are related structurally and functionally to the classical opioid system (see Henderson

Table II

Mu-receptor knockouts: delineation of cited literature in relation to different mouse strains

Kieffer's group (exon 2): Matthes et al. 1996; Kitchen et al. 1997; Gaveriaux-Ruff et al. 1998; Kitchen et al. 1998; Matthes et al. 1998; Slowe et al. 1999

Uhl's group (exon 1): Sora et al. 1997a; Sora et al. 1997b; Fuchs et al. 1998; Hosohata et al. 1998; Kitanaka et al. 1998; Li et al. 1998; Qui et al. 1998; Sora et al. 1998

Yu's group (exon 1): Tian et al. 1997

Pintar's group (exon 1): Schuller et al. 1997; King et al. 1998; Schuller et al. 1998; Schuller et al. 1999

Loh's group (exon 2 and 3): Loh et al. 1998; Roy et al. 1998a; Roy et al. 1998b

Note: For the five molecular genetics groups that have generated μ-knockout mice, the literature cited in this chapter is grouped according to the lead investigator to assist the reader in comparing responses in these differently derived knockouts. The site of gene disruption for each group is shown in parentheses.

and McKnight 1997; Meunier 1997). Given the clear involvement of the nociceptin/OFQ system in pain and analgesia, this chapter will also consider the information from relevant gene knockout studies. Mice deficient in the ORL1 receptor were first reported in 1997 (Nishi et al. 1997), and mice deficient in the endogenous peptide have recently been presented in abstract form (Jenck et al. 1998; Reinscheid et al. 1998).

Table III presents a summary of the first reports of the successful generation of opioid peptide and receptor knockout animals and the initial characterization of their phenotype. The generation of these knockout animals has provided us with new tools to investigate the opioid system. The major advantage of the knockout approach is the complete selectivity provided by removal of a gene-encoded protein, which is nearly impossible to achieve by the conventional use of pharmacological antagonists, antibodies, or even antisense oligonucleotide knockdown approaches. Nevertheless, it would be incorrect to assume that these animals provide definitive answers to questions previously unanswered by traditional pharmacology. The knockout mouse gives us an additional tool to address questions related to opioid system functioning and opioid sensitivity. Experiments with knockout mice are expanding our knowledge of the physiology, pathophysiology, and pharmacology of opioid systems and the potential tonic role of opioid peptides and receptors in regulating pain sensitivity and tolerance to opioid drugs. In addition, they are providing progress in addressing the long-standing de-

Table III
Opioid peptides and opioid receptors: successful gene deletions in mice

	References
Opioid Peptides	
β-Endorphin	Rubinstein et al. 1996
Proenkephalin	Konig et al. 1996; (King et al. 1998)
Prodynorphin	(Benoliel et al. 1998)
Nociceptin/OFQ	(Reinscheid et al. 1998; Jenck et al. 1998)
β-Endorphin/proenkephalin	(Wilson et al. 1998)
Opioid Receptors	
μ	Matthes et al. 1996; Sora et al. 1997; Tian et al. 1997; Loh et al. 1998; Schuller et al. 1999
κ	Simonin et al. 1998; (Zhang et al. 1998)
δ	(Zhu et al. 1997)
ORL1	Nishi et al. 1997

Note: The references listed are full papers that initially characterized the phenotype of the successfully generated knockout mice. (References in parentheses are abstracts.)

bates over receptor subtype heterogeneity and functional cooperativity between receptor subtypes. However, transgenic approaches have important limitations and caveats, which are outlined later in this chapter. This review primarily compares wild-type (+/+), normal, and homozygous (–/–) knockout mice. Additional information is becoming available from heterozygous (+/–) animals with deletion of only one copy of the gene and thus peptide or receptor levels that are typically 50% of the wild-type controls. These mice may well prove useful in studying diseases where receptor or peptide deficiencies are a feature, such as aging processes that often lead to downregulation of transmitter and receptor pools, or in the study of the pharmacodynamics of ligand–receptor interactions.

MU-OPIOID RECEPTOR KNOCKOUTS: WHAT IS CLEAR?

MORPHINE IS A MU-RECEPTOR AGONIST

To a pharmacologist, the statement that morphine exerts its analgesic activity by an action at the μ-opioid receptor is not entirely surprising, and all supraspinal and spinal analgesic models to date show complete loss of the analgesic activity of morphine in knockout mice (Matthes et al. 1996; Sora et al. 1997b; Loh et al. 1998; Schuller et al. 1999). What was perhaps unexpected is that even at doses approaching 100 mg/kg, morphine failed to elicit analgesia in knockout mice (Sora et al. 1997b; Schuller et al. 1999), and doses approaching 500 mg/kg were necessary to produce a 50% analgesic response (Loh et al. 1998). The receptor-binding studies both in brain homogenates (Paterson et al. 1983; Yeadon and Kitchen 1988) and on cloned receptors (Raynor et al. 1994) clearly indicate that morphine is only 50–100-fold selective for the μ receptor over the δ or κ receptor, so that some κ- or δ-opioid-receptor analgesia might have been anticipated in the μ-knockout mice. Clearly the knockout mouse points to the pivotal role the μ receptor plays in the analgesic responses to morphine and raises the issue of permissiveness in the functioning of δ- or κ-receptor systems. Virtually all other effects of morphine are abolished in μ-knockout mice, including reinforcing properties assessed by place-preference methods, withdrawal symptoms in chronically treated mice, hyperlocomotion, respiratory depression, immunosuppression, inhibition of gastrointestinal transit, and lethality (Matthes et al. 1996, 1998; Sora et al. 1997b; Tian et al. 1997; Gaveriaux-Ruff et al. 1998; Loh et al. 1998; Roy et al. 1998a,b). These data again emphasize the crucial role of the μ receptor for morphine's action. In relation to reward processes, a recent study showed that cocaine place preference is attenuated by 50% in μ-knockout mice (Sora et al. 1998). Thus, the μ-opioid receptor is also implicated in the rewarding properties of psychostimulant drugs, and earlier pharmacological evidence (see Koob 1992) would point to a common involvement of dopaminergic circuitry.

NORMAL EXPRESSION OF OPIOID PEPTIDES

Although no groups have performed quantitative analysis, in situ hybridization with probes directed to the precursors of the three opioid peptides indicates that the expression of these peptides in the brain is normal in μ-knockout mice (Matthes et al. 1996; Schuller et al. 1999). Thus, the loss of the μ receptor does not appear to cause any compensatory upregulation of endogenous opioid peptides, which suggests a lack of regulatory control on transcription of genes encoding the endogenous ligands. It also points to a lack of tonic functioning of the opioid system, a characteristic borne out by many other knockout studies. Alternatively, it could be that the endomorphins are the endogenous ligands for the μ receptor and that any compensation might be observed in the these novel peptides. However, changes in endomorphin levels in μ-knockout mice have yet to be investigated.

NORMAL DEVELOPMENT

All five groups that have generated μ-receptor knockout mice (Table II) reported normal gross development and body weight gain, with no noticeable neuroanatomical defects and no indication of lethality from the gene deletion. However, the more detailed developmental analysis of these animals has yet to be performed, although one group has already reported reduced mating activity, decreases in sperm count and motility, and smaller litter sizes in μ-knockout mice (Tian et al. 1997). In addition, increased cell proliferation in bone marrow and spleen points to enhanced hematopoiesis. Thus, subtle developmental changes in cell proliferation may have been missed. Substantial pharmacological evidence implicates the μ receptor in cell growth (Hauser et al. 1987, 1996), so further studies are warranted. However, one of the major limiting features of knockout studies is the inherent plasticity in the organism, and equally there may simply be developmental compensation following the gene deletion.

TONIC ROLE IN GASTROINTESTINAL TRANSIT

A tonic role for the μ receptor in regulating gastrointestinal (GI) function has been suggested because basal GI motility is lower in knockout mice compared to both heterozygous and wild-type animals (Roy et al. 1998b). One theory suggests that the system evolves with a reduced overall transit rate to compensate for the loss of μ-receptor inhibition of motility (Roy et al. 1998b). However, others have more recently reported a significant increase in GI transit in μ-knockout mice (Schuller et al. 1998), and suggest that this is due to loss of tonic regulation by μ agonists. The lack of effects of δ and κ agonists on GI transit in the μ-knockout mice again serve to confirm the μ receptor as the primary target for opioid regulation in the gut.

NO MU-RECEPTOR SUBTYPES DERIVED FROM ANOTHER GENE

Several of the earliest reports of μ-receptor knockout used homogenate binding to confirm a complete loss of μ receptors throughout the brain in knockout mice (Matthes et al. 1996; Sora et al. 1997b; Loh et al. 1998; Schuller et al. 1999) as well as absence of μ-receptor immunostaining (Sora et al. 1997b) and μ-receptor binding (I. Kitchen, unpublished observations) in the dorsal horn of the spinal cord. The issue of heterogeneity of the μ receptor (μ_1 and μ_2 subtypes) has been a matter of much contention (Pasternak and Wood 1986; Pasternak 1993). Use of the μ-knockout mouse has helped to resolve this matter. Long-exposure autoradiography in sagittal brain sections shows that no μ receptors are labeled with ^{3}H-DAMGO (Kitchen et al. 1997), a ligand that would bind all putative μ-receptor subtypes in μ-knockout mice. Thus, if μ-receptor subtypes exist, they must arise from the same gene. In this regard, evidence for splice variants has been reported (Zimprich et al. 1995).

MU-RECEPTOR KNOCKOUTS: WHAT IS NOT CLEAR?

TONIC ROLE IN REGULATING PAIN

Although the first μ-knockout animals showed no differences in pain sensitivity in the tail-flick and hot-plate thermal pain tests (Matthes et al. 1996), subsequent experiments from other μ-deficient mice indicate alteration in sensitivity to painful stimuli (Table IV). For example, one study reported shorter response latencies in both tail-flick and hot-plate tests in μ-knockout mice (Sora et al. 1997b). The possibility that these differences might reflect small differences in the testing temperature must be considered, as Sora et al. (1997b) failed to observe the hyperalgesia in the μ-knockout mouse when the temperature in the tail-flick assay was increased to 56°C. It is known that severity of stimulus markedly alters sensitivity to pain modulation by opioid drugs (Parsons and Headley 1989), and thus an endogenous involvement of the μ receptor in regulating pain sensitivity may well be dependent on stimulus as well as pain type. The most recent

Table IV
Basal pain sensitivity in opioid knockout mice

Gene Knockout	Thermal Supra-spinal	Thermal Spinal	Inflam-matory	Visceral	Pressure	SIA
μ receptor[1]	⇔ or ⇑	⇔ or ⇑	⇓	⇓	⇔	
δ receptor[2]		⇔				
κ receptor[3]	⇔	⇔	⇔ or ⇓	⇑	⇔	
ORL1 receptor[4]	⇔	⇔		⇔	⇔	
β-Endorphin[5]	⇔			⇔		0
Proenkephalin[6]	⇑	⇔	⇓			⇔
Prodynorphin[7]		⇓	⇔			
β-Endorphin/ proenkephalin[8]						⇔

Source: Data were derived from the following papers as indicated for each gene knockout by arabic superscripts: (1) Matthes et al. (1996), Sora et al. (1997b), Fuchs et al. (1998), Li et al. (1998), Qui et al. (1998); (2) Zhu et al. (1997); (3) Simonin et al. (1998), Zhang et al. (1998); (4) Nishi et al. (1997), Ueda et al. (1997), Mamiya et al. (1998); (5) Rubenstein et al. (1996); (6) Konig et al. (1996); (7) Benoliel et al. (1998); (8) Wilson et al. (1998).

Note: Basal pain sensitivity in thermal tests (hot-plate for supraspinal and tail-immersion or radiant heat tail-flick or thermal paw withdrawal for spinal pain), mechanical tests (tail or paw pressure), inflammatory tests (formalin, Freund's adjuvant, or carrageenan injection in hindpaw), visceral chemical tests (acetic acid writing), plus effects on stress-induced analgesia (SIA). ⇔ = no change; ⇑ = increased pain sensitivity (hyperalgesia); ⇓ = decreased pain sensitivity (hypoalgesia); 0 = abolition of SIA.

studies in the μ-knockout strain (which showed hyperalgesia in thermal tests) reported hypoalgesia in models of visceral pain (acetic acid writhing) (Li et al. 1998) and inflammatory pain (intraplantar Freund's adjuvant) (Qui et al. 1998), but no alterations in paw-pressure tests (Fuchs et al. 1998).

TONIC ROLE IN LOCOMOTION

Another area of literature divergence is in the modulation of locomotion. The first study of μ-receptor knockout reported a tendency to hypolocomotion in the knockout mice (Matthes et al. 1996). Subsequent studies showed a reduction in horizontal but not vertical locomotor activity (Tian et al. 1997), although Sora et al. (1997b) found no differences between genotypes using several tests of locomotor skills, including the accelerating rotarod. It is well known that locomotor deficits can give false changes in sensitivity to pain in tests that involve motor movement. Some of the inconsistency in the literature reports on basal nociception could reflect the disparity in reports of locomotor disturbances.

RESPONSES TO MORPHINE-6-GLUCURONIDE

One of the major metabolites of morphine, morphine-6-glucuronide (M6G), is also known to exert analgesic effects (Abbott and Palmour 1998), and may substantially contribute to pain relief in humans chronically treated with morphine (see Lehmann and Zech 1993). Schuller and co-workers (1997, 1999) reported that although μ-knockout mice showed abolition of analgesic responses to morphine, a substantial component of analgesic activity for both M6G and heroin was retained, which raised the possibility that a novel receptor mediates their analgesia, a proposal already advanced from pharmacological data (Rossi et al. 1996, 1997). Two other groups, however, have failed to observe any M6G analgesia in μ-knockout mice (Kitanaka et al. 1998; Loh et al. 1998), thus the existence of a novel receptor is a contentious issue. It is possible that responses to M6G are dependent on the type of gene disruption. A recent study has proposed the existence of sequences encoding for novel splice variants of the μ receptor (Schuller et al. 1999). This group has shown retention of M6G analgesia in Pintar's exon 1-disrupted μ knockouts, but not in the exon 2 knockouts generated by Kieffer's group (Matthes et al. 1996). This finding would also accord with a lack of M6G analgesia reported by Loh's group (1998), which disrupted exon 2 and exon 3, but it is still at odds with the failure to observe M6G analgesia in Uhl's exon 1-disrupted μ knockouts (Kitanaka et al. 1998). However, the possibility remains that a unique M6G receptor is encoded for by an alternative transcript from the MOR1 locus (Schuller et al. 1999), especially since the amount of exon 1 disruption will have a bearing on any alternative transcripts that might be produced.

FUNCTIONAL RESPONSES TO DELTA AND KAPPA AGONISTS

Another unresolved issue is whether functional activity of δ- and κ-receptor systems is altered in the μ-knockout animals. Certainly, much of the past work in pharmacology suggests interactions and cooperativity between opioid receptor subtypes, particularly for the μ and δ receptors (Heyman et al. 1989a,b). Although Matthes et al. (1996) reported absence of analgesic responses to the selective δ-opioid agonist BUBU in μ-knockout mice, a subsequent, more detailed investigation has revealed that activity of the δ receptor is only partially reduced in these animals (Matthes et al. 1998). This study showed normal functional coupling of the δ receptor on

GTPγS binding and in adenylyl cyclase inhibition assays, and reported normal responses to δ agonists in the mouse vas deferens bioassay. However, analgesic responses to deltorphin II, and more strikingly respiratory depression, were attenuated in the μ-knockout mice. In parallel studies, functioning of the κ-receptor system appeared normal. Another study showed a marked loss of analgesic responses to the δ agonist [D-Pen^2,D-Pen^5]enkephalin (DPDPE) (Sora et al. 1997a), while Matthes et al. (1998) showed only a modest attenuation, and others have failed to observe any modulation of analgesic responses to DPDPE in the μ-knockout mice (Loh et al. 1998). It is not possible to ascribe the disparity to differences in spinal or supraspinal pain tests, as all three groups used protocols to test both sites; however, the data of the Matthes group suggest that the dysfunction of δ-opioid systems is more pronounced at the spinal level. The possibility that DPDPE is not acting in a δ-selective manner should also be entertained, since in binding assays it is not as selective as the deltorphin peptides (Salvadori et al. 1991; Knapp and Yamamura 1992), and comparative studies of wild-type and μ-knockout mice show that DPDPE functionally activates both μ and δ receptors in GTP binding assays (Hosohata et al. 1998). Thus, DPDPE in wild-type mice can exert effects at μ receptors, which compromises the interpretation of the knockout data.

DOWNREGULATION OF DELTA- AND KAPPA-OPIOID RECEPTORS

One possible explanation for functional alterations in δ systems in the μ-knockout mice may reside in receptor loss. It is clear from the homogenate binding studies (Matthes et al. 1996; Sora et al. 1997b; Loh et al. 1998; Schuller et al. 1999) and in situ hybridization (Schuller et al. 1999) that there are no major compensatory changes in either δ- or κ-opioid receptors. Detailed quantitative autoradiographic mapping of δ and κ receptors in the brain of μ-knockout mice (Kitchen et al. 1997) show the overall decrement of δ and κ receptors to be little more than 10%. However, several discrete anatomical regions show downregulation of 30–40% for the δ receptor, which is significantly correlated with areas of high μ-receptor expression in wild-type mice. This is most striking in noncortical structures. Interestingly, parallel studies in κ-knockout mice show reciprocal increases in receptor binding in many of these structures, including the nucleus accumbens, the vertical limb of the diagonal band, the hypothalamus, and the preoptic area (Slowe et al. 1999). It is thus possible that some of the functional changes in responses to δ agonists that have been reported in μ-knockout mice reflect regional deficits in the expression of δ receptors. Our group is mapping other nonopioid receptors also involved in pain circuitry in both μ- and κ-

Table V
Summary of changes in expression of opioid and nonopioid
receptors in μ- and κ-opioid-receptor knockout mice assessed by
quantitative autoradiography

Receptor	μ Knockout	κ Knockout
μ	0	⇑
δ	⇓	⇑
κ	⇓	0
ORL1	⇔	⇔
A_1	⇓	
A_{2A}	⇔	

Note: ⇔ = no change; ⇑ = increased expression; ⇓ = decreased expression; 0 = complete abolition of binding. Some of the data are from Kitchen et al. (1997, 1998) and Slowe et al. (1999).

knockout mice. Table V summarizes the changes observed as of early 1999. In addition to decrements in δ receptors in the μ-knockout mice, adenosine A_1 receptors show significant downregulation throughout the brain. We need more quantitative information on both receptor expression and functional coupling to G proteins in the spinal cord, where significant pain modulation occurs. The data so far suggest some subtle alterations in opioid and nonopioid circuitry in the μ-deficient mice.

KAPPA-RECEPTOR KNOCKOUTS: WHAT IS CLEAR?

U50488H IS A KAPPA-1 AGONIST

In accordance with the observations for morphine in the μ-knockout mouse, the classical arylacetamide ligand U50488H, which has been designated a prototypic $κ_1$ agonist, has no effect in κ-knockout animals. Analgesic responses to U50488H are completely abolished, and hypolocomotor, salivation, and place aversion induced by this agonist are also markedly attenuated (Simonin et al. 1998). Interestingly, U50488H did induce a weak hypolocomotor response at the highest dose studied (20 mg/kg), and there was also some residual place-aversion response. These effects cannot be mediated by the μ receptor because the behavioral characteristic of a μ-receptor action is opposite to that observed. It raises a tempting speculation about an action at another opioid or nonopioid receptor site (Simonin et al. 1998). Recently a second group generated κ-knockout mice that also show loss of analgesic responses to U50488H (Zhang et al. 1998).

TONIC ROLE IN VISCERAL PAIN

Basal pain sensitivity has been assessed in thermal tests (tail immersion and hot-plate), mechanical tests (tail pressure), chemical visceral tests (acetic acid abdominal constriction), and inflammatory tests (formalin hindpaw test). There were no differences in sensitivity to the painful stimulus except for the acetic acid writhing test, where κ-knockout mice showed more than double the number of writhes compared to wild-type mice. This hyperalgesia is compatible with the previous pharmacological studies that implicated the κ receptor in the control of visceral pain (Tyers 1980; Schmauss et al. 1983).

NORMAL DEVELOPMENT, LOCOMOTION, AND OPIOID PEPTIDE AND RECEPTOR EXPRESSION

Similar to the μ knockouts, κ-knockout mice develop normally, have normal body weight, have no gross abnormalities, and exhibit normal maternal behavior. The only indication of developmental changes was a significant increase in litter size (Simonin et al. 1998). An interesting question will be whether more detailed developmental analysis reveals an important reproductive role of the κ receptor, since pharmacological studies have clearly shown the receptor to be instrumental in initiating the suckling process (Smotherman and Robinson 1992). Spontaneous locomotor behavior is also normal in the knockout mouse. As in the μ-knockout, there are no obvious compensatory changes in the expression of opioid peptides (Simonin et al. 1998), and full quantitative autoradiographic mapping shows no major changes in expression of μ- or δ-opioid receptors (Slowe et al. 1999). However, in common with the μ-receptor knockout, some region-specific disturbance of the δ receptor is observed, but in contrast to the μ-knockout, upregulation occurs (Slowe et al. 1999) (Table IV).

MORPHINE WITHDRAWAL IMPAIRED

The involvement of κ receptors in modulating μ-receptor responses again relates to potential interactions between the opioid receptor subtypes. Both analgesic and place-preference responses to morphine are normal in the κ-knockout mouse (Simonin et al. 1998). This finding accords with studies of κ agonists in μ-knockout mice (Matthes et al. 1998), and again points to a lack of interaction between μ and κ receptors in response to pain. The lack of modulation of reward is perhaps surprising, given that μ and κ agonists have opposing actions on mesolimbic dopaminergic neurons (Shippenberg et al. 1987). However, involvement of the κ receptor in the modulation of the dependence process is clear because morphine withdrawal responses are impaired in κ-knockout mice (Simonin et al. 1998).

NO KAPPA-1 RECEPTOR SUBTYPES DERIVED FROM ANOTHER GENE

Although only three genes have been cloned for the μ, δ, and κ receptors (Kieffer 1995), evidence from binding and autoradiographic studies suggests further receptor heterogeneity. For the κ receptor at least three subtypes (κ_1, κ_2, and κ_3) have been proposed (Zukin et al. 1988; Clark et al. 1989; Unterwald et al. 1991), although the pharmacological profile of the cloned receptor is most closely aligned with the κ_1 receptor, which recognizes arylacetamide ligands (Raynor et al. 1994). In addition, subtypes of the κ_1 receptor have been proposed (Clark et al. 1989; Rothman et al. 1989). Homogenate-binding experiments with the arylacetamide ligand CI-977 show complete loss of binding sites in the brain of the κ-knockout mouse (Simonin et al. 1998), and long-exposure autoradiography in sagittal brain sections confirms the lack of μ receptors labeled with the κ_1 ligand (Slowe et al. 1999). Thus, if κ_1-receptor subtypes exist, they must arise from the same gene. Clearly, any of the residual behavioral responses observed with U50488H are not due to κ_1-subtype activation.

KAPPA-1 RECEPTOR KNOCKOUTS: WHAT IS NOT CLEAR?

To date only one full paper reporting κ-opioid-receptor knockout has appeared in the literature, so the lack of contentious issues is not surprising. Nevertheless, several questions still need to be addressed.

KAPPA-RECEPTOR SUBTYPES

Arylacetamide ligands label only a proportion of the κ receptors labeled by benzomorphan ligands such as bremazocine or ethylketocyclazocine (Fowler and Fraser 1994), and the binding profile of the cloned receptor is consistent with high affinity for arylacetamides (Reisine and Bell 1993; Raynor et al. 1994), so it has been conventional to define the cloned receptor as κ_1. The putative additional population of κ receptors labeled with benzomorphans has been termed κ_2 (Tiberi et al. 1988; Zukin et al. 1988; Smith et al. 1989; Unterwald et al. 1991). The existence of additional κ-receptor subtypes is extremely contentious because the benzomorphans also label μ and δ receptors, and all binding studies must be conducted under conditions designed to suppress labeling of the other opioid subtypes. The κ-knockout mouse and mice deficient in μ and δ receptors have now provided a genetic tool to finally determine whether the putative $κ_2$ receptor arises from a gene not previously characterized. Current data from homogenate-binding and long-exposure autoradiographic studies suggest that virtually all binding of bremazocine can be explained by the labeling of μ and δ receptors (Kitchen et al. 1999). Finally, a recently published abstract reported retention of naloxone benzoylhydrazone analgesia in the κ-knockout mouse (Zhang et al. 1998). Whether this is due to an action at a putative $κ_3$ receptor or to its affinity for the ORL1 receptor (Noda et al. 1998) remains to be confirmed.

DELTA-RECEPTOR KNOCKOUTS: WHAT IS CLEAR AS MUD!

The phenotype of the δ-knockout mouse has at the time of writing only been published in abstract form. The animals show no evidence of δ-receptor binding labeled with DPDPE or deltorphin II and no alterations in κ- or μ-receptor binding, expression of opioid peptides, basal pain sensitivity, or morphine analgesia (Zhu et al. 1997). These findings seem clear; however, although there is no δ binding in these mice and spinal analgesia to DPDPE and deltorphin II is abolished, supraspinal analgesia still persists. The obvious interpretation is that this is a μ-mediated analgesia, and yet μ antagonists do not block this analgesia while δ antagonists are active. Other groups have now successfully generated δ-knockout mice, and time (and more experiments) will surely resolve these anomalies.

ORL1 KNOCKOUTS: WHAT IS CLEAR?

NO TONIC ROLE IN PAIN SENSITIVITY

In thermal (radiant heat tail-flick) and visceral (acetic acid writhing) pain tests, sensitivity to the noxious stimuli is normal in ORL1-knockout mice (Nishi et al. 1997). Lack of effects on pain sensitivity has also been reported for tail-pinch (Ueda et al. 1997) and hot-plate and foot-shock tests (Mamiya et al. 1998). Clearly this body of data suggests no tonic role for the ORL1 receptor in setting pain sensitivity in response to a variety of stimuli.

RESPONSES TO NOCICEPTIN/OFQ AND MORPHINE

Nociceptin/OFQ-induced hypolocomotion and hyperalgesia are abolished in the ORL1-knockout mice (Nishi et al. 1997). However, a tonic role for the

ORL1 receptor in locomotion can be discounted, as spontaneous locomotion was similar in all genotypes. Morphine analgesia is normal in the ORL1 knockouts (Nishi et al. 1997), but an interaction with the μ-opioid system is suggested by the attenuation of tolerance to morphine in ORL1-deficient mice (Ueda et al. 1997).

NALOXONE BENZOYLHYDRAZONE ANALGESIA IS MEDIATED BY THE ORL1 RECEPTOR

Naloxone benzoylhydrazone (NalBzoH) is a derivative of naloxone that produces analgesia. Evidence from ligand-binding studies suggests that it interacts with a novel opioid receptor named κ_3 (Clark et al. 1989; Cheng et al. 1992; Pan et al. 1995). However, in binding studies in cell systems expressing the ORL1 receptor, NalBzoH shows appreciable binding affinity, while in ORL1-knockout mice the analgesic activity of this compound is lost in both thermal and visceral pain tests (Noda et al. 1998). Further, nociceptin/OFQ-induced hypolocomotion was blocked by NalBzoH in wild-type mice, but both nociceptin/OFQ and NalBzoH were without effect in ORL1 knockouts. The gene knockout studies therefore strongly suggest that NalBzoH is an ORL1 antagonist rather than a ligand for a novel κ receptor.

DISRUPTION OF HEARING AND MEMORY

Mice deficient in the ORL1 receptor lack the ability to recover from intense sound exposure injury, which points to a tonic role for this receptor in the regulation of the auditory system (Nishi et al. 1997). Perhaps even more important is that removal of the ORL1 receptor produces mice with greater learning ability and better memory than wild-type controls, as evidenced by improved performance in water maze tests and passive avoidance tasks. At the cellular level, enhanced long-term potentiation in hippocampal slices is also observed in these animals, which implies that the nociceptin/OFQ system plays a negative role in both learning and memory processes (Manabe et al. 1998).

PROENKEPHALIN KNOCKOUTS: WHAT IS CLEAR?

Deletion of the proenkephalin gene has revealed some surprising alterations in pain and analgesic responses (Konig et al. 1996). Animals displayed enhanced sensitivity to pain in the hot-plate test, but there was no change in tail-flick latencies, indicating supraspinal but not spinal hyperalgesia. Animals receiving hindpaw injections of formalin did not show typical pain responses such as paw lifting and licking, but appeared agitated and shook their paws immediately after injection. In addition, mice displayed some locomotor deficits that appeared to be associated with anxiogenic behavior in maze performance tasks and aggressive behavior in "resident intruder" tests (Konig et al. 1996). Surprisingly, proenkephalin-deficient mice showed no alteration in swim-stress-induced analgesia using an experimental model recognized to operate via opioid receptors; enkephalins thus do not appear to be the substrates of stress-induced analgesic behavior. Despite this spectrum of behavior the animals are healthy, fertile, and have no gross abnormalities. Another group has now successfully generated proenkephalin-deficient mice that do not display tolerance to morphine but retain tolerance to the κ agonist U50488H, a feature also observed with δ-knockout mice (King et al. 1998). Thus, the proenkephalin/δ-receptor system is a requirement for pathways that mediate μ-receptor tolerance.

BETA-ENDORPHIN KNOCKOUTS: WHAT IS CLEAR?

Although β-endorphin was the first opioid knockout to be reported, the literature for this deletion is sparse. In both supraspinal and visceral pain tests, the basal pain sensitivity was unaltered, which suggests a lack of tonic control in the regulation of central and peripheral pain (Rubenstein et al. 1996). However, β-endorphin clearly mediates stress-induced analgesia, as the knockout mice show loss of opioid-mediated swim-stress-induced analgesia and a compensatory upregulated nonopioid stress-induced analgesia that is resistant to naloxone administration (Rubenstein et al. 1996). These data support the assertion made nearly 20 years ago that there is collateral inhibition between the opioid and nonopioid analgesic systems (Kirchgessner et al. 1982). Although these animals are equisensitive to systemically administered morphine, they are more sensitive to supraspinal than to spinal administration of this drug (Grisel et al. 1997), again suggesting compensatory changes in the pain/analgesic circuitry. As with the other opioid knockouts, development is relatively normal, with the exception of postpubertal weight gain (Konig et al. 1996).

Most recently, mice deficient in β-endorphin have been crossed with animals deficient in proenkephalin. Although we would expect these "double knockouts" to show loss of stress-induced analgesia, surprisingly, these analgesic responses were restored (Wilson et al. 1998). Perhaps the organism has compensatory mechanisms that are activated only by the double insult. The issue of plasticity limits the interpretations that can be made from gene knockout experiments.

PRODYNORPHIN KNOCKOUTS: WHAT IS CLEAR?

Only one abstract reporting this successful gene deletion has been published (Benoliel et al. 1998). Reduced thermal pain sensitivity is observed in the knockout mice and is more evident in males. Inflammatory hyperalgesia induced by carrageenan injection in the hindpaw did not differ between this genotype and wild-type controls, but analysis of locomotor behavior after inflammation revealed a decrease in activity, most pronounced in females (Benoliel et al. 1998). These initial gender differences are of interest because human studies indicate differences between the sexes in sensitivity to pain associated with different κ-receptor sensitivities (Gear et al. 1996).

NOCICEPTIN/OFQ KNOCKOUTS: WHAT IS CLEAR?

Again, only abstracts have reported animals deficient in nociceptin/OFQ (Jenck et al. 1998; Reinscheid et al. 1998). Preliminary data suggest normal neurological and behavioral characteristics but indicate increased anxiety and aggression under stressed conditions. There is also evidence of increased pain sensitivity and alterations in stress-induced analgesia.

LIMITATIONS OF OPIOID KNOCKOUT STUDIES

A knockout mouse is not the answer to all the problems that the traditional pharmacological approach has left unresolved. Rather, it is a complementary genetic tool that can provide new information, but in many instances may also provide us with new questions. There are limitations and problems in interpreting the phenotypic findings in transgenic animals (for a more detailed review see Gerlai 1996; Tecott et al. 1996; Crawley and Paylor 1997; Mogil and Grisel 1998). The most serious confounding factor in knockout studies is that the study animals lack the targeted gene not only during behavioral testing but throughout development. This prolonged absence of the gene may lead to any number of compensatory mechanisms that are part of the inherent plasticity of mammalian systems. Such compensation may lead to false negative or false positive phenotypes. The future use of inducible knockouts (Kuhn et al. 1995) in studies that will maintain temporal control of the gene disruption may eventually remove this major hurdle.

A second issue of concern is that most genes have multiple functions that may yield multiple consequences, which may in turn affect the behavioral function that is being tested. In turn, the ultimate behavioral change might be an indirect rather than a direct association with the deleted protein.

The third main problem arises from the almost universal use of the C57BL/6 mouse strain as a recipient genome for the cell lines derived from the 129/sv strain of mouse. The resulting knockout mice are thus a random mix of 129/sv and C57BL/6 alleles; the linked "hitchhiking" genes (Crusio 1996) are 129/sv alleles in knockout mice but C57BL/6 alleles in wild-type animals. In the pain field, the question has been raised as to whether the C57BL/6 mouse is representative of mice in general, given indications that it has a higher pain sensitivity than most other strains (Mogil and Grisel 1998). Another issue is that although gene-targeting strategies (i.e., different replacement or inactivation of exons) all lead to loss of the targeted protein, the genetic material that remains can give rise to alternatively spliced molecules with possible biological activity. In the opioid knockout studies this offers a possible explanation for some of the failures to replicate results in the μ-knockout mice that have been generated by several groups (Schuller et al. 1999). Finally, much of the pharmacological knowledge of opioids is based on studies in rats. Some of the data are not equivalent to data from mouse models, and many of the methods are more difficult to implement in mice. Thus, we may need to revisit traditional pharmacology because the successes of molecular genetics have given us knockout mice rather than knockout rats.

CONCLUDING REMARKS

Of all the opioid knockouts, the most controversy surrounds the responses observed in animals with μ-receptor deletions. A simple explanation would be that these gene deletions are being performed by several different groups, and as with all other areas of pharmacology, this can mean many permutations of results. Although I am sure there is some truth in this, disparities in the literature may be partly due to the molecular genetics used to generate these animals. Of particular note is the divergence in the data for M6G, and it is possible that the residual responses to this compound are only seen when disruption of the μ-receptor gene leaves functional exons that produce proteins that can respond to this drug (Schuller et al. 1999).

What have the opioid knockouts given us that is new? They undoubtedly add to our knowledge of the pharmacology and physiology of opioid system functioning. Some of the results confirm previous pharmacological experiments. This is partly because we are fortunate that opioid chemistry is sufficiently advanced that we have highly selective receptor agonists and some receptor-selective antagonists. This is not yet true for the ORL1 receptor, and ORL1 knockouts have instantaneously given us tools that precede successful medicinal chemistry.

The receptor knockouts are adding to the debate over cooperativity and functional interactions between opioid receptor subtypes, and point to μ/δ interactions rather than μ/κ cooperativity. Perhaps more importantly, the receptor knockouts are shedding new light on receptor subtype heterogeneity, particularly for μ and κ sites. Some opioid knockouts have given us new insights into the potential pathophysiology of opioid systems; in particular, the deletion of the ORL1 receptor gives new pointers to cognitive disease, and the deletion of proenkephalin raises issues concerning anxiogenesis.

Finally, what have the opioid knockouts told us about opioid sensitivity to date? It appears that κ and μ receptors regulate pain sensitivity and that enkephalins, dynorphins, and nociceptin/OFQ also contribute to the setting of pain thresholds. Moreover, this peptide and receptor modulation is extremely specific to pain types, and much more work needs to be done before modulatory circuitry can be drawn. It also appears that both enkephalins and the δ receptor are involved in pathways that mediate tolerance to μ opioids. Whether this is a significant clinical issue is still a matter of debate, but again it gives a new handle on how the system can be manipulated. Such information could be invaluable for clinical management of intractable pain.

Inevitably, when a field of study emerges and rapidly evolves, review articles quickly become dated. To be as up-to-date as possible, a number of publications are cited in abstract form, and the full papers are eagerly awaited. The compilation of the studies in this chapter serves purely as a snapshot and provides a template for the beginning of another review. I suspect, however, the next review of the opioid knockout literature will have a rather different title—"Opioid gene knockouts—new answers *and more* questions!"

ACKNOWLEDGMENTS

The work from the author's own laboratory cited in this review was supported by a European Community grant, EC BMH4-CT96-0510.

REFERENCES

Abbott RM, Palmour RM. Morphine-6-glucuronide: analgesic effects and receptor binding profile in rats. *Life Sci* 1998; 43:1685–1695.

Benoliel R, Faraday M, Apatov N, et al. Modulation of tonic nociceptive input in dynorphin knockout (KO) mice. *Soc Neurosci Abs* 1998; 24:1355.

Capecchi MR. Altering the genome by homologous recombination. *Science* 1989; 244:288–1292.

Cheng J, Roques BP, Gacel GA, Huang E, Pasternak GW. κ_3 opiate receptor binding in the mouse and the rat. *Eur J Pharmacol* 1992; 226:15–20.

Clark JA, Lui L, Price M, et al. Kappa opiate receptor multiplicity: evidence for two U50,488-

sensitive κ_1 subtypes and a novel κ_3 subtype. *J Pharmacol Exp Ther* 1989; 251:461–468.

Crawley JN, Paylor R. A proposed test battery and constellation of specific behavioural paradigms to investigate the behavioural phenotypes of transgenic and knockout mice. *Horm Behav* 1997; 31:197–211.

Crusio WE. Gene-targeting studies: new methods, old problems. *Trends Neurosci* 1996; 19:186–187.

Evans CJ, Keith DE, Morrison H, Magendzo K, Edwards RH. Cloning of a delta opioid receptor by functional expression. *Science* 1992; 258:1952–1955.

Fowler CJ, Fraser GL. μ-, δ-, κ-opioid receptors and their subtypes. A critical review with emphasis on radioligand binding experiments. *Neurochem Int* 1994; 24:401–426.

Fuchs PN, Roza C, Sora I, et al. Differential effects of μ, δ, and κ-opioid receptor agonists on the response to mechanical stimuli in μ-opioid receptor knockout mice. *Soc Neurosci Abs* 1998; 24:888.

Gaveriaux-Ruff C, Matthes HWD, Peluso J, Kieffer BL. Abolition of morphine-immunosuppression in mice lacking the μ-opioid receptor gene. *Proc Natl Acad Sci USA* 1998; 95:6326–6330.

Gear RW, Miaskowski C, Gordon NC, et al. Kappa-opioids produce significantly greater analgesia in women than in men. *Nat Med* 1996; 2:1248–1250.

Gerlai R. Gene-targeting studies of mammalian behavior: is it the mutation or the background genotype? *Trends Neurosci* 1996; 19:177–181.

Grisel JE, Mogil JS, Belknap JK, Low MJ. β-Endorphin knockout mice display altered analgesic responses to centrally administered opioid agonists. *Soc Neurosci Abs* 1997; 23:678.

Hauser KF, McLaughlin PJ, Zagon IS. Endogenous opioids regulate dendritic growth and spine formation in developing rat brain. *Brain Res* 1987; 416:157–161.

Hauser KF, Stiene-Martin A, Mattson MP, et al. μ-Opioid receptor-induced Ca^{2+} mobilization and astroglial development: morphine inhibits DNA synthesis and stimulates cellular hypertrophy through a Ca^{2+}-dependent mechanism. *Brain Res* 1996; 720:191–203.

Henderson G, McKnight AT. The orphan opioid receptor and its endogenous ligand—nociceptin/orphanin FQ. *Trends Pharmacol Sci* 1997; 18:293–300.

Heyman JS, Jiang Q, Rothman RB, Mosberg HI, Porreca F. Modulation of μ-mediated antinociception by δ agonists: characterisation with antagonists. *Eur J Pharmacol* 1989a; 169:43–52.

Heyman JS, Vaught JL, Mosberg HI, Hasseth RC, Porreca F. Modulation of μ-mediated antinociception by δ agonists in the mouse: selective potentiation of morphine and normorphine by [D-Pen^2,D-Pen^5]enkephalin. *Eur J Pharmacol* 1989b; 165:1–10.

Hosohata Y, Burkey TH, Sora I, et al. DPDPE stimulates G protein activity through μ- and δ-opioid receptors as determined in μ knockout mouse brain membranes. *Soc Neurosci Abs* 1998; 24:849.

Jenck F, Borroni E, Cesura AM, et al. OFQ knock-out mice: behavioral phenotype seems to indicate homeostatic compensation of OFQ functional deficits. *Soc Neurosci Abs* 1998; 24:201.

Kieffer BL. Recent advances in molecular recognition and signal transduction of active peptides: receptors for opioid peptides. *Cell Mol Neurobiol* 1995; 15:615–635.

Kieffer BL, Befort K, Gaveriaux-Ruff C, Hirth CG. The δ-opioid receptor: isolation of a cDNA by expression cloning and pharmacological characterisation. *Proc Natl Acad Sci USA* 1992; 89:12048–12052.

King M, Schuller AGP, Zhu J, et al. Requirement of enkephalin/delta receptor systems in morphine tolerance. *Soc Neurosci Abs* 1998; 24:524.

Kirchgessner AL, Bodnar RJ, Pasternak GW. Naloxazone and pain-inhibitory systems: evidence for a collateral inhibition model. *Pharmacol Biochem Behav* 1982; 17:1175–1179.

Kitanaka N, Sora I, Kinsey S, Zeng Z, Uhl GR. No heroin or morphine 6β-glucuronide analgesia in μ-opioid receptor knockout mice. *Eur J Pharmacol* 1998; 355:R1–R3.

Kitchen I, Slowe S, Matthes H, Kieffer B. Quantitative autoradiographic mapping of mu-, delta and kappa opioid receptors in knockout mice lacking the mu-opioid receptor gene. *Brain Res* 1997; 778:73–88.

Kitchen I, Hourani SMO, Slowe SJ, et al. ORL1, adenosine A_1 and A_{2A} receptor distribution in the brains of μ-knockout mice. *Soc Neurosci Abs* 1998; 24:524.

Kitchen I, Slowe S, Goody R, et al. Quantitative audioradiography in opioid knockout mice: receptor heterogeneity and subtype interactions. *Dolor* 1999; 14(Suppl 1):12.

Knapp RJ, Yamamura HI. Delta opioid receptor radioligands. *Biochem Pharmacol* 1992; 44:1687–1695.

Konig M, Zimmer AM, Steiner H, et al. Pain responses, anxiety and aggression in mice deficient in pre-proenkephalin. *Nature* 1996; 383:535–538.

Koob GF. Drugs of abuse: anatomy, pharmacology and function of reward pathways. *Trends Pharmacol Sci* 1992; 13:177–184.

Kuhn R, Schwenk F, Aguet M, Rajewsky K. Inducible gene targeting in mice. *Science* 1995; 269:1427–1429.

Lehmann KA, Zech D. Morphine-6-glucuronide, a pharmacologically active morphine metabolite: a review of the literature. *Eur J Pain* 1993; 14:28–35.

Li X-F, Sora I, Kinsey S, et al. Visceral chemical antinociception induced by opioid agonists in μ-opioid receptor knockout mice. *Soc Neurosci Abs* 1998; 24:848.

Loh HH, Liu H-C, Cavalli A, et al. μ Opioid receptor knockout mice: effects on ligand-induced analgesia and morphine lethality. *Mol Brain Res* 1998; 54:321–326.

Mamiya T, Noda Y, Nishi M, Takeshima H, Nabshima T. Enhancement of spatial attention in nociceptin/orphanin FQ receptor-knockout mice. *Brain Res* 1998; 783:236–240.

Manabe T, Noda Y, Mamiya T, et al. Facilitation of long-term potentiation and memory in mice lacking nociceptin receptors. *Nature* 1998; 394:577–581.

Mansour A, Khachaturian H, Lewis ME, Akil H, Watson SJ. Anatomy of CNS opioid receptors. *Trends Neurosci* 1988; 11:308–314.

Matthes HWD, Maldonado R, Simonin F, et al. Loss of morphine-induced analgesia, reward effect and withdrawal symptoms in mice lacking the μ-opioid receptor gene. *Nature* 1996; 383:819–823.

Matthes HWD, Smadja C, Valverde O, et al. Activity of the δ-opioid receptor is partially reduced, whereas activity of the κ-receptor is maintained in mice lacking the μ-receptor. *J Neurosci* 1998; 18:7285–7295.

Meunier J-C. Nociceptin/orphanin FQ and the opioid receptor-like ORL1 receptor. *Eur J Pharmacol* 1997; 340:1–15.

Meunier JC, Mollereau C, Toll L, et al. Isolation and structure of the endogenous agonist of opioid receptor-like ORL1 receptor. *Nature* 1995; 377:532–535.

Mogil JS, Grisel JE. Transgenic studies of pain. *Pain* 1998; 77:107–128.

Nishi M, Houtani T, Noda Y, et al. Unrestrained nociceptive response and disregulation of hearing ability in mice lacking the nociceptin/orphanin FQ receptor. *EMBO J* 1997; 16:1858–1864.

Noda Y, Mamiya T, Nabeshima T, et al. Loss of antinociception induced by naloxone benzoylhydrazone in nociceptin receptor-knockout mice. *J Biol Chem* 1998; 273:18047–18051.

Pan Y-X, Cheng J, Xu J, et al. Cloning and functional characterization through antisense mapping of a $κ_3$-related opioid receptor. *Mol Pharmacol* 1995; 47:1180–1188.

Parsons CG, Headley PM. Spinal antinociceptive actions of μ- and κ-opioids: the importance of stimulus intensity in determining 'selectivity' between reflexes to different modalities of noxious stimulus. *Br J Pharmacol* 1989; 98:523–532.

Pasternak GW. Pharmacological mechanisms of opioid analgesics. *Clin Neuropharmacol* 1993; 16:1–18.

Pasternak GW, Wood PJ. Minireview: multiple mu opiate receptors. *Life Sci* 1986; 38:1889–1898.

Paterson SJ, Robson LE, Kosterlitz HW. Classification of opioid receptors. *Br Med Bull* 1983; 39:31–36.

Qui C, Sora I, Ren K, Uhl G, Dubner R. Opioid receptor plasticity in mu opioid receptor knockout (MOR KO) mice following persistent inflammation. *Soc Neurosci Abs* 1998; 24:892.

Raynor K, Kong H, Chen Y, et al. Pharmacological characterization of the cloned κ-,δ- and μ-opioid receptors. *Mol Pharmacol* 1994; 45:330–334.

Reinscheid RK, Nothacker HP, Bourson A, et al. Orphanin FQ: a neuropeptide that activates an opioid-like G protein-coupled receptor. *Science* 1995; 270:792–794.

Reinscheid RK, Koster A, Montkowski O, Civelli O. The role of orphanin FQ (OFQ) in pain perception studies in OFQ-knock out mice. *Soc Neurosci Abs* 1998; 24:1009.

Reisine T, Bell GI. Molecular biology of opioid receptors. *Trends Neurosci* 1993; 16:506–509.

Rossi GC, Brown GP, Leventhal L, Yang K, Pasternak GW. Novel receptor mechanisms for heroin and morphine 6β-glucuronide analgesia. *Neurosci Lett* 1996; 216:1–4.

Rossi G, Leventhal L, Pan Y-X, et al. Antisense mapping of MOR-1 in rats: distinguishing between morphine and morphine-6β-glucuronide antinociception. *J Pharmacol Exp Ther* 1997; 281:109–114.

Rossier J. Opioid peptides have found their roots. *Nature* 1982; 298:221.

Rothman RB, Bykov V, De Costa BR, et al. Interaction of endogenous opioid peptides and other drugs with four kappa opioid binding sites in guinea pig brain. *Peptides* 1989; 11:311–331.

Roy S, Barke RA, Loh HH. Mu-opioid receptor-knockout mice: role of μ-opioid receptor in morphine mediated immune functions. *Mol Brain Res* 1998a; 61:190–194.

Roy S, Liu H-C, Loh HH. μ-Opioid receptor-knockout mice: the role of μ-opioid receptor in gastrointestinal transit. *Mol Brain Res* 1998b; 56:281–283.

Rubinstein M. Introduction of a point mutation into the mouse genome by homologous recombination in embryonic stem cells using a replacement type vector with a selectable marker. *Nucleic Acids Res* 1993; 21:2613–2617.

Rubinstein M, Mogil JS, Japon M, et al. Absence of opioid stress-induced analgesia in mice lacking β-endorphin by site-directed mutagenesis. *Proc Natl Acad Sci USA* 1996; 93:3995–4000.

Salvadori S, Marastoni M, Balboni G, et al. Synthesis and structure-activity relationships of deltorphin analogues. *J Med Chem* 1991; 34:1656–1661.

Schmauss C, Yaksh TL, Shimhigashi Y, et al. Differential association of spinal mu, delta and kappa opioid receptors with subcutaneous, thermal and visceral chemical nociceptive stimuli in the rat. *Life Sci* 1983; 33:653–656.

Schuller AGP, King M, Zhang J, et al. Heroin and M6G analgesia are retained in mu opioid receptor deficient mice. *Soc Neurosci Abs* 1997; 23:584.

Schuller AGP, King M, Sherwood AC, Pintar JE, Pasternak GW. M6G but not morphine inhibits GI transit in mu opioid receptor deficient mice. *Soc Neurosci Abs* 1998; 24:210.7.

Schuller AGP, King MA, Zhang J, et al. Retention of heroin and morphine-6β-glucuronide analgesia in MOR-1 exon 1 knockout mice insensitive to morphine: evidence for a novel MOR-1-related receptor. *Nature Neurosci* 1999; 2:151–156.

Shippenberg TS, Bals-Kubik R, Herz A. Motivational properties of opioids: evidence that an activation of δ-receptors mediates reinforcement processes. *Brain Res* 1987; 436:234–239.

Simonin F, Valverde O, Smaje C, et al. Disruption of the κ-opioid receptor gene in mice impairs hypolocomotor, analgesic and aversive actions of the selective κ-agonist U-50,488H and attenuates morphine withdrawal. *EMBO J* 1998; 17:886–897.

Slowe SJ, Simonin F, Kieffer B, Kitchen I. Quantitative autoradiography of μ-, δ, and κ₁ opioid receptors in κ-opioid receptor knockout mice. *Brain Res* 1999, in press.

Smith JAM, Hunter JC, Hughes J. Analysis of κ-opioid binding sites in the guinea-pig using [³H]bremazocine and [³H]U69593. *Adv Biosci* 1989; 75:49–52.

Smotherman WP, Robinson SR. Kappa opioid mediation of fetal responses to milk. *Behav Neurosci* 1992; 106:396–407.

Sora I, Funada M, Uhl GR. The μ-opioid receptor is necessary for [D-Pen²,D-Pen⁵]enkephalin-induced analgesia. *Eur J Pharmacol* 1997a; 324:R1–R2.

Sora I, Takahashi N, Funada M, et al. Opiate receptor knockout mice define μ receptor roles in endogenous nociceptive responses and morphine-induced analgesia. *Proc Natl Acad Sci USA* 1997b; 94:1544–1549.

Sora I, Li X-F, Kinsey S, et al. μ-Opioid receptor knockout mice: psychostimulant- and opiate-induced place preferences. *Soc Neurosci Abs* 1998; 24:996.

Tecott LH, Brennan TJ, Guh L. Gene targeting approaches to analyse neurotransmitter receptor function. *Sem Neurosci* 1996; 8:145–152.

Tian MT, Broxmeyer HE, Fan Y, et al. Altered hematopoiesis, behavior, and sexual function in mu opioid receptor-deficient mice. *J Exp Med* 1997; 185:1517–1522.

Tiberi M, Payette P, Mongeau R, Magnan J. [^{3}H]U69,593 binding in guinea-pig brain comparison with [^{3}H]ethylketocyclazocine binding at the κ-opioid sites. *Can J Physiol Pharmacol* 1988; 66:1368–1372.

Tyers MB. A classification of opiate receptors that mediate antinociception in animals. *Br J Pharmacol* 1980; 69:503–512.

Ueda H, Yamaguchi T, Tokuyama S, et al. Partial loss of tolerance liability to morphine analgesia in mice lacking the nociceptin receptor gene. *Neurosci Lett* 1997; 237:136–138.

Unterwald EM, Knapp C, Zukin RS. Neuroanatomical localization of κ$_1$ and κ$_2$ opioid receptors in rat and guinea-pig brain. *Brain Res* 1991; 562:57–65.

Wilson SG, Low MJ, Mogil JS. Compensatory mediation of intraperitoneal injection-related stress-induced analgesia in double β-endorphin/enkephalin knock-out mice. *Soc Neurosci Abs* 1998; 24:892.

Yeadon M, Kitchen I. Comparative binding of μ and δ selective ligands in whole brain and pons/medulla homogenates from rat: affinity profiles of fentanyl derivatives. *Neuropharmacology* 1988; 27:345–348.

Zadina JE, Ge L-J, Hackler L, Kastin AJ. A potent and selective endogenous agonist for the μ-opiate receptor. *Nature* 1997; 386:499–503.

Zhang J, King M, Pasternak GW, Pintar JE. Production and analgesic characterisation of KOR-1 deficient mice. *Soc Neurosci Abs* 1998; 24:525.

Zhu Y, King M, Schuller A, et al. Genetic disruption of the mouse delta opioid gene. *Soc Neurosci Abs* 1997; 23:584.

Zimprich A, Simon S, Hollt V. Cloning and expression of an isoform of the rat μ opioid receptor (rMOR 1B) which differs in agonist induced desensitization from rMOR 1. *FEBS Lett* 1995; 359:142–146.

Zukin RS, Eghbali M, Olive D, Unterwald EM, Tempel A. Characterization and visualisation of rat and guinea-pig κ-opioid receptors: evidence for κ$_1$ and κ$_2$ opioid receptors. *Proc Natl Acad Sci USA* 1988; 85:4061–4065.

Correspondence to: Ian Kitchen, PhD, Pharmacology Research Group, School of Biological Sciences, University of Surrey, Guildford, Surrey, GU2 5XH, United Kingdom. Tel: 44-1483-879734; Fax: 44-1483-576978; email: i.kitchen@surrey.ac.uk.

Part IV

Opioid Sensitivity of Different Chronic Pain States—Answers and Questions from the Clinic

Opioid Sensitivity of Chronic Noncancer Pain,
Progress in Pain Research and Management,
Vol. 14, edited by Eija Kalso, Henry J. McQuay,
and Zsuzsanna Wiesenfeld-Hallin, IASP Press,
Seattle, © 1999.

18

The Debate over Opioids and Neuropathic Pain

Michael C. Rowbotham

*Pain Clinical Research Center and Mount Zion Pain Management Center,
University of California, San Francisco, California, USA*

As recently as a decade ago, the prevailing view held opioids to be useless as long-term therapy for chronic neuropathic pain. Despite a lack of prospectively gathered evidence to support such pessimism, it was believed that pain was rarely relieved, analgesia would soon be lost to tolerance, and addiction would occur in a high proportion of patients (Maruta et al. 1979; Pagni 1984; Portenoy et al. 1990; Wall 1990). Beginning in the early 1980s, this view was challenged by uncontrolled and mostly retrospective reports that opioids were effective as long-term therapy for nonmalignant pain (including neuropathic pain) with a low risk of addiction (Porter and Jick 1980; Taub 1982; France et al. 1984; Portenoy and Foley 1986; Urban et al. 1986; Watson et al. 1988).

In 1988, Arnér and Meyerson set off a lively debate with an article entitled "Lack of analgesic effect of opioids on neuropathic and idiopathic forms of pain" (Arnér and Meyerson 1988a). In it they presented the results of a randomized, double-blind, placebo controlled trial of intravenous (i.v.) opioids in patients with nociceptive visceral pain, neuropathic pain, and idiopathic pain. The protocol for the study was exceedingly complex. Simply summarized, three groups of patients underwent a series of blinded infusions of various opioids and saline placebo. Fifteen patients had chronic "nociceptive" pain of visceral origin. In six of these patients, their treating physicians had previously discontinued the mixed agonist/antagonist pentazocine by the parenteral route for fear of supporting or inducing addiction. This group received 4–8 infusions of placebo or the mixed agonist/antagonist buprenorphine. If "efficient" pain relief was demonstrated with the active drug, it was considered justified to sanction long-term treatment with sublingual buprenorphine. The 12 patients with neuropathic pain were all scheduled for placement of electrodes for deep brain stimulation. The purpose of the opioid and placebo infusions were to help plan the stimulation target and to see if opioids should be instituted as an alternative, or supplementary therapy. All of the neuropathic patients had long histories of "severely incapacitating pain which had resisted all previous treatments," including nerve blocks, peripheral pain surgery, opioids, and in most cases anticonvulsants and tricyclic antidepressants. Four of the neuropathic patients were still on high doses of opioids. The neuropathic group received 15 mg of morphine or placebo on at least four occasions. If significant pain reduction was reported, the effect was reversed with i.v. naloxone. The 21 patients suffering from idiopathic pain received a variety of different opioids, with a total of between 4 and 13 active or placebo infusions. The nociceptive group reported dramatic pain reduction with opioid infusion (87% reduction in pain measured on a visual analogue scale [VAS]) compared to saline placebo (17% reduction). The neuropathic and idiopathic pain groups did not experience pain relief from opioids.

Shortly after the Arnér and Meyerson paper appeared, Howard L. Fields strongly criticized the experimental design, patient selection, and data analysis in a letter to the editor of the journal *Pain* (Fields 1988). The data analysis scheme failed to specify precisely how the results of all the different infusions were averaged, and the results table for the neuropathic group did not even provide numerical data. In addition, the pain rating scales, the number of postopioid ratings, the total number of infusions and drugs administered, and the time interval between infusions were all variable within and among the three groups. The neuropathic patients had already proven refractory to nearly every treatment available, including opioids. Doses were not adjusted upwards for neuropathic patients already on opioids, and side effects were not produced with the opioid doses used. Further, those neuropathic patients that did experience pain relief had the effects reversed with naloxone, an unpleasant procedure not carried out in the other groups. Patient selection and the purpose of the infusions also differed in that the neuropathic patients were scheduled to undergo placement of brain stimulation electrodes, while in the other groups the purpose of the infusions was to determine whether long-term opioid therapy should be instituted as a primary treatment modality. Fields wrote that it may be correct that neuropathic pain is less responsive to opioids or that most patients with neuropathic pain do not respond to opioids. However, he strongly emphasized that the results of the Arnér and Meyerson study did not exclude the possibility that opioids are effective for neuropathic pain, and proposed that the study publication should not prompt physicians to withhold opioid therapy. In their response, Arnér and Meyerson (1988b) agreed that it would be unfortunate if opioids were withheld from patients in whom analgesia was produced. They further replied that "It may seem premature to base a conclusion concerning the lack of effect of opioids in chronic neuropathic pain on such a small group of patients. We would have hesitated to do so were it not for the fact that the outcome of the tests just confirmed our experience over the years with a larger number of such patients—an experience that we share with others."

In a 1988 article that gained little attention compared to the Arnér and Meyerson paper, Max and colleagues reported the results of a four-session crossover study comparing single oral doses of codeine (120 mg), clonidine, ibuprofen, and placebo in patients with postherpetic neuralgia (Max et al. 1988). The drug with the highest incidence of side effects, clonidine, also had the highest incidence of pain relief. Codeine produced side effects, but was no better than placebo at relieving pain. The authors concluded that the presence of side effects may enhance reported analgesia by suggesting to subjects that they received an active drug.

In 1990, Portenoy and colleagues published a comprehensive review of the concept of opioid responsiveness supported by data from uncontrolled infusions of various opioids in patients with neuropathic pain, primarily of malignant origin. They proposed a continuum of opioid responsiveness in which patients with neuropathic pain may simply require higher drug doses to experience analgesia. In a supportive accompanying editorial, *Pain* editor Patrick D. Wall noted the strong opposition of the authors to the conclusions of Arnér and Meyerson and provided a historical perspective: "A real triumph of medicine in the past 50 years has been to re-establish a proper place for the ancient therapy of narcotics in the treatment of pain" (Wall 1990). Wall lamented that doctors and scientists had allowed themselves to "join a mass hysteria which confused the tremendous benefits of narcotics for the patient in pain with the social abuse of the same compounds."

In 1991, Arnér and Meyerson responded again to the controversy surrounding their 1988 paper by acknowledging the somewhat provocative phrasing of the paper's title and stating that nowhere in that article did they suggest that patients in pain should be deprived of an open trial of opioids. On the contrary, they stated that this was part of their daily practice with all cancer-related pain and a number of other forms of pain. They pointed out that the Portenoy et al. paper conveys the message that there is little evidence supporting the resistance of neuropathic pain to opioids, but fails to admit there is actually no systematic, controlled study demonstrating that such pain *does* respond to opioids. Arnér and Meyerson defended their use of low doses of i.v. morphine to test the opioid responsivity of neuropathic pain because they wanted to keep analgesia separate from sedation. *Pain* editor Ronald Dubner summarized the state of affairs in the same issue through an editorial comment entitled "A call for more science, not more rhetoric, regarding opioids and neuropathic pain" (Dubner 1991). He drew an analogy with the chronology of research on the analgesic efficacy of antidepressants in pain associated with diabetic neuropathy and postherpetic neuralgia. Early anecdotal observations and open-trial studies had suggested that tricyclic antidepressants were clinically effective, but it was not known whether their effects were related to analgesia, mood changes, or sedative properties. Subsequent blinded trials with active and inactive placebos had been able to satisfactorily answer these questions by studying relatively homogeneous populations of patients. Dubner called for prospective, controlled trials in homogeneous groups of neuropathic pain patients.

NEUROPATHIC PAIN IS OPIOID RESPONSIVE

CONTROLLED STUDIES OF I.V. OPIOID ADMINISTRATION

Controlled evidence showing that neuropathic pain could indeed be opioid responsive came from two studies published in 1991. In the first, Rowbotham and colleagues (1991) reported the results of a three-session, double-blind crossover study comparing 1-hour i.v. infusions of 0.3 mg/kg of morphine (average total dose of 19.2 mg), 5 mg/kg of lidocaine (average total dose of 316 mg), and matching saline placebo in 19 patients with established postherpetic neuralgia (PHN). Pre-infusion pain intensity VAS ratings were moderate, averaging 49 mm. The composite infusion pain intensity ratings were 29.8 mm for the lidocaine, 32.6 mm for the morphine, and 43.6 mm for the placebo sessions. Both active drugs were significantly different from placebo ($P = 0.04$ for morphine, $P = 0.02$ for lidocaine), but lidocaine was not significantly different from morphine. The pain-relief VAS scale ratings were highest for the morphine sessions, 44.9 mm, compared to 38.5 mm for the lidocaine sessions and 22.2 for the placebo sessions. The morphine–placebo comparison was highly significant ($P = 0.01$), and the lidocaine–placebo comparison approached statistical significance ($P = 0.06$). Eleven subjects chose the morphine session as best, 10 of whom also experienced either a normalization of subjective cutaneous sensation or a loss of painful hypersensitivity following the morphine infusion. The change in pain intensity ratings was correlated with morphine blood level at the end of the infusion. Side effects were not correlated with pain relief for either active drug. In this study, morphine was given in a large enough dose to fully test the hypothesis that neuropathic pain could respond to opioids. The study was not designed to compare different types of chronic pain on opioid responsivity, or to determine whether morphine was better than other available therapies or if opioids were a useful long-term therapy for PHN.

In the second study, Kupers and colleagues (1991) reported the effect of i.v. morphine 0.3 mg/kg and saline placebo in a two-session crossover study. They hypothesized that the primary reason that patients with neuropathic pain consumed opioids long term was for their mood-changing effects. Therefore, they used a modification of the McGill Pain Questionnaire to train subjects to distinguish between affective (unpleasantness) and sensory (intensity) components of their ongoing pain and separately rate these two dimensions on a 101-point rating scale. Six of their subjects had neuropathic pain of central nervous system (CNS) origin, eight had neuropathic pain of peripheral nervous system (PNS) origin, and six had idiopathic chronic pain. The group with PNS-origin neuropathic pain was somewhat atypical; two had low back pain that had not responded to previous therapy and two had brachial plexus avulsions. Affective pain ratings decreased significantly in both groups of neuropathic pain patients, but sensory pain ratings were unchanged. The group with idiopathic pain demonstrated no change in either aspect of pain. Of 14 neuropathic pain subjects, half had prior experience with less potent opioids. The opioid-naive subjects had a nonsignificantly greater response to morphine on both sensory and affective pain relief scales. The major criticism of this study is the small sample size.

Preliminary results of a two-session, random-order, double-blind study of i.v. fentanyl in 23 patients with postherpetic neuralgia have been presented in poster form by Wilsey and colleagues (1997). Fentanyl was infused over 90 minutes at gradually increasing infusion rates to a total of 5.4 µg/kg. Compared to saline placebo, fentanyl significantly reduced overall pain intensity, allodynia severity, and area of skin surface demonstrating allodynia. Most descriptors of neuropathic pain were reduced by fentanyl. Fentanyl effects on pain intensity and subjective pain relief ratings were not correlated with alterations in symptom checklist items and VAS scales of dysphoria/euphoria, anxiety/relaxation, and confusion/alertness. However, suppression of the response to heat pain in nonpainful skin was significantly correlated with pain reduction from fentanyl, which is persuasive evidence of a specific analgesic effect of opioids in chronic neuropathic pain.

The largest study reported to date is the two-session crossover trial reported by Dellemijn and Vanneste (1997). In 50 patients with different types of neuropathic pain (primarily of PNS origin), they compared the analgesic effect of i.v. fentanyl with either saline placebo or the benzodiazepine diazepam. Diazepam was included as a control agent in the belief that it would modulate the subject's emotional experience of pain without producing intrinsic analgesic effects. Each infusion lasted a total of 5 hours, fentanyl at a rate of 5 $\mu g \cdot kg^{-1} \cdot h^{-1}$ and diazepam at a rate of 0.2 $\mu g \cdot kg^{-1} \cdot h^{-1}$. As with the study by Kupers and colleagues (1991), pain was rated on 101-point scales of unpleasantness and intensity. Fentanyl reduced both dimensions of pain to a nearly identical degree, with peak effects at 4 hours after the start of the infusion. Maximum pain reduction with fentanyl was 65% compared to 15–20% for control infusions. Results showed that saline and diazepam were completely ineffective on both pain scales, but that diazepam produced nearly as much sedation as did fentanyl. The Dellemijn and Vanneste study is especially important because the inclusion of a benzodiazepine allowed them to specifically control for the sedating effects of opioids. Their study provides compelling evidence in favor of a specific analgesic effect of opioids on both the intensity and the unpleasantness of pain.

CONTROLLED STUDIES OF ORAL OPIOID ADMINISTRATION

The results of two prospective, placebo-controlled trials of oral opioids for neuropathic pain appeared in the same issue of the journal *Neurology* in 1998 (Harati et al. 1998; Watson and Babul 1998). The drugs studied, oxycodone and tramadol, together comprise a significant percentage of the oral opioid market in the United States. Oxycodone is a typical μ-opioid agonist of moderate potency. Tramadol is an atypical drug that shows low-affinity binding to μ-opioid receptors and weak inhibition of norepinephrine and serotonin reuptake. Tramadol is approved for use in the United States by the Food and Drug Administration (FDA) for "moderate to moderately severe" pain. The importance of mechanisms other than μ-opioid-receptor binding in overall pain reduction is still undetermined.

Watson and Babul (1998) described a random-order crossover trial of twice-daily controlled-release oxycodone in 50 patients with PHN. The 45% of subjects with prior opioid experience (typically acetaminophen combined with codeine or oxycodone) abstained from all opioid use for at least 7 days before study entry. At randomization, subjects began with either placebo or 10 mg oxycodone twice a day; the drug dose was titrated at weekly intervals up to a maximum of 30 mg twice a day. A total of 38 subjects completed the trial (dropout rate = 24%). Outcome data for efficacy in the 12 dropouts was not reported; the statistical analysis was carried out on data from completing subjects only. A separate analysis comparing opioid-experienced subjects with opioid-naive subjects was not performed. Completing subjects received a mean total daily oxycodone intake of 45 mg. Daily diary pain intensity scores were significantly lower during oxycodone treatment than during placebo treatment by the second week of the 4-week treatment period. Overall pain intensity during the last week of treatment was 54 mm on a VAS during treatment with placebo and 35 mm during treatment with oxycodone ($P = 0.0001$). VAS scores for steady pain, brief pain, and skin pain were all significantly lower during the last week of oxycodone treatment than during placebo treatment. Similarly, pain-relief category ratings and disability scores significantly favored oxycodone. Mean pain-relief ratings on a 6-point scale were "moderate" with oxycodone compared to "slight" with placebo. Not surprisingly, significantly more adverse events were reported during oxycodone therapy, particularly constipation, nausea, and sedation. Despite the greater reduction of pain during oxycodone therapy, there were no treatment differences on the Beck Depression Inventory or on any of the six scales of the Profile of Mood States. Given the steady dose escalation during a treatment period of only 4 weeks, tolerance was not expected and was not evident.

Harati and coworkers (1998) reported the results of a multicenter, randomized, placebo-controlled trial of parallel design in 131 subjects with chronic neuropathic pain due to distal symmetric diabetic neuropathy. After 21 days off tricyclic antidepressants or anticonvulsants and 7 days off shorter-acting analgesics, subjects were treated with either tramadol or placebo for 6 weeks. Subjects were allowed to titrate up to a maximum of 400 mg/day, and were required to use a minimum of 100 mg/day during the last 4 weeks of the treatment period. A total of 82 subjects completed the study (dropout rate = 37%), taking a mean dose of 210 mg/day of tramadol. There were more "adverse event" dropouts in the tramadol group, and more "lack of efficacy" dropouts in the placebo group. In contrast to the Watson and Babul study, the data analysis was based on all drug-exposed subjects not lost to follow-up ($n = 127$). Subjects treated with tramadol had significantly less pain and greater pain relief at all time points from day 14 of treatment to day 42 at the end of the treatment period. Pain intensity on a 5-point Likert scale was reduced from 2.5 to 1.4, compared to a change from 2.6 to 2.2 for those subjects assigned to placebo ($P < 0.001$). Pain-relief ratings were similar to those in the Watson and Babul study. Tramadol produced "moderate" relief, compared to "slight" relief with placebo. Sleep, current health perception, psychological distress, and overall role-functioning scales were not improved with tramadol therapy, but scales of physical and social functioning showed significant improvement in the tramadol group. The data was not presented in a way that would allow analysis for development of tolerance. Compared to the Watson and Babul study, Harati et al. provide more convincing proof of efficacy because of the larger sample size, a more conservative efficacy analysis using all drug-exposed subjects, and a longer treatment period.

OPIOID THERAPY FOR NEUROPATHIC PAIN IN PERSPECTIVE

At least for neuropathic pain of peripheral nerve origin in the form of postherpetic neuralgia and diabetic neuropathy, we now have the same chronology of proof for opioids and neuropathic pain that was described for antidepressants by Dubner in his 1991 editorial. Case reports have been followed by controlled trials demonstrating longer-term efficacy of oral opioids. The i.v. infusion studies have demonstrated that opioid analgesia is not caused by side effects. It would be fair to state that the opioid responsivity of chronic neuropathic pain of peripheral nervous system origin is now better validated than that of any other type of chronic nonmalignant pain. For example, longer-term opioid trials for chronic musculoskeletal pain have had mixed results. A prospective controlled trial of codeine in osteoarthritis of the hip showed no benefit over a 4-week treatment period and a very high dropout rate (Kjaersgaard-Andersen et al. 1990). A controlled trial of oral morphine for chronic musculoskeletal pain showed modest benefit that was almost completely lost by the end of the 9-week treatment period (Moulin et al. 1996). Animal research has indirectly promoted the belief that chronic neuropathic pain is somehow less opioid responsive than is non-neuropathic chronic pain. However, there are no data comparing patient groups with chronic neuropathic and non-neuropathic pain of nonmalignant origin who are matched for disease chronicity, age, and pain severity and treated with opioids under identical double-blind conditions.

We still lack data on the relative opioid responsivity of the many subtypes of chronic neuropathic pain. In his landmark book, *The Management of Pain*, John J. Bonica (1953) observed that thalamic pain and other central pain states appeared unresponsive to opioids. Pagni and others have also presented anecdotal evidence in favor of this view (Pagni 1984; Hammond 1991). Preliminary data from double-blind, placebo-controlled studies conducted in our laboratory indicate that pain of CNS origin is indeed less responsive to opioids than pain of PNS origin. My personal suspicion is that the unresolved problem of how to treat central pain has colored our thinking about opioids and neuropathic pain in general. Some patients with thalamic pain, for example, make a strong impression on the pain practitioner with their strikingly abnormal neurological examinations, profound suffering, and utter failure to respond to all therapies. Leijon and Boivie (1989) were able to demonstrate that amitriptyline was effective in a very small group of patients with post-stroke pain. Otherwise, there is no published controlled evidence in favor of any drug category for central pain, and little effort has been made in the form of organized clinical trials to study this group more carefully.

The concept of a continuum of opioid responsiveness in which many chronic neuropathic pain patients obtain relief at clinically tolerated doses of opioids is no longer controversial. But what is opioid responsiveness? Conversely, what evidence is needed to convincingly demonstrate that an individual patient's pain is opioid resistant? Henry McQuay's eloquent review in Chapter 24 of this volume makes it clear that testing individual patients is very different than demonstrating efficacy in a particular syndrome. Judgments of pain relief and adverse effects need to be balanced, and outcome measures must be appropriate for the larger question being tested. If the goal is to demonstrate that a particular type of neuropathic pain can be reduced in intensity, or that abnormal sensory examination findings can be altered, the i.v. infusion studies by Dellemijn and Vanneste (1997) and Wilsey et al. (1997) are satisfactory. If the goal is to determine that patients with chronic neuropathic pain will lead better, more productive lives through pain control from regular intake of opioids, we have a long way to go. McQuay also makes the point that best clinical judgment remains superior to high technology. Our studies of i.v. opioid challenges show statistically significant, but modest predictive power for the results of subsequent oral opioid therapy under double-blind conditions. Techniques need to be developed that can be reliably used in individual patients to distinguish between nonspecific sedative or placebo effects and true opioid analgesia.

Modern clinical medicine is all about relative risk versus relative benefit. It remains to be determined how effective opioids are compared to other therapies for neuropathic pain. For postherpetic neuralgia and diabetic neuropathy, three medication classes have proven effective in double-blind controlled studies with sufficiently large groups of subjects for adequate statistical power and treatment periods of 4–8 weeks. The three medications, tricyclic antidepressants, opioids, and the anticonvulsant gabapentin (McQuay et al. 1996; Backonja et al. 1998; Harati et al. 1998; Rowbotham et al. 1998; Watson and Babul 1998) have shown roughly equivalent results in both the placebo groups and the active treatment groups. With active therapy, overall pain intensity reduction averages 30–40%, pain relief is "moderate," and about 50% of drug-exposed subjects experience satisfactory pain relief. No large-scale, random-assignment studies have directly compared opioids with proven nonopioid therapies to determine whether differences in long-term efficacy, side effect profiles, and risks of long-term use are meaningful. Crossover studies exposing subjects in random order to all three types of medications would be particularly useful to determine what proportion of patients who fail to respond to antidepressants and gabapentin would have a satisfactory response to opioids, and vice versa. As long as physicians reject opioids through fear of scrutiny by regulatory agencies (Joranson 1995) and pressure from other physicians and health insurance organizations, opioids will continue to be used only when other medications fail. For opioids more than any other type of pain therapy, the attitudes and beliefs of the patient and his or her social network, the prescribing physician, and society at large must all be taken into account. It is not enough to simply demonstrate that pain is reduced. For opioids to become a first-line medication for chronic neuropathic pain, it must be prospectively demonstrated that the ratio of risks to benefits of chronic opioid therapy are at least as favorable as for any other therapy.

REFERENCES

Arnér S, Meyerson BA. Lack of analgesia effect of opioids on neuropathic and idiopathic forms of pain. *Pain* 1988a; 33:11–23.
Arnér S, Meyerson BA. Reply to Howard L. Fields on 'Can opiates relieve neuropathic pain?' *Pain* 1988b; 35:366–367.
Arnér S, Meyerson BA. Genuine resistance to opioids—fact or fiction? *Pain* 1991; 47:116–118.
Backonja M, Beydoun A, Edwards KR, et al. Gabapentin for the symptomatic treatment of painful neuropathy in patients with diabetes mellitus. *JAMA* 1998; 280:1831–1836.
Bonica JJ. *The Management of Pain*. Philadelphia: Lea and Febiger, 1953.
Dellemijn PL, Vanneste JA. Randomized double-blind active-placebo-controlled crossover trial of intravenous fentanyl in neuropathic pain. *Lancet* 1997; 349:753–758.
Dubner R. A call for more science, not more rhetoric, regarding opioids and neuropathic pain. *Pain* 1991; 47:1–2.
Fields HL. Can opiates relieve neuropathic pain? *Pain* 1988; 35:365.
France RD, Urban BJ, Keefe FJ. Long-term use of narcotic analgesics in chronic pain. *Soc Sci Med* 1984; 19:1379–1382.
Hammond DL. Do opioids relieve central pain? In: KL Casey (Ed). *Pain and Central Nervous System Disease: The Central Pain Syndromes*. New York: Raven Press, 1991, pp 233–241.
Harati Y, Gooch C, Swenson M, et al. Double-blind randomized trial of tramadol for the treatment of the pain of diabetic neuropathy. *Neurology* 1998; 50:1842–1846.
Joranson DE. State medical board guidelines for treatment of intractable pain. *Am Pain Soc Bull* 1995; 5:1–4.
Kjaersgaard-Andersen P, Nafei A, Skov O, et al. Codeine plus paracetamol versus paracetamol in longer-term treatment of chronic pain due to osteoarthritis of the hip. A randomised, double-blind, multi-centre study. *Pain* 1990; 43:309–318.
Kupers RC, Konings H, Adriaensen H, Gybels JM. Morphine differentially affects the sensory and affective pain ratings in neurogenic and idiopathic forms of pain. *Pain* 1991; 47:5–12.
Leijon G, Boivie J. Central post-stroke pain: a controlled trial of amitriptyline and carbamazepine. *Pain* 1989; 36:27–36.
Maruta T, Swanson DW, Finlayson RE. Drug abuse and dependency in patients with chronic pain. *Mayo Clin Proc* 1979; 54:241–244.
Max MB, Schafer SC, Culnane M, Dubner R, Gracely RH. Association of pain relief with side effects in postherpetic neuralgia: a single-dose study of clonidine, codeine, ibuprofen and placebo. *Clin Pharmacol Ther* 1988; 43:363–371.
McQuay HJ, Tramèr M, Nye BA, et al. A systematic review of antidepressants for neuropathic pain. *Pain* 1996; 68:217–227.

Moulin DE, Iezzi A, Amireh R, et al. Randomized trial of oral morphine for chronic non-cancer pain. *Lancet* 1996; 347:143–147.

Pagni CA. Central pain due to spinal cord and brainstem damage. In: Wall PD, Melzack R (Eds). *Textbook of Pain,* Edinburgh: Churchill Livingstone, 1984, pp 481–496.

Portenoy RK, Foley KM. Chronic use of opioid analgesics in non-malignant pain: report of 38 cases. *Pain* 1986; 25:171–186.

Portenoy RK, Foley KM, Inturrisi CE. The nature of opioid responsiveness and its implications for neuropathic pain: new hypotheses derived from studies of opioid infusions. *Pain* 1990; 43:273–286.

Porter J, Jick H. Addiction rare in patients treated with narcotics. *N Engl J Med* 1980; 302:123.

Rowbotham MC, Reisner-Keller LA, Fields HL. Both intravenous lidocaine and morphine reduce the pain of postherpetic neuralgia. *Neurology* 1991; 41:1024–1028.

Rowbotham MC, Harden N, Stacey B, Bernstein P, Magnus-Miller L. Gabapentin for the treatment of post-herpetic neuralgia. *JAMA* 1998; 280:1837–1842.

Taub A. Opioid analgesics in the treatment of chronic intractable pain of non-neoplastic origin. In: Kitihata LM, Collins JD (Eds). *Narcotic Analgesics in Anesthesiology.* Baltimore: Williams and Wilkins, 1982, pp 199–208.

Urban BJ, France RD, Steinberger EK, Scott DL, Maltbie AA. Long-term use of narcotic/antidepressant medication in the management of phantom limb pain. *Pain* 1986; 24:191–196.

Wall PD. Neuropathic pain. *Pain* 1990; 43:267–268.

Watson CPN, Babul N. Efficacy of oxycodone in neuropathic pain: a randomized trial in postherpetic neuralgia. *Neurology* 1998; 50:1837–1841.

Watson CPN, Evans RJ, Watt VR, Birkett N. Post-herpetic neuralgia: 208 cases. *Pain* 1988; 35:289–297.

Wilsey BL, Davies PS, Rowbotham MC. Changes in pain, mood, and sensation from i.v. fentanyl in patients with PHN. *Abstracts, 16th Annual Scientific Meeting, American Pain Society,* October, 1997.

Correspondence to: Michael C. Rowbotham, MD, UCSF Pain Clinical Research Center, 1701 Divisadero Street, Suite 480, San Francisco, CA 94115, USA. Fax: 415-885-7855.

Opioid Sensitivity of Chronic Noncancer Pain,
Progress in Pain Research and Management,
Vol. 14, edited by Eija Kalso, Henry J. McQuay,
and Zsuzsanna Wiesenfeld-Hallin, IASP Press,
Seattle, © 1999.

19

Opioids and Painful
Peripheral Neuropathy

Gary J. Bennett

*Department of Neurology, MCP Hahnemann University,
Philadelphia, Pennsylvania, USA*

There is considerable debate over the question, "Do opioids work for neuropathic pain?" I believe that the controversy has several causes. First, we confront two related but clearly distinct issues: "Do opioids have any efficacy for neuropathic pain?" and "Are opioids useful medicines for the control of neuropathic pain?" Clearly, it is possible for opioids to have efficacy, but nonetheless to be impractical as therapeutic agents because the doses that are required are too high to be well tolerated. Second, the question treats neuropathic pain as a single phenomenon, when it is actually a multidimensional problem composed of many different kinds of abnormal pain (e.g., heat-hyperalgesia, mechano-allodynia, cold-allodynia, spontaneous lancinating pain, and spontaneous burning pain) that may result from various underlying mechanisms. Third, the question is imprecise unless the route of administration is specified, as neuropathy may alter one or more of the endogenous neural substrates upon which a therapeutic opioid acts.

DO OPIOIDS HAVE *ANY* EFFICACY AGAINST
PAINFUL PERIPHERAL NEUROPATHY?

The answer to this question is clearly, "Yes, in at least some cases." When neuropathic pain is measured while patients receive an intravenous infusion of an opioid, the pain decreases (Portenoy et al. 1990; Rowbotham et al. 1991). However, not all neuropathy patients respond (Arnér and Meyerson 1988), perhaps because intolerable doses would be required. When pain is measured while normal human subjects experiencing neuropathic-like hyperalgesia and allodynia (produced by an intradermal injection of

capsaicin) receive an intravenous infusion of an opioid, the hyperalgesia
and allodynia symptoms decrease (Park et al. 1995; Sethna et al. 1998).
Intrathecal (i.t.) opioids are clearly effective in many patients with peripheral neuropathy (Krames 1996). Both systemic and i.t. opioids are effective
against at least some kinds of abnormal pain in experimental animals with
painful peripheral neuropathy.

DO OPIOIDS HAVE *USEFUL* EFFICACY AGAINST
PAINFUL PERIPHERAL NEUROPATHY?

Opioids are often prescribed for neuropathy patients, but clinical opinion is divided on this practice. In common with questions about using opioids
for chronic pain in general (for review, see Portenoy 1994), some clinicians
fear addiction and tolerance from chronic opioid use ("Sure, the patient would
get pain relief, but he would rapidly develop tolerance and then I would have a
pain patient *and* an addict to treat!"). Few randomized clinical trials have
tested the efficacy of opioids for the long-term relief of painful peripheral neuropathy. Over the course of a month, oxycodone has been shown to be effective
for the control of postherpetic neuralgia (Watson and Babul 1998). Harati et al.
(1998) have shown tramadol to be effective in patients with painful diabetic
neuropathy treated for 6 weeks. These studies are encouraging, but they do
not prove whether opioids are truly effective for long-term treatment.

I make it a practice to ask neuropathy patients about the effects of their
opioid use. Three replies are remarkably common (note that I am not their
prescribing physician, that they are always informed that I am not any kind
of physician, and that it is my habit to speak with them in the absence of
their physician): (1) "I save my pills for emergencies—times when the pain
is unbearably bad," (2) "The opioid does not really stop the pain, it just
takes the edge off it," and (3) "I save my pills for bedtime." The last reply
reveals what I believe is a very under-appreciated problem—the neuropathy
patient suffers from lack of sleep almost as much as from pain (opioids, of
course, are very effective sedatives).

DOES NEUROPATHIC PAIN SIMPLY
REQUIRE HIGHER DOSES?

It is often said that patients with painful peripheral neuropathy require
doses of opioids that are so high (either initially because of the supposed
refractoriness of neuropathic pain, or subsequently because of tolerance)
that long-term efficacy is simply impossible. These concerns are mostly

obviated when the i.t. route is used. But very high i.t. doses are sometimes required (Krames 1996), and (at least for upper extremity pain and a cervical delivery site) the threat of respiratory depression is real. Moreover, the installation and maintenance of an i.t. delivery system are very expensive, and problems with the indwelling cannula frequently occur.

The possibility that human neuropathic pain is relieved only by doses of an opioid that are higher than those a physician is accustomed to prescribing is unproven, but not unreasonable. A direct comparison of opioid efficacy against "spontaneous" ongoing pain in patients with neuropathic versus inflammatory pain has not been performed. Such a trial would be difficult to carry out, because even pains with equal intensity might be of fundamentally different quality (neuropathy patients frequently insist that there is something unnatural about their pain). But in the case of stimulus-evoked pains (i.e., hyperalgesia and allodynia), we can speculate that there may be a simple explanation. For example, if a given dose of an opioid normally raises the pain threshold by 1 unit of measure, but the patient's hyperalgesia or allodynia is equal to a 3-unit decrease in the normal pain threshold, then it would obviously take more opioid to restore the hyperalgesic pain threshold to a normal or hypoalgesic level.

Interestingly, it is rather difficult to demonstrate an opioid analgesic effect against the acute pain threshold in the normal human subject (Gracely et al. 1979). Another noteworthy feature is that relative to normal acute pain, opioid efficacy seems to increase in inflammatory pain (see Hylden et al. 1991 and other chapters in this volume for discussion).

Data from animal models of painful peripheral neuropathy are consistent on at least one point: morphine is less effective when given by the i.t. route. The dose-response function for reducing heat-evoked pain shifts to the right by 4–6-fold (Yamamoto and Yaksh 1992; Lee et al. 1995; Mao et al. 1995; Ossipov et al. 1995; Chung and Na 1996; Nichols et al. 1997; Wegert et al. 1997). As Yamamoto and Yaksh (1992) noted, the rightwards-shifted dose-response curve is nearly parallel with the normal curve. Evidence also suggests a marked decrease in opioid efficacy with the intracerebroventricular route of administration (Wegert et al. 1997). However, the story is unclear for opioids given systemically. Using the chronic constriction injury (CCI) model (Bennett and Xie 1988) and intravenous administration, Lee et al. (1994) showed an increased efficacy for morphine and μ-, δ-, and κ-receptor-specific agonists. Using the spinal nerve transection model (Kim and Chung 1992) and intraperitoneal administration, Wegert et al. (1997) showed a decrease in efficacy. The reason for the discrepant results with systemically administered opioids is unknown; perhaps peripheral opioid receptors play a more important role in the CCI model.

ARE THE DIFFERENT KINDS OF NEUROPATHIC PAIN DIFFERENTIALLY SENSITIVE TO OPIOIDS?

I know of no human data that relate to this question, but work with experimental animals clearly shows that many drugs, including opioids, differentially affect different symptoms. Results from the CCI model alone show that at least six kinds of drugs have very pronounced differential efficacy against different abnormal pains: opioids (including morphine and μ-, δ-, and κ-specific agonists; Lee et al. 1994), NMDA-receptor antagonists (dextrorphan and magnesium ion; Tal and Bennett 1994; Xiao and Bennett 1994), gabapentin (Xiao and Bennett 1996), zincotide (an N-type calcium channel blocker; Xiao and Bennett 1995), clonidine (Kayser et al. 1995), and felbamate (Imamura and Bennett 1995). For example, consider the following results obtained in CCI rats with systemic dosing (Lee et al. 1994; Tal and Bennett 1994): Dextrorphan: complete reversal of heat-hyperalgesia; zero effect on mechano-hyperalgesia. Opioids: near zero effect on heat-hyperalgesia; complete reversal of mechano-hyperalgesia.

Clearly, different kinds of abnormal pain respond differentially to different drugs, which indicates that the mechanisms underlying different kinds of abnormal pain also vary, at least in part. There may even be different pathological mechanisms for the same symptom. As noted above, Lee et al. (1994) found that morphine and receptor-subtype-specific agonists were very effective against mechano-allodynia in CCI rats. In the Kim and Chung (1992) spinal nerve transection model, mechano-allodynia is very resistant to systemic and i.t. morphine, even at doses that cause severe side effects (Yamamoto and Yaksh 1992; Mao et al. 1995; Ossipov et al. 1995; Chung and Na 1996; Nichols et al. 1997; Wegert et al. 1997). Evidence indicates that the mechano-allodynia seen in the Kim and Chung model is a response to input from low-threshold mechanoreceptive Aβ afferents (Na et al. 1993). The mechano-allodynia seen in the Kim and Chung model and that seen in the CCI model have nearly identical time courses and severity (Kim et al. 1997). But the CCI model's mechano-allodynia cannot possibly be a response to input from low-threshold mechanoreceptive Aβ afferents, because all (or very nearly all) of these fibers are interrupted at the level of the constriction (Munger et al. 1992). Thus, what appears to be the identical symptom is produced by different mechanisms and responds to different drugs. If rats are this complicated, then our human patients are likely to be at least as complicated.

IS NEUROPATHIC PAIN ASSOCIATED WITH A CHANGE IN THE NEURAL CIRCUITRY UPON WHICH A THERAPEUTIC OPIOID ACTS?

No human data relate to this question, but data from animals with experimental painful peripheral neuropathy give an interesting answer: "There are enormous changes, but they do not seem to explain anything!"

In the normal subject (human or animal), a systemic injection of an opioid produces its effect via interactions with multiple sites in the brain and spinal cord. The relative contribution of each site of action is not known with exactness, but evidence suggests that the spinal site is paramount. Now consider the case of a subject (human or animal) with inflammatory pain. First, the relative contributions of the brain and spinal sites may not be the same. Second, there may be entirely different sites of action (or new substrates at the same sites). This possibility is supported by the leftwards shift of i.t. μ and δ (but not κ) agonists in rats with inflammatory hyperalgesia (Hylden et al. 1991). At the very least, we must now consider a de novo opioid action upon receptors on primary afferent neurons, which acquire efficacy only in the inflammatory state. For inflammatory pain, the bulk of the evidence still supports the great importance of the spinal site of action, but in animals at least, the primary afferent site seems to play a significant role as well (Stein 1993). But now consider the case of a subject (human or animal) with painful peripheral neuropathy. Is the spinal site of action still of paramount importance? We do not know. Do injured or intact neighboring afferents acquire a functional opioid sensitivity? We do not know. Are entirely new regions of the brain involved in pain processing? Evidence suggests that they are (Iadarola et al. 1998).

Finally, in the case of painful peripheral neuropathy we must consider the possibility that at least some of the mechanisms producing pain are fundamentally unlike those that produce normal acute pain or inflammatory pain. A great deal of evidence supports this hypothesis. Many drugs have little or no effect against normal acute pain, but suppress at least some kinds of neuropathic pain (e.g., tricyclic antidepressants, NMDA-receptor antagonists, α_2-adrenergic agonists, broad-spectrum calcium channel blockers, N-type calcium channel blockers, sodium channel blockers, and anti-epileptics of diverse chemistry and mechanisms of action: felbamate, gabapentin, lamotrigine, and topiramate). Conversely, while NSAIDs are wonderfully effective against inflammatory pain, they are devoid of activity against neuropathic pain. Moreover, Malmberg et al. (1997) have shown that a mutation that disrupts the function of cyclic adenosine monophosphate (cAMP)-dependent protein kinase markedly decreases acute and postinflammatory pain, but has no effect on painful peripheral neuropathy.

Animals with painful peripheral neuropathy show greatly increased levels of synthesis of endogenous enkephalin and dynorphin in the spinal cord dorsal horn (Draisci et al. 1991). One might hypothesize that this reflects an increased activity of endogenous pain-controlling circuitry, and that the increase is at or near the physiological maximum of the system's efficacy. Therapeutic opioids would thus be relatively ineffective because the system that they work on is already operating at its limit (i.e., a ceiling effect). But this cannot be the case for enkephalin, because inflammation increases it even more, and i.t. δ and μ agonists have a leftwards (not a rightwards) potency shift in inflammatory pain (Hylden et al. 1991). Inflammation causes an even larger increase in the level of dorsal horn dynorphin, but the dose response of a κ agonist does not change in inflammatory pain (Hylden et al. 1991).

Stevens et al. (1991) have shown that large changes in binding occur at μ, δ, and κ sites in the spinal dorsal horn of rats with an experimental painful peripheral neuropathy. These changes are very complex; they evolve over time and differ from one area of the spinal gray to another, and even involve the opposite side. The relevance of such changes for the opioid responsiveness of neuropathic pain is unknown.

CONCLUSION

"Do opioids work for neuropathic pain?" is a poorly stated question. We should clearly separate the issue of efficacy from that of practical efficacy. If there is any efficacy at all, even if only at intolerably high doses, then we can try many things to increase the therapeutic ratio. Of course, if there is no efficacy at all, we can look elsewhere. We should realize that the endogenous substrate for opioid analgesia is a complex interaction among several sites of drug action, and that this substrate is not the same when we compare normal subjects, patients with inflammatory pain, and patients with painful peripheral neuropathy. Results obtained in patients when using systemic administration are not comparable to those obtained with i.t. dosing. We should stop considering neuropathic pain as a unitary phenomenon; it very clearly is not. Different kinds of neuropathic pain in humans are very likely to be differentially sensitive to drugs (they clearly are in experimental animals). This indicates that our clinical trials must be better. It makes no sense to ask the patient to "Rate your pain intensity"; instead, we should be measuring drug effects on each symptom separately. It is not difficult, for example, to obtain ratings of the intensity of mechano-allodynia evoked by a standardized touch stimulus, or to measure the size of the patient's allodynic area. It is likely that in the future we will treat the neuropathic pain patient with a combination of drugs, each targeted toward a particular symptom. This will be no different than the combination drug approach that typifies today's treatment of hypertension.

REFERENCES

Arnér S, Meyerson BA. Lack of analgesic effect of opioids on neuropathic and idiopathic forms of pain. *Pain* 1988; 33:11–23.

Bennett GJ, Xie Y-K. A peripheral mononeuropathy in rat that produces disorders of pain sensation like those seen in man. *Pain* 1988; 33:87–107.

Chung JM, Na HS. Effects of systemic morphine on neuropathic pain behaviors in an experimental rat model. *Analgesia* 1996; 2:151–156.

Draisci G, Kajander KC, Dubner R, Bennett GJ, Iadarola MJ. Up-regulation of opioid gene expression in spinal cord evoked by experimental nerve injuries and inflammation. *Brain Res* 1991; 560:186–192.

Gracely RH, Dubner R, McGrath PA. Narcotic analgesia: fentanyl reduces the intensity but not the unpleasantness of painful tooth pulp sensations. *Science* 1979; 203:1261–1263.

Harati Y, Gooch C, Swenson M, Edelman S, Greene D, et al. Double-blind randomized trial of tramadol for the treatment of the pain of diabetic neuropathy. *Neurology* 1998; 50:1842–1846.

Hylden JKL, Thomas DA, Iadarola MJ, Nahin RL, Dubner R. Spinal opioid analgesic effects are enhanced in a model of unilateral inflammation/hyperalgesia: possible involvement of noradrenergic mechanisms. *Eur J Pharmacol* 1991; 194:135–143.

Iadarola MJ, Berman KF, Zeffiro TA, et al. Neural activation during acute capsaicin-evoked pain and allodynia assessed with PET. *Brain* 1998; 121:931–947.

Imamura Y, Bennett GJ. Felbamate relieves several abnormal pain sensations in rats with an experimental painful peripheral neuropathy. *J Pharmacol Exp Ther* 1995; 275:177–182.

Kayser V, Desmeules J, Guilbaud G. Systemic clonidine differentially modulates the abnormal reactions to mechanical and thermal stimuli in rats with peripheral mononeuropathy. *Pain* 1995; 60:275–285.

Kim KJ, Yoon,YW, Chung JM. Comparison of three rodent neuropathic pain models. *Exp Brain Res* 1997; 113:200–206.

Kim SH, Chung JM. An experimental model for peripheral neuropathy produced by segmental spinal nerve ligation in the rat. *Pain* 1992; 50:355–363.

Krames E. Intraspinal opioid therapy for chronic nonmalignant pain: current practice and clinical guidelines. *J Pain Symptom Manage* 1996; 11:333–352.

Lee SH, Kayser V, Desmeules J, Guilbaud G. Differential action of morphine and various opioid agonists on thermal allodynia and hyperalgesia in mononeuropathic rats. *Pain* 1994; 57:233–240.

Lee YW, Chaplan SR, Yaksh TL. Systemic and supraspinal, but not spinal, opiates suppress allodynia in a rat neuropathic pain model. *Neurosci Lett* 1995; 186:1–4.

Malmberg AB, Brandon EP, Idzerda RL, et al. Diminished inflammation and nociceptive pain with preservation of neuropathic pain in mice with a targeted mutation of the type I regulatory subunit of cAMP-dependent protein kinase. *J Neurosci* 1997; 17:7462–7470.

Mao J, Price DD, Mayer DJ. Experimental mononeuropathy reduces the antinociceptive effects of morphine: implications for common intracellular mechanisms involved in morphine tolerance and neuropathic pain. *Pain* 1995; 61:353–364.

Munger BL, Bennett GJ, Kajander KC. An experimental painful peripheral neuropathy due to nerve constriction. I. Axonal pathology in the sciatic nerve. *Exp Neurol* 1992; 118:204–214.

Na HS, Leem JW, Chung JM. Abnormalities of mechanoreceptors in a rat model of neuropathic pain possible involvement in mediating mechanical allodynia. *J Neurophysiol* 1993; 70:522–528.

Nichols ML, Lopez Y, Ossipov MH, Bian D, Porreca F. Enhancement of the antiallodynic and antinociceptive efficacy of spinal morphine by antisera to dynorphin A (1–13) or MK-801 in a nerve-ligation model of peripheral neuropathy. *Pain* 1997; 69:317–322.

Ossipov MH, Lopez Y, Nichols ML, Bian D, Porreca F. The loss of antinociceptive efficacy of spinal morphine in rats with nerve ligation injury is prevented by reducing spinal afferent drive. *Neurosci Lett* 1995; 199:83–86.

Park KM, Max MB, Robinovitz E, Gracely RH, Bennett GJ. Intradermal capsaicin as a model of chronic neuropathic pain: effects of ketamine, alfentanil, and placebo. *Pain* 1995; 63:163–172.

Portenoy RK. Opioid therapy for chronic nonmalignant pain: current status. In: Fields HL, Liebeskind JC (Eds). *Pharmacological Approaches to the Treatment of Chronic Pain. Progress in Pain Research and Management*, Vol. 1. Seattle: IASP Press, 1994, pp 247–287.

Portenoy RK, Foley KM, Inturrisi CE. The nature of opioid responsiveness and its implications for neuropathic pain: new hypotheses derived from studies of opioid infusions. *Pain* 1990; 43:273–286.

Rowbotham MC, Reisner-Keller LA, Fields HL. Both intravenous lidocaine and morphine reduce the pain of postherpetic neuralgia. *Neurology* 1991; 41:891–902.

Sethna N, Liu M, Gracely R, Bennett GJ, Max M. Analgesic and cognitive effects of intravenous ketamine-alfentanil combinations vs. either drug alone after intradermal capsaicin in normal subjects. *Anesth Analg* 1998; 86:1250–1256.

Stein C. Peripheral mechanisms of opioid analgesia. *Anesth Analg* 1993; 76:182–191.

Stevens CW, Kajander KC, Bennett GJ, Seybold VS. Bilateral and differential changes in spinal mu, delta, and kappa binding in rats with a painful, unilateral neuropathy. *Pain* 1991; 46:315–326.

Tal M, Bennett GJ. Neuropathic pain sensations are differentially sensitive to dextrorphan. *Neuroreport* 1994; 5:1438–1440.

Watson CP, Babul N. Efficacy of oxycodone in neuropathic pain: a randomized trial in postherpetic neuralgia. *Neurology* 1998; 50:1837–1841.

Wegert S, Ossipov MH, Nichols ML, et al. Differential activities of intrathecal MK-801 or morphine to alter responses to thermal and mechanical stimuli in normal or nerve-injured rats. *Pain* 1997; 71:57–64.

Xiao W-H, Bennett GJ. Magnesium suppresses abnormal pain responses via a spinal site of action in rats with an experimental peripheral neuropathy. *Brain Res* 1994; 666:168–172.

Xiao W-H, Bennett GJ. Synthetic omega-conopeptides applied to the site of nerve injury suppress neuropathic pains in rats. *J Pharmacol Exp Ther* 1995; 274:666–672.

Xiao W-H, Bennett GJ. Gabapentin has an anti-nociceptive effect mediated via a spinal site of action in a rat model of painful peripheral neuropathy. *Analgesia* 1996; 2:267–273.

Yamamoto T, Yaksh TL. Studies on the spinal interaction of morphine and the NMDA antagonist MK-801 on the hyperesthesia observed in a rat model of sciatic mononeuropathy. *Neurosci Lett* 1992; 135:67–70.

Correspondence to: G.J. Bennett, PhD, Department of Neurology, MCP Hahnemann University, Broad and Vine Street (Mail Stop 423), Philadelphia, PA 19102-1192, USA. Fax: 215-762-3161; email: bennettg@auhs.edu.

Opioid Sensitivity of Chronic Noncancer Pain,
Progress in Pain Research and Management,
Vol. 14, edited by Eija Kalso, Henry J. McQuay,
and Zsuzsanna Wiesenfeld-Hallin, IASP Press,
Seattle, © 1999.

20

Efficacy of Peripheral Opioid Analgesia in Inflammatory Pain: Evidence from Clinical Studies

Michael Schäfer

Department of Anesthesiology and Critical Care Medicine, Benjamin Franklin University Hospital, Free University of Berlin, Berlin, Germany

New scientific evidence has challenged the traditional distinction between two commonly used classes of analgesics, the nonsteroidal anti-inflammatory drugs (NSAIDs) and the opioids. Until recently, the NSAIDs have been classified as "peripheral" analgesics because their main action, inhibition of cyclooxygenase and subsequently of prostaglandin synthesis, has been understood to occur exclusively at the peripheral site of injury and inflammation (Hardman et al. 1996). In contrast, the opioids have been classified as "central" analgesics, because their main action, inhibition of the conductance of painful stimuli through activation of opioid receptors, has been understood to occur exclusively within the central nervous system (CNS) (Hardman et al. 1996). According to recent experimental studies, this clear-cut distinction between the two classes of analgesics is no longer justified. Prostaglandins are also released within the spinal cord and contribute to a state of hyperalgesia that can be reduced by the intrathecal administration of NSAIDs (Malmberg and Yaksh 1992). On the other hand, opioid receptors have been identified on peripheral nerve endings of primary afferent neurons, and their activation by local administration of opioid agonists produces potent analgesia in animals and humans (Stein 1995). Thus, both classes of analgesics appear to have both a central and peripheral site of action.

These findings open up new therapeutic approaches for the treatment of pain. Local administration of systemically ineffective doses of opioids at the site of a painful injury results in potent analgesia without serious central side effects such as sedation, respiratory depression, euphoria, dependence, and addiction. This chapter focuses on the analgesic efficacy of peripheral opioids in human inflammatory pain. It compares results from controlled clinical studies with key findings from experimental studies, presents preliminary clinical results on the use of local opioids in chronic inflammatory pain such as arthritis, and suggests future research strategies. This chapter will not provide an extensive review of the current clinical literature on local opioid treatment, since two excellent reviews have recently been published (Kalso et al. 1997; Stein et al. 1997).

EXPERIMENTAL STUDIES: KEY FINDINGS

While the early reports on the peripheral analgesic effects of opioids were somewhat anecdotal, recent experimental studies have systematically applied the pharmacological criteria of opioid receptor specificity to demonstrate peripheral opioid analgesia (Stein 1993). These animal studies used quaternary compounds (compounds that do not enter the CNS) (Rios and Jacob 1983) or compared local versus systemic administration (Stein et al. 1989) to show that the analgesic effects of locally applied opioids are mediated by a peripheral mechanism and not by systemic absorption of the drug into the circulation. Furthermore, it was demonstrated that the peripheral analgesic effects are dose-dependent, stereospecific, and reversed by opioid-receptor antagonists, and thus are opioid-receptor specific. These analgesic effects are most prominent under inflammatory conditions and increase with the duration of inflammation (Schäfer et al. 1995; Zhou et al. 1998). Depending on the specific characteristics of the experimental inflammatory agent (e.g., carrageenan, Freund's adjuvant), ligands for all three opioid receptors can be effective, producing potent analgesia (Stein et al. 1989; Nagasaka et al. 1996). Finally, peripheral analgesic effects of opioids have been described for conditions such as somatic pain (Stein et al. 1993), and visceral pain (Burton and Gebhart 1998), in the acute and chronic inflammatory state. In addition, recent experimental evidence indicates the analgesic efficacy of topical opioid treatment with loperamide, a μ-opioid agonist that does not cross the blood–brain barrier (Nozaki-Taguchi and Yaksh 1999). The results of these pharmacological studies are consistent with those of other studies that have identified mRNA (Mansour et al. 1994; Minami et al. 1995; Schäfer et al. 1995) and cellular proteins of opioid receptors in primary afferent neurons by use of an anti-idiotypic antibody (Stein et al. 1990), a radiolabeled ligand (Hassan et al. 1993), and antisera against the cloned μ-, δ- and κ-opioid receptors (Dado et al. 1993; Ji et al. 1995; Zhang et al. 1998).

CLINICAL STUDIES

ACUTE PAIN

How do clinical studies examining the analgesic effects of locally applied opioids relate to the findings from experimental studies? In the first controlled clinical trial, attenuation of postoperative pain by an intra-articular (i.a.) injection of morphine was investigated in patients undergoing arthroscopic knee surgery (Stein et al. 1991). Patients receiving 1 mg i.a. morphine had significantly lower pain scores (determined by the visual analogue scale [VAS], numerical rating scale, and McGill Pain Questionnaire) than those receiving i.a. saline (control). Mean requirements for supplemental analgesics were lower in the i.a. morphine group than in the i.a. saline group. To ensure that analgesic effects were not due to systemic absorption, patients in the control group received in addition to i.a. saline an intravenous (i.v.) injection of 1 mg morphine, which was not effective. Thus, the analgesic effect of i.a. morphine seems to be exclusively due to a peripheral mechanism. This finding has been recently supported by an elegant study by Koppert and colleagues (1999), who used a peripheral model of UV-B-induced hyperalgesia and the technique of "i.v. regional analgesia" in 11 volunteers. UV-B irradiation produced a local skin inflammation with signs of erythema and hyperalgesia on both forearms. The next day, 4 mg of morphine hydrochloride in 40 mL saline 0.9% (0.04% solution) was injected i.v. after a tourniquet was inflated to 250 mm Hg around the upper arm. Calibrated heat and phasic mechanical stimuli were used to test for nociceptive responsiveness. Regional i.v. administration of morphine (but not saline 0.9%) into the forearm resulted in a significant increase of heat pain thresholds in inflamed but not in normal skin areas. Tests for regional plasma levels of morphine and its metabolites, morphine-3- and morphine-6-glucuronide, in the forearm detected high levels of morphine but no metabolites. In contrast, neither morphine nor its metabolites were detected in the systemic circulation. Five minutes after the release of the tourniquet, morphine and metabolites, mainly morphine-3-glucuronide, were detected systemically. These findings indicate that analgesic effects of regional i.v. morphine to heat stimuli are elicited exclusively by peripheral mechanisms. Moreover, these clinical findings are similar to previous experimental findings in that an inflammatory process seems to facilitate the peripheral action of opioids. The findings are also consistent with recent observations in patients undergoing dental surgery (Likar et al. 1998). Administration of 1 mg morphine together with the local anesthetic into the submucous site of the painful tooth produced prolonged and better pain relief than did saline after dental surgery in patients who presented with acute inflammatory tooth pain (Likar et al. 1998). Supplemental morphine was not effective in patients who were scheduled for elective dental surgery and thus had no apparent inflammation (R. Likar et al., unpublished data).

The most consistent results for local opioid analgesia have come from clinical trials examining the analgesic efficacy of i.a. morphine with a study protocol similar to the first published report (Stein et al. 1991). Interestingly, studies using higher doses of morphine did not show greater pain reduction compared to others using smaller doses (Stein et al. 1991; Joshi et al. 1993; McSwiney et al. 1993). Only three studies compared different doses of i.a. morphine alone, and showed no dose-dependency of analgesic effects. In one study, the two doses chosen (0.5 and 1 mg i.a. morphine) were too similar to detect a statistically significant difference in postoperative analgesia (Stein et al. 1991). Another study examined doses of 2 and 4 mg i.a. morphine, but failed to include a control group receiving i.a. saline. Since pain intensity scores were already very low in the group with 2 mg i.a. morphine, further decreases with the higher dose of 4 mg i.a. morphine could not be detected (Juelsgaard et al. 1993). A third study showed higher pain scores with 2 mg compared to 1 mg i.a. morphine; however, the authors had no explanation for this surprising result (Allen et al. 1993). Studies that used different doses of morphine together with bupivacaine (Heine et al. 1994; Laurent et al. 1994) are not comparable because postoperative analgesic effects might be influenced by the local anesthetic. A recent clinical trial compared three doses of i.a. morphine against i.a. saline under randomized, double-blind conditions following a standardized protocol (Likar et al. 1999). Patients were excluded if the arthroscopy was only diagnostic and no therapeutic interventions were performed. The results showed that increasing doses of i.a. morphine were associated with decreasing pain intensity (measured by VAS) and supplemental analgesic consumption (piritramide administered by a patient-controlled analgesia device). Thus, as in the experimental findings, analgesic effects of i.a. morphine increased dose-dependently under standardized conditions. The demonstration of a peripheral and dose-dependent effect suggests that morphine acts specifically on opioid receptors within the knee joint. This hypothesis is supported by the fact that patients who received 0.04 mg i.a. naloxone together with 1 mg i.a. morphine had higher pain scores than did patients receiving 1 mg i.a. morphine alone (Stein et al. 1991). Taken together, dose-dependency and antagonism by naloxone of local analgesic effects of i.a. morphine suggest that these effects are opioid-receptor specific. In fact, opioid receptors have recently been identified by autoradiography on peripheral sensory nerve terminals in human synovial tissue (Lawrence et al. 1992; Stein et al. 1996).

One clinical trial investigated whether local opioid treatment can effectively relieve acute visceral pain (Duckett et al. 1997). This is particularly interesting, since experimental literature on the analgesic effects of opioids in visceral pain models is continuing to grow (Burton and Gebhart 1998). Fifty-two children undergoing ureteral reimplantation were randomized to receive postoperatively one of three concentrations of intravesical morphine (0.05, 0.375, or 0.5 mg/mL) as a continuous infusion. Pain intensity was assessed with a Baker-Wong faces scale. Patients reported greater pain intensity in the group with 0.05 mg/mL than in the 0.375 and 0.5 mg/mL groups on the first two days postoperatively. No differences were noted on the third postoperative day, on which the continuous morphine drip was removed. This is the first clinical report on the analgesic efficacy of local morphine treatment in visceral pain states. It is intriguing that morphine, predominantly a μ-opioid-receptor agonist, is effective in relieving visceral pain in humans, since experimental studies (mainly in rats) point to a major role of κ agonists rather than μ agonists (Sengupta et al. 1996). However, this discrepancy may be explained by species differences. Further clinical trials are needed to corroborate these findings. In general, local opioid treatment appears to be effective in somatic as well as visceral pain. In addition, new experimental evidence of the analgesic efficacy of topically applied opioids (Nozaki-Taguchi and Yaksh 1999) seems to be supported by preliminary clinical experiences (Back and Finlay 1995; Krajnik and Zylicz 1997).

Ever-increasing evidence from experimental and clinical studies by various research groups has demonstrated the analgesic efficacy of peripheral opioids, but clinical studies still present conflicting results. The major reasons for this controversy were outlined in the review by Kalso et al. (1997): (1) The analgesic assay lacks sensitivity due to the fact that pain scores are too low. This may result from an analgesic regimen that combines spinal, epidural, or general anesthesia with high doses of opioids whose effects continue into the postoperative period. Another problem may be that the pain stimulus intensity of the interventions is too low, for example, diagnostic arthroscopy versus arthroscopic surgical interventions (e.g., anterior cruciate ligament repair). (2) The analgesic assay lacks internal sensitivity, i.e., the opioid effect is compared neither to a standard analgesic (e.g., local anesthetic) (positive control) nor to a placebo (negative control). (3) The site and mode of local administration can influence the result. A review by Picard et al. (1997) indicated that incisional, perineural, intrapleural, and intraperitoneal administrations are less promising routes for local treatment with opioids due to pharmacokinetic or pharmacodynamic shortcomings. For example, intrapleural and intraperitoneal substances may be quickly absorbed, and opioid receptors may not be coupled to G proteins and thus may not be functionally active during their axonal transport to the peripheral nerve ending. Also, the perineural sheath may be an impenetrable barrier for certain drugs under normal conditions, but may be disrupted under inflammatory conditions (Antonijevic et al. 1995). Future clinical studies should take into account these important considerations to ensure that the results are not due to errors in the study design but are based on solid scientific evidence.

CHRONIC PAIN

While peripheral opioids seem to be effective in acute pain, a completely new approach is to examine their efficacy in chronic pain states such as arthritis. The rationale for this approach is based on experimental findings that local analgesic effects of opioids and the number of opioid receptors that are axonally transported to the peripheral nerve ending increase according to the duration of inflammation (Antonijevic et al. 1995; Zhou et al. 1998). In a crossover study (Likar et al. 1997), patients with osteoarthritis of the knee joint suffering from an acute pain attack were randomly assigned to an i.a. injection of either 1 mg morphine or saline 0.9%. Additional pain medication (diclofenac) was available at all times, and the amount of analgesic intake was recorded. After 7 days, patients crossed over to the opposite treatment. Patients who received a single injection of 1 mg i.a. morphine had significantly lower pain scores than did patients receiving saline 0.9%. The surprising finding was that the analgesic effect lasted up to 7 days, so that results in the second phase could not be analyzed statistically. Interestingly, pain scores in the group of patients who crossed over to 1 mg i.a. morphine also decreased. These findings confirm case reports about the efficacy of i.a. opioids together with local anesthetics in chronic pain patients (Khoury et al. 1994). The long duration of analgesic effects of i.a. morphine is surprising and cannot solely be explained by a direct action of opioids on the opioid receptors of peripheral sensory neurons, i.e., a decrease in the excitability and propagation of action potentials of these neurons (McFadzean 1988).

Anti-inflammatory effects of opioids have been described (Carr 1991; Binder and Walker 1998), and opioid receptors have been identified on various immune cells (Hassan et al. 1993; Gaveriaux et al. 1995). Thus, local opioids could, in addition to their action on sensory neurons, also act on resident immune cells and result in decreased secretion of cytokines, a downregulation of adhesion molecule expression, and a reduced migration of immune cells into the injured tissue (Wilson et al. 1998). The combination of analgesic and presumed anti-inflammatory effects of local opioids could be most advantageous in the therapy of arthritis, since its goals are the relief of pain, the reduction of inflammation, and the maintenance of functional activity (Lipsky 1998). However, future studies must investigate whether the therapeutic effect of local opioid treatment is comparable to or even better than standard treatment for arthritis (NSAIDs, steroids, etc.). Stein et al. (1996) conducted a preliminary study to compare i.a. injection of morphine with an i.a. standard steroid treatment and with placebo (saline 0.9%) in patients suffering from osteoarthritis or rheumatoid arthritis. The i.a. morphine treatment seemed to be superior to the steroid or saline treatment, underscoring the efficacy of local opioids in arthritic pain. Further controlled clinical studies with greater numbers of patients are necessary to prove the efficacy of this approach.

A serious limitation of local opioid treatment is the requirement for repeated i.a. injections, which carry risks such as bleeding, infection, or eventual cartilage breakdown. On the other hand, systemically applied opioids have serious central side effects. These risks could be avoided with new opioid compounds that act exclusively at peripheral opioid receptors and do not cross the blood–brain barrier.

SUMMARY

Increasing evidence shows that opioid receptors are present on sensory neurons outside the CNS, and that activation of these receptors by local opioid therapy results in experimental as well as clinically relevant pain relief. This is a radical change in our traditional thinking about opioid pharmacology and therapy. Analgesic effects following the systemic administration of opioids can thus be explained by activation not only of central but also of peripheral opioid receptors. Since the local analgesic effects of opioids are most effective under inflammatory conditions, possibly due to combined analgesic and anti-inflammatory effects, their use in chronic inflammatory pain states such as arthritis may be an alternative to conventional therapy. The possibility of peripherally selective opioid compounds that are devoid of typical central side effects such as sedation, respiratory depression, euphoria, and addiction, is an exciting prospect. Pharmaceutical companies are developing such compounds, some of which have already entered preclinical trials (Barber et al. 1994). Thus, new drugs with fewer side effects may be available for patients with arthritis in the near future.

ACKNOWLEDGMENTS

This work was supported by a grant from the International Anesthesia Research Society.

REFERENCES

Allen GC, Amand MA, Lui ACP, et al. Postarthroscopy analgesia with intra-articular bupivacaine/ morphine. *Anesthesiology* 1993; 79:4169–4172.

Antonijevic I, Mousa SA, Schäfer M, et al. Perineurial defect and peripheral opioid analgesia in inflammation. *J Neurosci* 1995; 15:165–172.

Back IN, Finlay I. Analgesic efficacy of topical opioids on painful skin ulcers. *J Pain Symptom Manage* 1995; 10:493.

Barber A, Bartoszyk GD, Bender HM, et al. A pharmacological profile of the novel, peripherally-selective κ-opioid receptor agonist, EMD 61753. *Br J Pharmacol* 1994; 113:1317–1327.

Binder W, Walker JS. Effect of the peripherally selective kappa-opioid agonist, asimadoline, on adjuvant arthritis. *Br J Pharmacol* 1998; 124:647–654.

Burton MB, Gebhart GF. Effects of kappa-opioid receptor agonists on response to colorectal distention in rats with and without acute colonic inflammation. *J Pharmacol Exp Ther* 1998; 285:707–715.

Carr DJ. The role of endogenous opioids and their receptors in the immune system. *Proc Soc Exp Biol Med* 1991; 198:710–720.

Dado RJ, Law PY, Loh HH, et al. Immunofluorescent identification of a delta (δ)-opioid receptor on primary afferent nerve terminals. *Neuroreport* 1993; 5:341–344.

Duckett JW, Cangiano T, Cubina M, et al. Intravesical morphine analgesia after bladder surgery. *J Urol* 1997; 157:1407–1409.

Gaveriaux C, Peluso J, Simonin F, Laforet J, Kieffer B. Identification of kappa- and delta-opioid receptor transcripts in immune cells. *FEBS Lett* 1995; 369:272–276.

Hardman JG, Limbird LE, Molinoff PB, et al. (Eds). Goodman and Gilman's *The Pharmacological Basis of Therapeutics,* 9th ed. New York: McGraw-Hill, 1996.

Hassan AHS, Ableitner A, Stein C, et al. Inflammation of the rat paw enhances axonal transport of opioid receptors in the sciatic nerve and increases their density in the inflamed tissue. *Neuroscience* 1993; 55:185–195.

Heine MF, Tillet ED, Tsueda K, et al. Intra-articular morphine after arthroscopic knee operation. *Br J Anaesth* 1994; 73:413–415.

Ji RR, Zhang Q, Law PY, et al. Expression of mu-, delta-, and kappa-opioid receptor-like immunoreactivities in rat dorsal root ganglia after carrageenan-induced inflammation. *J Neurosci* 1995; 15:8156–8166.

Joshi GP, McCarroll SM, O'Brian TM, et al. Intra-articular analgesia following knee arthroscopy. *Anesth Analg* 1993; 76:333–336.

Juelsgaard P, Dalsgaard J, Felsby S, et al. Analgesic effect of 2 different doses of intra-articular morphine after ambulatory knee arthroscopy. A randomized, prospective, double-blind study. *Ugeskr Laeger* 1993; 155:4169–4172.

Kalso E, Tramèr MR, Carroll D, et al. Pain relief from intra-articular morphine after knee surgery: a qualitative systemic review. *Pain* 1997; 71:127–134.

Khoury GF, Garland DE, Stein C. Intraarticular opioid-local anesthetic combinations for chronic joint pain. *Middle East J Anaesthesiol* 1994; 12:579–585.

Koppert W, Likar R, Geisslinger G, et al. Peripheral antihyperalgesic effect of morphine to heat, but not mechanical, stimulation in healthy volunteers after ultraviolet-B irradiation. *Anesth Analg* 1999; 88:117–122.

Krajnik M, Zylicz Z. Topical morphine for cutaneous cancer pain. *Palliat Med* 1997; 11:325.

Laurent SC, Nolan JP, Pozo JL, et al. Addition of morphine to intra-articular bupivacaine does not improve analgesia after day-case arthroscopy. *Br J Anaesth* 1994; 72:170–173.

Lawrence AJ, Joshi GP, Michalkiewicz A, Blunnie WP, Moriarty DC. Evidence for analgesia mediated by peripheral opioid receptors in inflamed synovial tissue. *Eur J Clin Pharmacol* 1992; 43(4): 351–355.

Likar R, Schäfer M, Paulak F, et al. Intraarticular morphine analgesia in chronic pain patients with osteoarthritis. *Anesth Analg* 1997, 84:1313–1317.

Likar R, Sittl R, Gragger K, et al. Peripheral morphine analgesia in dental surgery, *Pain* 1998; 76:145–160.

Likar R, Kapral S, Steinkellner H, et al. Dose-dependency of intraarticular morphine analgesia. *Br J Anaesth* 1999, in press.

Lipsky PE. Rheumatoid arthritis. In: Braunwald E, Fauci AS, Hauser SL (Eds). *Harrison's Principles of Internal Medicine,* 14th ed. New York: McGraw-Hill, 1998, pp 1880–1888.

Malmberg AB, Yaksh TL. Hyperalgesia mediated by spinal glutamate or substance P receptor blocked by spinal cyclooxygenase inhibition. *Science* 1992; 257:1276–1279.

Mansour A, Fox CA, Burke S, et al. Mu, delta, and kappa opioid receptor mRNA expression in the rat CNS: an in situ hybridization study. *J Comp Neurol* 1994; 350:412–438.

McFadzean I. The ionic mechanisms underlying opioid actions. *Neuropeptides* 1998; 11:173–180.

McSwiney MM, Joshi GP, Kenny P, et al. Analgesia following arthroscopic knee surgery. A controlled study of intra-articular morphine, bupivacaine or both combined. *Anesth Intens Care* 1993; 21:201–203.

Minami M, Maekawa K, Yabuuchi K, et al. Double in situ hybridization study on coexistence of mu-, delta-, and kappa-opioid receptor mRNAs with preprotachykinin A mRNA in the rat dorsal root ganglion. *Brain Res Mol Brain Res* 1995; 30:203–210.

Nagasaka H, Awad H, Yaksh TL. Peripheral and spinal actions of opioids in the blockade of the autonomic response evoked by compression of the inflamed knee joint. *Anesthesiology* 1996; 85:808–816.

Nozaki-Taguchi N, Yaksh TL. Characterization of the antihyperalgesic action of a novel peripheral mu-opioid receptor agonist—loperamide. *Anesthesiology* 1999; 90:225–234.

Picard PR, Tramèr MR, McQuay HJ, et al. Analgesic efficacy of peripheral opioids (all except intra-articular): a qualitative systematic review of randomized controlled trials. *Pain* 1997; 72:309–318.

Rios L, Jacob JJ. Local inhibition of inflammatory pain by naloxone and its N-methyl quaternary analogue. *Eur J Pharmacol* 1983; 96:277–283.

Schäfer M, Imai Y, Uhl GR, et al. Inflammation enhances peripheral mu-opioid receptor-mediated analgesia, but not mu-opioid receptor transcription in dorsal root ganglia. *Eur J Pharmacol* 1995; 279:165–169.

Sengupta JN, Su X, Gebhart GF. Kappa, but not mu or delta, opioids attenuate responses to distention of afferent fibres innervating the rat colon. *Gastroenterology* 1996; 111:968–980.

Stein C. Peripheral mechanisms of opioid analgesia. *Anesth Analg* 1993; 76:182–191.

Stein C. Mechanisms of disease: the control of pain in peripheral tissue by opioids. *N Engl J Med* 1995; 332:1685–1690.

Stein C, Millan MJ, Shippenberg TS, et al. Peripheral opioid receptors mediating antinociception in inflammation. Evidence for involvement of mu-, delta- and kappa-receptors. *J Pharmacol Exp Ther* 1989; 248:1269–1275.

Stein C, Hassan AHS, Przewlocki R, Gramsch C, Peter K, et al. Opioids from immunocytes interact with receptors on sensory nerves to inhibit nociception in inflammation. *Proc Natl Acad Sci USA* 1990, 87:5935–5939.

Stein C, Comisel K, Haimerl E, et al. Analgesic effect of intraarticular morphine after arthroscopic knee surgery. *N Engl J Med* 1991; 325:1123–1126.

Stein C, Pflüger M, Yassouridis A, et al. No tolerance to peripheral morphine analgesia in presence of opioid expression in inflamed synovia. *J Clin Invest* 1996, 98:793–799.

M. SCHÄFER

Stein C, Schäfer M, Cabot PJ, et al. Peripheral opioid analgesia. *Pain Rev* 1997; 4:171–185.
Wilson JL, Walker JS, Antoon JS, et al. Intercellular adhesion molecule-1 expression in adjuvant arthritis in rats: inhibition by kappa-opioid agonists but not by NSAID. *J Rheumatol* 1998; 25:499–505.
Zhang Q, Schäfer M, Elde R, et al. Effects of neurotoxins and hindpaw inflammation on opioid receptor immunoreactivities in dorsal root ganglia. *Neuroscience* 1998; 85:281–291.
Zhou L, Zhang Q, Stein C, et al. Contribution of opioid receptors on primary afferent versus sympathetic neurons to peripheral opioid analgesia. *J Pharmacol Exp Ther* 1998; 286:1000–1006.

Correspondence to: Michael Schäfer, Department of Anesthesiology and Critical Care Medicine, Free University of Berlin, Hindenburgdamm 30, D-12200 Berlin, Germany. Fax: 49-30-8445-4469; email: mischaefer@medizin.fu-berlin.de.

Opioid Sensitivity of Chronic Noncancer Pain,
Progress in Pain Research and Management,
Vol. 14, edited by Eija Kalso, Henry J. McQuay,
and Zsuzsanna Wiesenfeld-Hallin, IASP Press,
Seattle, © 1999.

21

Opioids in Ischemic Pain

Jan Persson

Pain Section, Department of Anaesthesia and Intensive Care, Karolinska Institute, Huddinge University Hospital, Stockholm, Sweden

Pain is a signal to the organism of potential tissue damage. An inadequate blood supply to part of the body is a very obvious such threat and would thus be expected to generate significant pain. Many relatively common types of pain encountered in the clinic are in fact ischemic in nature.

Cardiac pain is the most common type of ischemic pain, at least in the developed countries. Therapy for myocardial infarction is mainly directed at treating the ischemia by using vasodilatation and thrombolysis, rather than treating the symptoms of pain, as such. The degree of pain relief obtained from thrombolysis is often used to monitor the success of the treatment, and so analgesic drugs can be regarded as confounding elements. Nevertheless, opioids are frequently used to alleviate cardiac pain when analgesia is imperative.

Pain due to a compromised blood supply to the abdominal organs is also a common clinical entity. The pain is sometimes iatrogenic, following therapeutic embolization. Many of the underlying mechanisms are shared with cardiogenic pain (Bonica 1990: Chapter 3). Somatic ischemic pain is also a source of substantial clinical pain problems. Chronic occlusive arterial disease, mainly in the form of arteriosclerosis obliterans, is the most frequent type.

In an organ deprived of an adequate blood supply, hypoxia will develop and the pH will drop, partly due to the formation of lactic acid. Inflammatory mediators such as histamine, acetylcholine, phosphorylcreatine, serotonin, potassium, and bradykinin will accumulate. These changes in the *milieu interieur* would be expected to activate nociceptors in the tissue (Mills et al. 1989). The mechanisms underlying ischemic pain have not yet been completely elucidated and probably differ for cardiac, intestinal, deep somatic (muscular), and superficial somatic (cutaneous) pain. Furthermore, many of the clinical pain manifestations may be referred from the tissue suffering ischemia (Bonica 1990: Chapters 3, 7). The skin could also be a main source of pain in patients with ischemic rest pain in the extremities (Dormandy 1996).

When the ischemia is chronic, i.e., prolonged or recurrent, changes in central neuronal function may also play a significant role, contributing to what has been called "pathological pain" (Woolf and Thompson 1991; Coderre et al. 1993).

ISCHEMIC PAIN MECHANISMS

Lewis and colleagues performed seminal work on ischemic pain mechanisms in humans almost 70 years ago (Lewis et al. 1931). They found that the pain of patients with intermittent claudication due to occlusive arterial disease in one leg could be mimicked in the healthy leg by a combination of induced ischemia and muscular activity in that leg. Up to 20 minutes of additional ischemia induced prior to exercise made no difference in the time it took for pain to develop after starting to exercise. Lewis therefore postulated the accumulation of a stable algogenic substance, "factor P," which he thought must be produced by muscular activity during ischemia.

Following Lewis, experimental ischemic muscle pain in human subjects has often been studied using the tourniquet technique. In this model, a tourniquet is applied to the upper arm and inflated above the arterial pressure. Before or after inflation, the forearm muscles are exercised (Sternbach 1983; Maurset et al. 1991). Factors such as the pattern of force and the timing of the muscular contractions play an unclear role. The amount of energy expended by the muscles and the frequency of the contractions seem to govern the development of pain, whereas the force of contractions plays a minor role (Mills et al. 1982).

Issberner and co-workers (1996) compared the effect of the tourniquet technique with that of an intramuscular infusion of an acid phosphate buffer in humans. They concluded that pain from ischemic contractions is generated by the same mechanisms as in the acidic infusion, i.e., an algogenic action of protons, and thus proposed that protons are Lewis's "factor P."

Using a similar technique, Steen and co-workers (1995) infused an acidic buffer into the skin of human volunteers and concluded that the pain from human tissue acidosis results from a nonadapting excitation of a relatively constant population of nociceptors. Working on a preparation of the skin and saphenous nerve of rats, Steen also found a distinct subpopulation of mechano- and heat-sensitive polymodal C-units with stimulus-related responses that increased with proton concentration and according to the time course of the pH change (Steen et al. 1992).

There is thus quite a strong case that the accumulation of protons initiates nociception in ischemic somatic pain, although the mechanisms underlying the pain of ischemic muscular contractions are still the subject of controversy. Candidates for the role of initiating stimulus are protons, lactic acid, potassium ions, PGE_2, and bradykinin (Mense 1993). It has been shown that ischemia alone (for periods up to 1 hour) is not an effective stimulus for the activation of muscle group III and IV afferents, thought to mediate nociception. However, the combination of muscular contractions and ischemia strongly excites nociceptive neurons, mostly those in group IV. The time course of activation follows that of the pain experienced by human volunteers when performing ischemic muscular contractions (Mense and Stahnke 1983; Mense 1993).

Referred pain mechanisms have been known to be important contributors to the symptoms of patients with deep somatic or visceral pathology since the time of H. Head, over 100 years ago (Bonica 1990: Chapter 7). In patients with peripheral occlusive arterial disease, hyperalgesia in the calf and foot ("myalgic spots") paralleled intermittent claudication, but blood flow to the calf showed no correlation with the claudication. Injection of procaine in the hyperalgesic areas also increased the distance patients were able to walk (Arcangeli et al. 1976).

Long-standing ischemia also induces changes in central nociceptive processing. Increased sensitivity and enlarged receptive fields of nociceptive dorsal horn neurons have been demonstrated in rats after 60 minutes of hindlimb ischemia (Sher and Mitchell 1990).

Unlike ischemic pain in the extremities, cardiac pain is visceral and therefore is often vague, diffuse, poorly localized, and generally referred (Hammermeister 1990). The intensity, quality, and localization of the pain in myocardial ischemia do not allow the clinician to discriminate between angina pectoris with and without myocardial infarction (Eriksson et al. 1994). Furthermore, the duration and severity of myocardial ischemia are not sufficient to explain the occurrence of pain (Maseri 1987). Mediators such as bradykinin, prostaglandins, protons, potassium, and substance P may activate or sensitize cardiac nociceptors. Adenosine is a strong candidate. Depending on the pattern of ischemia-induced release and spatiotemporal summation, adenosine appears to stabilize or sensitize afferent cardiac nerves, resulting either in silent or painful ischemia. The mediators listed above may enhance the activity of the adenosine-sensitized afferent nerves (Sylvén 1997).

Poole and colleagues (1987) studied the mechanisms involved in intestinal ischemic pain. They used hydraulic occluders on the celiac and superior mesenteric arteries of dogs to achieve a 50% reduction in flow. This decreased the mean intestinal intramural pH, measured by tonometry, from 7.33 to 7.11. Instilling dairy cream into the stomach further reduced the pH to 7.03. Patients with occlusion of the mesenteric arteries may experience an exacerbation of their pain when eating, and Poole's results indicate that low pH is one of the mechanisms generating pain in splanchnic ischemia. Nociceptive afferents sensitive to intestinal ischemia have been identified as a subpopulation of sympathetic C-fiber afferents. The structural and functional differences that distinguish ischemically sensitive and insensitive sympathetic C-fiber endings are largely unknown, however (Pan and Longhurst 1996).

OPIOID EFFECTS IN ISCHEMIC PAIN

Clinical and experimental studies of opioid effects on ischemic intestinal pain are lacking, probably because the causes of abdominal pain are often unclear and a homogeneous study population would be difficult to find. Furthermore, we lack experimental pain models in humans for this type of pain.

Considering the morbidity and impact of ischemic heart disease, the number of controlled studies that focus on opioid effects is surprisingly small, and there are few recent studies. One study compared morphine with indoprofen (a nonsteroidal anti-inflammatory drug) in a double-blind randomized study (Bressan et al. 1985). Forty patients with acute myocardial infarction received indoprofen 400 mg intravenously (i.v.) or morphine 10 mg intramuscularly (i.m.). Pain was assessed on a 4-degree scale. There was no significant difference in the average analgesic response to the two drugs as measured by pain intensity difference (PID) scores, which were 2.3 and 1.9 for indoprofen and morphine, respectively. The proportion of responding patients in the indoprofen group was greater than in the morphine group at all observation times.

Pentazocine, postulated to be a κ agonist and a μ antagonist, has been compared with pethidine (Maurer et al. 1970). One hundred patients with a diagnosis of acute myocardial insufficiency or acute myocardial infarction and severe precordial pain were administered pentazocine 40 mg or pethidine 100 mg in a double-blind randomized protocol. Maurer's team assessed pain by noting the time required to obtain pain relief at four time points during the first hour, and found no difference between the two groups. Four patients in each group did not have satisfactory pain relief at 1 hour. While the pain measurement was not up to modern standards, the study is still of interest because of the receptor profiles of the respective drugs.

Another study compared buprenorphine (considered to be a partial agonist at the μ receptor) with a pure μ agonist, diamorphine (Hayes et al. 1979). In a randomized double-blind protocol, 120 patients with chest pain due to suspected myocardial infarction that required analgesia were given buprenorphine 0.3 mg i.v. or diamorphine 5 mg i.v. The time, degree, and duration of pain relief were monitored using a visual analogue scale (VAS). Five minutes after administration of the respective drug, the percentage of pain relief was significantly lower in the buprenorphine group than in the diamorphine group. From 15 minutes to 6 hours after administration, however, there were no significant differences in pain relief between the groups. During the 6 hours, 12 and 16 patients in the buprenorphine and diamorphine groups, respectively, had incomplete pain relief.

Conventional μ agonists have also been compared. Nielsen et al. (1984) selected 275 patients with suspected acute myocardial infarction (AMI) requiring analgesic intervention and administered morphine 10 mg, nicomorphine 10 mg, or pethidine 75 mg in a randomized double-blind protocol at intervals of 30 minutes or longer as needed. The first two injections were given i.v. and the following subcutaneously (s.c.). If the patients were not pain free for at least 3 hours after the third dose, the dose was increased by 50%. Analgesia was rated on a 0–3 point scale. All three analgesics provided equal pain relief. Additional analgesic treatment was required after 24 hours by 30–45% of the AMI patients and by 10–20% of patients who later were considered not to have AMI.

In spite of the fact that ischemic limb pain is common and often unsatisfactorily controlled with opioids, very few clinical studies have addressed this type of pain,. The opioid effect was rarely the focus in the few existing studies. In one experimental pain study, six female volunteers exercised their left forearm muscles for 2 minutes with a handgrip strengthener, and a tourniquet was then applied to the upper arm and inflated to 100 mm Hg above systolic blood pressure (Maurset et al. 1989). Ketamin 0.3 mg/kg or pethidine 0.7 mg/kg were given as a 2-minute infusion using an i.v. cannula in the opposite arm when the tourniquet was inflated, and pain was rated on a VAS scale 5 minutes after the infusion. Either placebo or naloxone 1.6 mg was also administered 5 minutes before inflation of the cuff for a total of four randomized administrations. Pethidine was half as effective as ketamine at these doses, and the effect of pethidine was partly antagonized by naloxone (a μ antagonist).

In another study using the tourniquet method, adenosine 70 $\mu g \cdot kg^{-1} \cdot min^{-1}$ lowered the sum of pain scores (SPS) as much as morphine 0.1 mg/kg i.v and ketamine 0.1 mg/kg i.v. (Segerdahl et al. 1994). Combining adenosine with morphine or ketamine significantly lowered the number of subjects reaching a VAS score of 100 compared with morphine or ketamine given alone.

Pentazocine, postulated to be a κ agonist and a μ antagonist, was compared with morphine and pethidine in patients suffering from ischemic lower-extremity pain (Taylor 1971). Eighteen patients with arterial insufficiency in a lower limb were given pentazocine 45 mg, morphine 15 mg, and pethidine 100 mg consecutively in a randomized, double-blind order. The drugs were injected i.m. as required up to four times a day, and each drug was given for 2 days. Pain was then assessed on a 4-degree scale. Before treatment three patients scored 2 (moderate), six scored 3 (severe), and nine scored 4 (very severe) pain. Following treatment, the mean reduction in pain score was 2.17 for morphine, 1.82 for pethidine, and 2.17 for pentazocine. The differences were not statistically significant. No pain relief was reported by one patient when receiving morphine, two when receiving pethidine, and two when receiving morphine.

The abovementioned study by Maurset and co-workers (1989) inspired a clinical study in patients with ischemic rest pain (Persson et al. 1998). Nine patients with pain in the lower limb were enrolled, but one patient required an acute amputation half-way through the study, so only eight patients completed the protocol (Table I). Reconstructive vascular surgery had been performed on all of them, but no further surgery was possible in any of them. All the patients had been taking opioids with unsatisfactory pain relief (previously prescribed analgesics were discontinued during the study period).

Table I
Profile of eight patients who participated in a study of
ischemic pain in the lower extremity

Patient No.	Age (y), Gender	Weight (kg)	Medical/Surgical History	Opioid Medication*
1	81, M	78	Prostate cancer	Ketobemidone 5 mg q.l.
2	80, M	80	Diabetes mellitus, stroke, myocardial infarction	Slow-release morphine 30 mg q.n.; ketobemidone 5 mg q.l.
3	67, M	77	Atrial fibrillation	Ketobemidone 5 mg q.l.
4	81, F	50	Angina, hypertension	Ketobemidone 5 mg q.l.
5	61, F	58	Chronic low back pain, hypertension	Morphine 10 mg q.n.; buprenorphine 0.2 mg q.l.
6	75, F	53	Thyroidectomy	Morphine 10 mg q.l.
7	65, F	50	Hyperlipidemia, stroke	Buprenorphine 0.2 mg q.l.
8	72, F	40	Goiter operation	Morphine 10 mg q.4 h.

Source: Persson et al. (1998).
Abbreviations: q.l. = as much as desired; q.n. = every night; q.4 h. = every 4 hours.
* Medications are those prescribed prior to entry into the study.

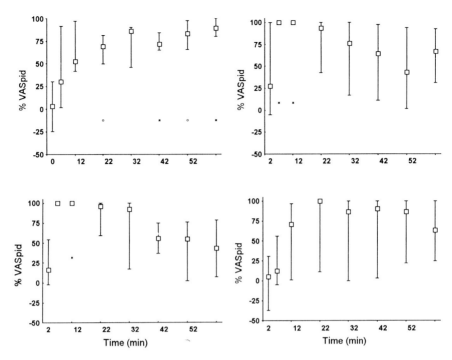

Fig. 1. VAS pain ratings expressed as the pain intensity difference from baseline as a percentage (% VASpid) plotted as a function of time for ketamine at (a) 0.15 mg/kg (upper left), (b) 0.30 mg/kg (upper right), and (c) 0.45 mg/kg (lower left), and (d) for morphine at 10 mg (lower right). The boxes indicate median values and the bars indicate the 25th–75th percentiles; open circles indicate outliers and asterisks denote extremes. Reprinted with permission from Persson et al. (1998).

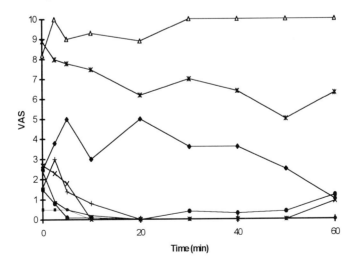

Fig. 2. Individual VAS pain ratings for all eight patients after morphine 10 mg was given as a 5-minute i.v. infusion.

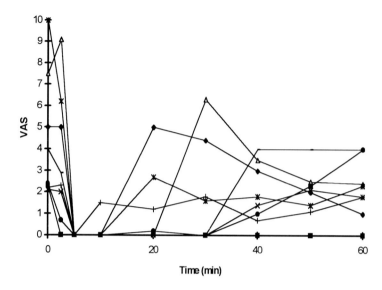

Fig. 3. Individual VAS pain ratings for all eight patients after ketamine 0.45 mg/kg was given as a 5-minute i.v. infusion.

Care was taken to ensure that the pain rated was of the ischemic type. The following criteria were used: (1) angiography and ankle blood pressure showed signs of occluded distal arteries, and (2) pain in the foot, ankle, and/ or calf that was (a) accentuated or provoked by muscular activity of the leg or elevation of the foot and (b) relieved by lowering the foot. If the patients had ulcers on their feet, neuropathy, or other identifiable distinct sources of pain, they were required to be able to distinguish between the different types.

The patients received racemic ketamine hydrochloride (Ketalar; Parke-Davis) 0.15, 0.3, 0.45 mg/kg and morphine hydrochloride (Pharmacia) 10 mg in a double-blind randomized design on four separate days at least 1 day apart. They were instructed to rate the sensory dimension of their pain as distinct from the affective dimension. VAS ratings were obtained at 0, 2.5, 5, 10, 20, 30, 40, 50, and 60 minutes. Pain intensity differences were then calculated as a percentage of the value at the start of the session (Fig. 1).

The variation in the morphine pain ratings was considerable (Fig. 2). A group of good responders (five patients), and a group of poor responders (three patients) could be identified. The good responders reported complete pain relief at 20 minutes. Two of the poor responders (patients 1 and 3) reported no analgesic effect from morphine, and even rated increased pain at 20 minutes. The third poor responder (patient 5) had a VAS pain intensity increase of 30% at 20 minutes. All three poor responders also had high baseline pain scores, patients no 3 and 5 the highest of all. In the ketamine 0.45 mg/kg session all the patients became pain free at the time of peak effect at 5 minutes (Fig. 3). The analgesic effect of ketamine 0.45 mg/kg and morphine 10 mg at the time of their peak effects (5 and 20 minutes, respectively) was not significantly different ($P < 0.10$, Wilcoxon test). It is interesting to note, however, that the three patients with complete pain relief from ketamine but poor pain relief from morphine had high pain scores. This can be compared to reports that differences in analgesic potency among different drugs may not be detectable if the pain intensity is low (Bjune et al. 1996). Part of the explanation for the patients' indeterminate reports concerning opioid efficacy might therefore be the varying intensity of pain. The prescribed opioids could conceivably control the low-grade pain but not the more intense bouts. Since cutaneous pain often responds poorly to opioids (Samuelsson et al. 1995), skin pain may be a contributing factor to the total experience of pain (Dormandy 1996).

CONCLUSIONS

The pain-generating mechanisms in ischemic pain are complex and not completely understood. Referred pain and central sensitization are important factors in all types of ischemic pain. In somatic tissue, cutaneous pain components may play a role; an important initiating factor seems to be the accumulation of protons in ischemia. In cardiac ischemic pain, the duration and severity of myocardial ischemia are not sufficient factors to explain the occurrence of pain. Several pain mediators may be involved, but adenosine appears to play a key role. In intestinal ischemic pain, the pain-generating mechanisms have not been extensively studied, but ischemia-sensitive nociceptive afferents have been identified.

Opioid effects in ischemic pain have been scantily investigated. In peripheral ischemia, there are indications of a limited analgesic effect of standard doses when the pain is intense. In ischemic cardiac pain there are few studies, particularly recent ones, of opioid effects. In the published studies, different opioids provide essentially equal pain relief, but a subgroup of patients do not respond to standard doses. It is not known whether the poor effect of standard opioid doses that has been observed is due to reduced opioid responsiveness or to insufficient doses. The response to opioids in ischemic intestinal pain has not been studied.

To conclude, scientific knowledge concerning the effect of opioids in ischemic pain is meager. Further research is needed in order to elucidate ischemic pain mechanisms in different organ systems. Clarifying the issues of opioid responsiveness, choice of opioid, and dosing regimes in ischemic pain will also require a great deal of clinical research.

ACKNOWLEDGMENTS

This work was supported in part by the Swedish Cancer Fund (3948-B97-01XAB) and the Swedish Medical Research Council (grant no. 3902).

REFERENCES

Arcangeli P, Digiesi V, Ronchi O, Dorigo B, Bartoli V. Mechanisms of ischaemic pain in peripheral occlusive arterial disease. In: Bonica JJ, Albe-Fessard D (Eds). *Advances in Pain Research and Therapy,* Vol. 1. New York: Raven Press, 1976.

Bjune K, Stubhaug A, Dodgson MS, Breivik H. Additive analgesic effect of codeine and paracetamol can be detected in strong, but not moderate, pain after Caesarean section. Baseline pain-intensity is a determinant of assay-sensitivity in a postoperative analgesic trial. *Acta Anaesthesiol Scand* 1996; 40:399–407.

Bonica JJ. In: Bonica JJ (Ed). *The Management of Pain.* Philadelphia: Lea and Febiger, 1990.

Bressan MA, Constantini M, Klersy C, et al. Analgesic treatment in acute myocardial infarction: a comparison between indoprofen and morphine by a double-blind randomized pilot study. *Int J Clin Pharmacol Ther Toxicol* 1985; 23:668–672.

Coderre T J, Katz J, Vaccarino AL, Melzack R. Contribution of central neuroplasticity to pathological pain: review of clinical and experimental evidence. *Pain* 1993; 52:259–285.

Dormandy JA. Prostanoid drug therapy for peripheral arterial occlusive disease—the European experience. *Vasc Med* 1996; 1:155–158.

Eriksson B, Vuorisalo D, Sylvén C. Diagnostic potential of chest pain characteristics in coronary care. *J Int Med* 1994; 235(5):473–478.

Hammermeister KE. Cardiac and aortic pain. In: Bonica JJ (Ed). *The Management of Pain.* Philadelphia: Lea and Febiger, 1990.

Hayes MJ, Fraser AR, Hampton JR. Randomised trial comparing buprenorphine and diamorphine for chest pain in suspected myocardial infarction. *BMJ* 1979; 2:300–302.

Issberner U, Reeh PW, Steen KH. Pain due to tissue acidosis: a mechanism for inflammatory and ischemic myalgia? *Neurosci Lett* 1996; 208:191–194.

Lewis T, Pickering GW, Rothschild P. Observations upon muscular pain in intermittent claudication. *Heart* 1931; 15:359–383.

Maseri A. Mechanisms of ischaemic cardiac pain and significance of silent myocardial ischaemia. *Acta Cardiol* 1987; 3:153–159.

Maurer B, Murnaghan D, Hickey N, Mulcahy R. Pentazocine in the relief of acute cardiac pain. *Acta Cardiol* 1970; 29:157–164.

Maurset A, Skoglund LA, Hustveit O, Øye I. Comparison of ketamine and pethidine in experimental and postoperative pain. *Pain* 1989; 36:37–41.

Maurset A, Skoglund LA, Hustveit O, Klepstad P, Øye I. A new version of the ischaemic tourniquet pain test. *Methods Find Exp Clin Pharmacol* 1991; 13(9):643–647.

Mense S. Nociception from skeletal muscle in relation to clinical muscle pain. *Pain* 1993; 54:241–289.

Mense S, Stahnke M. Responses in muscle afferent fibres of slow conduction velocity to contractions and ischemia in the cat. *J Physiol* 1983; 342:383–397.

Mills KR, Newham DJ, Edwards RHT. Force, contraction frequency and energy metabolism as determinants of ischaemic muscle pain. *Pain* 1982; 14:149–154.

Mills KR, Newham DJ, Edwards RHT. Muscle pain. In: Wall PD, Melzack R (Eds). *Textbook of Pain.* Edinburgh: Churchill Livingstone, 1989.

Nielsen JR, Pedersen KE, Dahlstrøm CG, et al. Analgetic treatment in acute myocardial infarction. *Acta Med Scand* 1984; 215:349–354.

Pan H-L, Longhurst JC. Ischaemia-sensitive sympathetic afferents innervating the gastrointestinal tract function as nociceptors in cats. *J Physiol* 1996; 492(Pt 3):841–850.

Persson J, Hasselström J, Wiklund B, et al. The analgesic effect of racemic ketamine in patients with chronic ischemic pain due to lower extremity arteriosclerosis obliterans. *Acta Anaesthesiol Scand* 1998; 42:750–758.

Poole JW, Sammartano RJ, Boley SJ. Hemodynamic basis of the pain of chronic mesenteric ischaemia. *Am J Surg* 1987; 153:171–175.

Samuelsson H, Malmberg F, Eriksson M, Hedner T. Outcomes of epidural morphine treatment in cancer pain: nine years of clinical experience. *J Pain Symptom Manage* 1995; 10(2):105–112.

Segerdahl M, Ekblom A, Sollevi A. The influence of adenosine, ketamine, and morphine on experimentally induced ischemic pain in healthy volunteers. *Anesth Analg* 1994; 79:787–791.

Sher GD, Mitchell D. N-Methyl-D-aspartate receptors mediate responses of rat dorsal horn neurones to hindlimb ischaemia. *Brain Res* 1990; 522:55–62.

Steen KH, Reeh PW, Anton F, Handwerker HO. Protons selectively induce lasting excitation and sensitization to mechanical stimulation of nociceptors in rat skin in vitro. *J Neurosci* 1992; 12(19):86–95.

Steen KH, Issberner U, Reeh PW. Pain due to experimental acidosis in human skin: evidence for non-adapting nociceptor excitation. *Neurosci Lett* 1995; 199(19):29–32.

Sternbach RA. The tourniquet pain test. In: Melzack (Ed). *Pain Measurement and Assessment.* New York: Raven Press, 1983, pp 27–31.

Sylvén C. Neurophysiological aspects of angina pectoris. *Z Kardiol* 1997; 86(Suppl 1):95–105.

Taylor I. Clinical trial comparing pentazocine with pethidine and morphine in severe ischaemic limb pain. *Br J Clin Pract* 1971; 25(1):27–30.

Woolf C J, Thompson WN. The induction and maintenance of central sensitisation is dependent on N-methyl-D-aspartic acid receptor activation; implications for the treatment of post-injury pain hypersensitivity states. *Pain* 1991; 44:293–299.

Correspondence to: Jan Persson, MD, PhD, Pain Section, Department of Anesthesia and Intensive Care, Karolinska Institute, Huddinge University Hospital, HS-14186 Huddinge, Sweden. Tel: 46-85858000; Fax: 46-87795424; email: jan.persson@anaesth.hs.sll.se.

Opioid Sensitivity of Chronic Noncancer Pain,
Progress in Pain Research and Management,
Vol. 14, edited by Eija Kalso, Henry J. McQuay,
and Zsuzsanna Wiesenfeld-Hallin, IASP Press,
Seattle, © 1999.

22

Opioids for Chronic Musculoskeletal Pain

Peter J.D. Evans

Pain Management Centre, Charing Cross Hospital, London, United Kingdom

The use of analgesics is widespread in the community for applications ranging from "hangover" to migraine. Most analgesics can be obtained as over the counter preparations. Many are used to treat musculoskeletal problems, which may be acute (sprains and strains) or chronic (osteoarthritis and chronic low back pain).

Most analgesic compounds are based on aspirin or acetaminophen. However, manufacturers have attempted to improve efficacy by including small quantities of opioid analgesics such as codeine and dextropropoxyphene. Such additives have rarely improved the quality of pain relief, but have often produced improved satisfaction for patients due to sedation or mild euphoria. The use of such compounds has been considered "low risk"; abuse potential is minimal and incidence of toxicity is low, except when an overdose is intentionally taken. Although the volume of prescriptions is known, little information is available concerning consumption and use. Clinical experience suggests that the long-term harmful effects of these compounds are minimal and that there is considerable tolerance to consumption. Patients regularly take more than the recommended daily maximum dose.

The use of opioids for the control of cancer pain is fully acknowledged and endorsed. Nevertheless, problems of delivery and accessibility persist for some cancer patients (Stjernsward 1991). Data on the role of such drugs in chronic nonmalignant pain, largely collected from retrospective studies, are conflicting. Some reports advocate the use of opioids (Boukoums et al. 1992), while others suggest that chronic administration leads to reductions in performance, impairment of cognition, and exacerbation of psychological problems or illness behavior (Maruta et al. 1979; Turner et al. 1982).

Of major concern for all physicians are the procedures necessary for prescribing controlled drugs and complying with national regulatory requirements (Hill 1991; Clarke and Sees 1993). Physicians may be understandably reluctant to prescribe such compounds for patients with nonmalignant pain, where the organic disease process may be ill defined and where life expectancy is normal. However, such a view is scientifically unsound and reflects erroneous beliefs and values, although influential papers have sustained such views by supporting the notion that psychological dependence and addiction are problematic (Kolb 1925; Rayport 1954). Later publications citing legal action against physicians who prescribed opioids to patients with nonmalignant pain helped to reinforce the view that the chronic administration of opioids in this population is dangerous (Tennant and Uelman 1983).

This chapter will focus on chronic musculoskeletal pain and particularly on chronic low back pain in addressing several fundamental questions related to the role of narcotic analgesics: What is the epidemiology of opioid administration in chronic pain? Are opioids efficacious? What are the myths and misconceptions? What are the problems? Which are the best agents? What are appropriate management guidelines?

CHRONIC MUSCULOSKELETAL PAIN

Chronic musculoskeletal pain is very much a nonspecific term that relates to a whole range of problems associated with mechanical injury to the muscles, vertebrae, and nerves (Table I). The common characteristics are recurrent pain, disability, and dysfunction. Several "red flag" problems, such as paralysis or acute root and cord compression, could require immediate surgical intervention. However, the management of most other musculoskeletal problems is conservative.

Opinions have changed dramatically on the management of acute low back pain. Early mobilization is seen as a key indicator to recovery (Clinical

Table I
Common causes of chronic low back pain

Prolapsed intervertebral disk
Osteoarthritis
Fibromyalgia
Ligament strain
Root entrapment
Myofascial syndrome
Lumbar facet syndrome
Postsurgical scarring
Arachnoiditis
Spinal stenosis

Standards Advisory Group 1994), and so the use of powerful analgesics in the acute phase has much to commend it. However, many treatment options (ranging from acupuncture to epidurals) are available in the early phase that are known to have beneficial effects.

The combination of a nonsteroidal anti-inflammatory drug (NSAID), an opioid analgesic, and a simple muscle relaxant can prove to be an extremely effective combination in the first few days post "disk prolapse." For most patients the problem is self-limiting and the physician does not have to ask, "How long is it safe to continue with such a combination?"

Fewer than 2% of patients have symptoms that last beyond 12 months (Nachemson 1979). These tend to be the patients who eventually seek help at pain management centers, along with those for whom surgical intervention has failed and others with largely untreatable problems such as arachnoiditis and spinal stenosis. They form a heterogeneous group with a predominance of females, for whom continued opioid administration poses potential risks.

THE EPIDEMIOLOGY OF OPIOID ADMINISTRATION IN CHRONIC PAIN

Sadly, there is a lack of information relating to opioid analgesic consumption among chronic pain sufferers. A few surveys have looked at "self-selected" groups attending pain clinics (Table II), which may not be representative of the general population. Evans (1985) suggested that 1 in 10 chronic pain patients were regularly taking opioids and that 1 in 5 patients with back pain were consuming these drugs. Jamison and colleagues (1994) suggested that the frequency was even higher; when they included all analgesics that contained any amount of an opioid, then over 50% of patients

Table II
Drug use in chronic pain patients

Evans (1983)†	%	Jamison et al. (1994)‡	%
Over the counter analgesics	47	Over the counter analgesics	35
NSAIDs	13	NSAIDs	28
Antidepressants	3	Antidepressants	56
Opioids (cancer pain)	8	Benzodiazepines	24
Opioids (noncancer pain)	10	Muscle relaxants	25
		Sleeping tablets	18
		Other drugs	37

†717 chronic pain patients.
‡109 chronic pain patients.

were using such compounds. Paradoxically, many of these patients were prescribed such drugs prior to their attendance at the pain clinic, and so we must question the effectiveness of such medication.

Sorenson and colleagues (1992) used a questionnaire to evaluate the use of opioids outside hospitals in Denmark. Their sample of 480,000 represented almost 10% of the Danish population. During 1 month they noted that 0.2% of the sample used strong analgesics. Of the acute conditions for which the drugs were prescribed, back pain represented 23% and trauma 17%. Twenty-nine percent of those requiring chronic administration were suffering from chronic low back pain.

It is possible that the wider exposure and greater awareness among physicians of the role of opioid drugs in chronic pain will increase usage. A review from the United States of 403 patients attending a pain clinic suggested that 19% were using narcotic analgesics (Chabal et al. 1997). This view is echoed by a study from Australia demonstrating that over a 10-year period the quantity of opioids dispensed in that country for nonmalignant pain had increased five-fold (Bell 1997).

ARE OPIOIDS EFFICACIOUS?

Various retrospective studies have tried to answer this question (Table III). Unfortunately, the results are far from reliable and suggest an efficacy of between 20% and 88%. If we accept the notion of "some benefit," then at least half of the patients exposed to opioids received some benefit. However, all the studies were retrospective analyses, they often had small samples, and all were subjected to various levels of bias.

The socioeconomic impact of chronic pain is enormous (Linton 1998) and relates to patient and health care factors (Table IV). Portenoy and Foley (1986), in a review of 38 patients on long-term therapy, 25% of whom were suffering from low back pain, found that opioids were efficacious. Patients

Table III
Efficacy of orally administered opioids in
chronic nonmalignant pain

Reference	Sample	Good Relief	Partial Relief
Taub 1982	313	†	
Evans 1983	106	18%	48%
Portenoy and Foley 1986	38	30%	34%
Tennant and Uelman 1986	52	88%	12%
Zenz et al. 1992	100	51%	28%

†Few details; all gained benefit.

Table IV
Socioeconomic factors in chronic low back pain

Patient-Related Factors	Health-Care-Related Factors
Disability	Excessive demands
Depression	Medication abuse
Loss of employment	Inappropriate interventions
Withdrawal from social interaction	Litigation
Disturbance of family dynamics	

remained stable on opioid therapy and did not require alternative support, whereas all had previously failed to show respond to other therapies. Sixty-three percent reported acceptable or good pain relief with the long-term opioid regime. Jamison et al. (1994) reviewed 112 individuals who were taking various opioid combinations, 45% of whom were suffering from low back pain; 83% of patients reported that the drugs "were moderately beneficial in relieving pain."

Moulin et al. (1996), in a well-designed 9-week randomized crossover study, were less convinced about efficacy. The study involved doses of morphine of up to 120 mg per day. The authors concluded that such a dosage might confer analgesic benefit, but was unlikely to offer psychological or functional improvement; since the pain was multifactorial, they felt that a comprehensive treatment strategy was required. They hypothesized that use of an agent perceived as a "powerful pain killer" would tend to encourage passivity and make patients less compliant with other aspects of the treatment program.

The use of other agents has been explored in the management of chronic pain. Tramadol hydrochloride, an aminocyclohexanol derivative, has increased in popularity as it is a safe alternative to morphine. For pain of a skeletal or arthritic nature it has proved to be as effective as NSAIDs, even though 30% of patients discontinued the drugs due to side effects (Rauck et al. 1994). A randomized double-blind crossover study comparing tramadol with diclofenac in 54 patients evaluated treatment efficacy, activities of daily living, and patient preference. There were no overall differences, although the incidence of mild side effects was higher in the tramadol group (Pavelka et al. 1995). Other studies suggest that this drug has a useful role in chronic musculoskeletal pain. A double-blind crossover study compared the efficacy of tramadol with that of pentazocine in patients with osteoarthritis of the hips and or knees, and showed that tramadol was the more effective therapy as assessed by pain scores. The drug was also more effective at reducing morning stiffness. However, adverse events were recorded in 78% of the patients during the tramadol phase, and there were several withdrawals (Bird et al. 1995).

It has been suggested that for chronic nonmalignant pain a "start low, go slow" approach should be adopted to reduce traditional opioid side effects. (Bamigbade and Langford 1998). Arkinstall et al. (1995) investigated 46 patients, most of whom suffered from back problems, and demonstrated good efficacy for controlled-release codeine as compared to placebo. Ninety-three percent of the sample requested long-term, open-label treatment with controlled-release codeine at the completion of the study. The incidence of side effects was appreciably higher in the active group, but did not preclude use of the drug.

Transdermal fentanyl has also been used in chronic back pain patients. The use of a patch reduced the need for frequent medication. In an open-label study of 50 patients, all of whom had been regularly taking oral opioids, a 3-day 25 µg/h patch proved effective in 86% of patients (Simpson et al. 1997).

Buprenorphine has also been explored as a possible agent. The mixed agonist/antagonist properties of this drug have influenced its usefulness. In some patients it produces no effect at all, while in others the powerful side effects of nausea, sweating, and headache have curtailed usage. In one open study, only 15% of patients with chronic nonmalignant pain were able to use the drug without difficulty (Evans 1983). Low back pain was the primary diagnosis in half the patients. In another study using tramadol at doses up to 600 mg per day, even less relief was achieved in a group of patients whose only complaint was musculoskeletal pain. Very few patients wished to continue taking the drug at the end of the study, citing side effects and no pain relief (Volger et al. 1996). This lack of efficacy is not uncommon in chronic nonmalignant pain, due in part to the nature of opioid responsiveness.

OPIOID RESPONSIVENESS

The variability in response to opioid analgesics may be partly due to the inherent characteristics of chronic pain as perceived by the patient. The inconsistent results in chronic pain contrast with a generally good response to opioids in postoperative pain. The concept has evolved that certain types of pain, typically neuropathic, are unresponsive to opioids (Arnér and Meyerson 1988) or respond at a level too close to sedation or toxicity for safety (Portenoy et al. 1990). Arnér and Myerson (1988) also suggested that elevation in mood following opioid administration accounts for the benefits achieved in those patients with neuropathic pain. This opinion has been questioned by Jadad and colleagues (1992), who noted that neuropathic pain was generally less responsive than nociceptive pain. In their study of 13 patients, they reported that elevations in mood did not occur in the absence of a reduction in pain intensity.

Chronic musculoskeletal pain may well comprise nociceptive, neuro-pathic, and behavioral pain elements, and this variability may contribute to the relatively poor response to long-term opioid administration. Schofferman (1993), who divided low back pain patients into three categories, adopted a similar view. Type 1 patients were "typical" chronic pain patients with pain and disability far out of proportion to the peripheral stimulus. He felt that in this group, where psychological factors were significant, long-term opioids did more harm than good. In contrast, he believed that opioids had a useful place in the other two groups comprising nociceptive and neuropathic pain patients.

DOSE

Few data exist on the appropriate dose levels of opioids needed for treating chronic pain. It is widely recognized that individual variation in dose requirement is enormous in postoperative pain; the same probably per-tains in chronic pain. However, the treatment goals are very different; in acute pain, total pain relief is the object, while in chronic pain opioids provide a more supportive role. Retrospective studies demonstrate a wide range of dosage (Table V), and given that the period of delivery may be long and that tolerance may develop, this discrepancy is not surprising. But it leaves the clinician no nearer deciding what, if any, is the appropriate starting dose or at what point an alternative strategy should be adopted.

The pragmatic approach would be to adopt the view that if the patient is satisfied and there is a reduction in consulting behavior as a consequence of starting opioid therapy, then the dose is right. As a first principle it would be reasonable to start low and build up the dose over a matter of weeks. Pa-tients will very quickly react if the analgesic is not helpful, side effects will soon be reported, and therapy will be rejected. It is unlikely that patients will continue to comply with therapy if benefit is not felt quickly.

Chronic musculoskeletal pain patients tend to be young and ambulant,

Table V
Reported starting dose and range of opioids used in chronic nonmalignant pain

Reference	Drug	Starting Dose	Final Dose	Duration
Taub 1982	Methadone	10 mg	40 mg	Up to 6 y
France et al. 1984	Methadone	3 mg	20 mg	Max. 22 mo
Urban et al. 1986	Methadone	10 mg	20 mg	Max. 26 mo
Zenz et al. 1992	Morphine	20 mg	2 g	Max. 4 y
Arkinstall et al. 1995	CR codeine	200 mg	600 mg	Max. 304 d
Moulin et al. 1996	CR morphine	30 mg	120 mg	6 wk
Simpson et al. 1997	Fentanyl	25 µg/h	100 µg/h	1 mo

and will reject drugs with central side effects such as nausea, dizziness, and drowsiness. In patients who become tolerant to chronic administration, opioids should be seen as adjuvant therapy. Many patients who take narcotic analgesics for chronic pain will attend pain management centers to seek additional measures of pain relief such as alternative medications, physical therapy, or surgical procedures (Evans 1981).

WHAT ARE THE MYTHS AND MISCONCEPTIONS?

TOLERANCE

Tolerance is a pharmacological expression that indicates the need to increase the dose with time to produce a similar effect. This characteristic of opioids will be observed in all patients, but it is probably not a significant problem. Surprisingly, the dose of analgesic does not tend markedly to escalate in patients with chronic benign back pain. Studies demonstrate that opioids can be administered for long periods at relatively constant dosage. Brown et al. (1996), reviewing 566 case studies, confirmed that chronic opioid analgesic therapy for chronic low back pain was safe and effective. The authors did not observe the receptor saturation and metabolite toxicity associated with the wild acceleration in dosage often necessary in cancer patients. Rather, back pain patients tend to use opioids as an adjunct, and when efficacy starts to fail, they look to alternative therapies rather than increasing the opioid dose, perhaps because of the public misconception of risk and fear of addiction.

ADDICTION

Much has been said about addiction, which relates to the behavior of individuals, particularly drug-seeking activity. I have found that only a small percentage of patients on opioid analgesics will exhibit activity related to drug abuse (Evans 1981). In a review of 717 patients with chronic pain in whom 130 were taking narcotic analgesics, only 9 (16%) demonstrated addictive behavior.

A review of 24 papers by Fishbain et al. (1992) found that many had used poor diagnostic criteria; only seven of the studies used adequate criteria. Within this group the incidence of drug abuse, dependence, and addiction ranged from 3.2% to 18.9%. The authors concluded that addictive behavior was not common in the general chronic pain population.

Examples from postoperative pain studies using large samples (Medina and Diamond 1977; Porter and Jick 1980; Perry and Heidrich 1982) indicate that addiction is almost nonexistent. McQuay (1997) suggested that it is a "red herring." I completely concur with his view that the medical use of opioids does not create street addicts.

Although it can be difficult to gauge addiction in patients who are experiencing chronic pain, it probably does occur. Perhaps those with a "dependent" personality and those already encountering difficulties with other kinds of medication such as benzodiazepines and antidepressants may be more at risk. It is recognized, for instance, that one of the facets of good pain management is medication detoxification (Halpen 1982; Buckley et al. 1986). However, total withdrawal from medication is not necessarily a treatment goal.

Chronic pain patients behave differently from drug abusers (street addicts), whose levels of functioning and general well-being are impaired by substance use. Those with chronic pain tend to gain improved levels of function through the adequate and judicious use of medication, including narcotic analgesics. In the chronic pain patient taking long-term opioids, physical dependence and tolerance should be expected, but the maladaptive behavior associated with addiction should not be seen. Sees and Clark (1993) suggested that these behavioral changes should be considered a diagnostic indicator of addiction. However, doubt has been cast on this view by a recent study that used the parameters of the *Diagnostic and Statistic Manual of Mental Disorders* (third edition). Chabal and colleagues (1997) used five measures of abuse criteria in a sample of 76 patients taking prescription opioids, and found that 21 subjects (28%) met three or more of the criteria. None of these patients differed in any measurable way from those in whom no evidence of abuse was present. The authors determined that neither the history, pretreatment psychological tests, nor previous medication abuse assisted in predicting those at risk.

In such patients it may well be the case that addiction is used to reinforce pain and make more plausible the request for help (Savage 1993). Such a possibility cannot be ignored when only one drug is effective and only by one route of administration. In the United Kingdom this phenomenon is most commonly observed in the management of sickle cell pain and chronic pancreatitis, where patients will demand only pethidine (meperidine) by intramuscular injection.

Perhaps there are recognizable characteristics (Table VI) that can assist physicians in making decisions. When a drug fails to work or patients frequently demand increasing doses, it is all too easy to blame the patient and ignore possible changes in the underlying condition. Portenoy (1994) suggests that three types of aberrant phenomena characterize addiction: loss of control over drug use, compulsive drug use, and continued use despite harm.

Table VI
Opioid addiction: potential behavioral characteristics

Nonaddictive Behavior	Possible Addictive Behavior
Aggressive complaints	Selling drugs
Preferring specific analgesics	Forging prescriptions or "borrowing" drugs
Increasing dosage without consent	Injecting oral formulations
Demonstrating anxiety about changes in therapy	Abuse of other medications
	Resistance to change
Reporting psychic effects of drugs	Seeking drugs from several clinicians
	Failure to maintain work or other activity

To conclude, addiction to prescription opioids does occur; despite its low incidence, it should not be overlooked.

RESPIRATORY DEPRESSION

Any individual given a standard dose of an opioid will exhibit a shift in the CO_2 dose-response curve, which indicates respiratory depression. In post-operative pain management, such depression is always a significant risk factor (Etches et al. 1989). There is a fine balance between the sedative and depressant effects of opioids and the stimulus produced by nociceptive pain. Such effects should also be observed in those with chronic benign pain but are rarely, if ever, reported. Severe respiratory depression has been observed in cancer patients who have received effective nerve blocks that abolished the nociceptive stimulus (Hanks et al. 1981).

So why is the depressive effect not observed in, for example, back pain sufferers? The answer is four-fold. First, clinicians tend not to look for the problem and do not perform the tests. Second, the average dose of opioid administered is relatively small or is built up over a prolonged period of time. Third, the nature of chronic pain is fundamentally different; patients are not expecting complete freedom of pain and do not "dose up" accordingly. Fourth, while the nociceptive element of back pain remains significant, the other components—neuropathic pain and emotional factors such as anger, distress, and frustration—continue to provide a strong stimulus to offset any depressive effects.

WHAT ARE THE PROBLEMS?

SIDE EFFECTS

Of the narcotic drugs currently available for chronic use, none is devoid of significant and troublesome side effects. The situation is aggravated because many back pain sufferers remain ambulant and are thus liable to the additional problems of dizziness and unsteadiness. The principal side effects are well described, as are the possible remedies. For many patients it becomes a "trade-off" between the quality of pain relief achieved and the severity of the side effects. It has been suggested that there is a differential tolerance for some side effects and that feelings of dysphoria, euphoria, clouding of the mind, nausea, and sedation resolve fairly quickly while others such as constipation, sweating, and reduced libido tend to remain (Shannon and Baranowski 1997).

In reality, the principal side effects cause patients the greatest concern and constitute the single most important factor that determines withdrawal from use. Many studies report a high incidence of problems (Evans 1983; Pavelka et al. 1995). Some drugs have a higher profile for troublesome side effects, and attempts to alter the pharmacological design have not met with particularly encouraging results. Drugs such as pentazocine produce poor-quality analgesia and a high incidence of dysphoria. Even powerful agents such as buprenorphine do not necessarily show better results; problems such as sickness, sweating, and headaches persist.

DEPENDENCE

Pharmacological dependence is always perceived as a problem, but in reality never seems to be an issue in chronic noncancer pain. Chronic back pain patients who are offered opioids soon recognize whether the drug will be useful. They may experience immediate side effects, in which case this pharmacological approach may be ill considered, and experimentation with other drugs is rarely rewarding. In contrast, when the drug is perceived to be useful it is likely that the patient has an incurable problem, and long-term therapy will be the treatment goal. In these patients dependence, and for that matter tolerance, can be recognized, and the clinician can work with the patient to monitor the problem. Experience in pain management suggests that provided the patient is motivated to stop using an opioid and it proves to be the right therapeutic decision, then withdrawal poses no problems.

WHICH ARE THE BEST AGENTS?

Over the years prescribing practices have shifted from more addictive, short-acting analgesics to the longer-acting, slow-release compounds (Table VII). These aid in administration, but do not necessarily reduce risk. In cancer pain the emphasis has been to provide sustained, high-quality anal-

Table VII
Comparison of types of analgesics showing
percentage used to control chronic nonmalignant pain

Evans (1983)	%	Jamison et al. (1994)	%
Dipipanone	36	Codeine compounds	27
Pethidine	23	CR morphine*	19
Dextromoramide	20	Oxycodone	18
Levorphanol	5	Methadone	15
Methadone	5	Oral morphine	10
Others	11	Fentanyl	1
		Codeine	3
		Others	7

*CR = controlled release.

gesia. A range of controlled-release/slow-release compounds of the traditional drugs has appeared. In addition, numerous routes have been explored, from intrathecal to transdermal delivery; all have their devotees and detractors. A basic principle is that drugs for chronic nonmalignant pain such as back pain should offer ease of delivery with minimal follow-up visits to adjust medication. There is little evidence to support the use of implantable delivery systems or intrathecal pumps in this patient group. At best, such techniques should be considered experimental (Maron and Loeser 1996); in the available studies, sample sizes have been small and efficacy has been low (Yoshida et al. 1996).

Of the available choices, the four most popular compounds have been dihydrocodeine, tramadol hydrochloride, buprenorphine, and methadone. Where these drugs have proved unacceptable, the most popular recent choice has been sustained-release morphine. It is too soon to fully appreciate the role of transdermal fentanyl, although its use has been reported (Simpson 1997). Combination drugs have not generally proved popular because of their fixed nature. However, the combination of papaveretum and aspirin (Aspav) as an effervescent mixture has a long tradition in the United Kingdom. The drug is not long acting, but does offer short periods of good quality pain relief, which is often what patients prefer.

THE CLIMATE FOR CHANGE

Perhaps the most difficult issue concerning opioid administration in chronic problems such as low back pain has been the attitude of clinicians. There has been considerable resistance to use of these compounds to treat nonmalignant pain. Fears of addiction have produced a generation of doctors who have actively avoided giving opioids (Savage 1993). An American review by Cherkin et al. (1995) that looked at physician preference in the management of acute sciatica concluded that physicians would consider narcotic analgesics only 20% of the time. The respondents felt that physical therapies, NSAIDs, and muscle relaxants were of greater value. The study also suggested that physicians over 50 years old were more likely to have a positive attitude toward long-term opioid administration.

A similar type of review that polled specialist pain clinicians within the United Kingdom was more positive (Coniam 1989). The author reported that 62% of clinicians prescribed opioids for nonmalignant pain; the principal indication was the failure of other forms of treatment. However, these physicians also reported a high incidence of problems; they noted intolerable side effects in 64% of patients, and opioid tolerance in 34%.

Turk et al. (1994) examined prescribing practices within various disciplines and noted that opioids were often used but that prescribing practices varied greatly. Rheumatologists and family practitioners were most likely to prescribe these drugs, while surgeons and neurologists were more likely to emphasize functional improvement instead of attempting to ameliorate symptoms. A further study (Turk and Okifuji 1997) looked at patients attending a multidisciplinary pain clinic. They found that physicians' practice in prescribing opioids appeared to be most influenced by patients' nonverbal communications of pain distress and suffering and least influenced by the duration of pain, demographic factors, pain severity, and objective physical pathology.

A positive change has undoubtedly occurred in the extended role of opioids in chronic nonmalignant pain. Nevertheless, pressure by governmental agencies to contain such use is likely to be sustained, particularly as the borders between "hard" and "soft" drugs become blurred by the introduction of cannabinoids into medical practice (Hirst et al. 1998).

APPROPRIATE MANAGEMENT GUIDELINES

The practice of medicine is becoming more prescriptive with the introduction of care pathways, protocols, and clinical guidelines. The use of opioids will often be an "end stage" in the decision-making process, so it is probably appropriate than clinicians should develop some policy for the administration of these drugs. There is consensus on the need for guidelines, although considerable variation on how they should be adopted. Good communication with the patient and informed consent are probably as robust legally as any formal written contract.

Table VIII
Protocol for use of opioids in chronic
nonmalignant pain

Do not use as first line of therapy
Define the scope of therapy
Assess opioid sensitivity
Obtain informed consent
Agree on an "end point" for therapy
Regularly monitor dose and effects
Ensure single prescriber policy
Use slow-release preparations
Use least "addictive" compounds

In an ideal world every patient should at least have an intravenous opioid challenge prior to starting therapy. But is such a challenge sufficient? Certainly not, because too many factors can influence the response a patient will make to any single intervention, be it an injection, an oral drug, or a physical therapy (Schug et al. 1991). An opioid challenge may not be able to predict the suitability of the drug or the patient's propensity to side effects, but could give a measure of the sensitivity of the pain to the drug. Jadad et al. (1992) used patient-controlled analgesia techniques to assess responsiveness; although this process is laborious and time consuming, it is potentially very valuable in assessing opioid applicability in difficult cases.

For most patients, the gentle introduction of an opioid at low dosage by mouth will offer the most straightforward approach. Patients will soon report intolerable side effects, and such a simple trial is easy to administer in an outpatient setting. The guidelines outlined in Table VIII offer sound principles on which to base therapy and provide a robust framework within which administration of opioids can be tailored to meet the patients' needs.

CONCLUSION

Narcotic analgesics have a useful role in chronic low back pain. Their use is increasing as myths and false assumptions have less influence on clinicians. They are far from being a solution and will primarily assist in the reduction of nociceptive pain, which may only constitute a small portion of the overall pain problem. The introduction of opioids into the treatment plan should be on sound evidence-based principles, and casual administration should be deprecated.

Long-acting oral preparations remain the preferred choice, and inject-able agents should at all times be avoided. A trial of planned therapy seems preferable to isolated diagnostic tests such as the intravenous injection of opioids, which may be difficult to interpret, given the complexity of factors contributing to opioid responsiveness. Early demonstration of improvement and subsequent maintenance of improvement over several weeks would provide sound justification for continuation of therapy.

REFERENCES

Arkinstall W, Sandler A, Goughnour B, et al. Efficacy of controlled-release codeine in chronic non-malignant pain: a randomised, placebo controlled clinical trial. *Pain* 1995; 62:169–178.

Arnér S, Meyerson BA. Lack of analgesic effect of opioids on neuropathic and idiopathic forms of pain. *Pain* 1988; 33:11–23.

Bamigbade TA, Langford RM. The clinical use of tramadol hydrochloride. *Pain Rev* 1998; 5:155–182.

Bell JR. Australian trends in opioid prescribing for chronic non-cancer pain, 1986–1996. *Med J Aust* 1997; 167:26–29.

Bird HA, Hill J, Stratford ME, Fenn GC, Wright V. A double-blind cross-over study comparing the analgesic efficacy of tramadol with pentazocine in patients with osteoarthritis. *J Drug Dev Clin Res* 1995; 7:181–188.

Boukoms AJ, Masand P, Murray GB, et al. Chronic non-malignant pain treated with long-term oral narcotic analgesics. *Ann Clin Psychiatry* 1992; 4:185–192.

Brown RL, Fleming MF, Patterson JJ. Chronic opioid analgesic therapy for chronic low back pain. *J Am Board Fam Pract* 1996; 9:191–204.

Buckley FP, Sizemore WA, Charlton JE. Medication management in patients with chronic non malignant pain: a review of a drug withdrawal programme. *Pain* 1986; 26:153–165.

Chabal C, Erjavec MK, Jacobson L, Mariano A, Chaney E. Prescription opiate abuse in chronic pain patients: clinical criteria, incidence and predictors. *Clin J Pain* 1997; 13:150–155.

Cherkin DC, Deyo RA, Wheeler K, Ciol AC. Physician views about treating low back pain. *Spine* 1995; 20:1–10.

Clark HW, Sees KL. Opioids, chronic pain and the law. *J Pain Symptom Manage* 1993; 8:297–305.

Clinical Standards Advisory Group. 1. *Back Pain.* Report on a CSAG Committee. London: HMSO, 1994.

Coniam SW. Prescribing opioids for chronic pain in non-malignant disease. In: Twycross RG (Ed). *The Edinburgh Symposium on Pain Control and Medical Education.* Royal Society of Medical Services International Congress and Symposium Series No 149, 1989, pp 205–210.

Etches RC, Sandler AN, Daley MD. Respiratory depression and spinal opioids. *Can J Anaesthesiol* 1989; 36:165–185.

Evans PJD. Narcotic addiction in patients with chronic pain. *Anaesthesia* 1981; 36:597–602.

Evans PJD. Opiates in the management of chronic pain. In: Bullingham RES (Ed). *Clinics in Anaesthesiology—Opiate Analgesia.* Philadelphia: WB Saunders, 1983, pp 71–94.

Evans PJD. A simple rating system for assessing treatment outcome in chronic pain patients. In: Fields HL, Dubner R, Cervero F (Eds). *Advances in Pain Research and Therapy,* Vol. 9. New York: Raven Press, 1985.

Fishbain DA, Rosomoff HL, Rosomoff RS. Drug abuse, dependence, and addiction in chronic pain patients. *Clin J Pain* 1992; 8:77–85.

France RD, Urban BJ, Keef FJ. Long term use of narcotic analgesics in chronic pain. *Soc Sci Med* 1984; 19:1379–1382.

Halpen L. Substitution-detoxification and the role in the management of chronic benign pain. *J Clin Psychiatry* 1982; 43:10–14.

Hanks GW, Twycross RG, Lloyd JW. Unexpected complication of successful nerve block. *Anaesthesia* 1981; 36:37–39.

Hill CS. Influence of regulatory agencies on the treatment of pain and standards of medical practice for the use of narcotics. *Pain Digest* 1991; 1:7–12.

Hirst RA, Lambert DG, Notcutt WG. Pharmacology and potential therapeutic uses of cannabis. *Br J Anaesth* 1998; 81:77–84.

Jadad AR, Carroll D, Glynn CJ, Moore RA, McQuay HJ. Morphine responsiveness of chronic pain: double-blind randomised crossover study with patient-controlled analgesia. *Lancet* 1992; 339:1367–1371.

Jamison RN, Anderson KO, Peeters-Asdourian C, Ferrante FM. Survey of opioid use in chronic non-malignant pain patients. *Reg Anaesth* 1994; 19:225–230.

Kolb L. Types and characteristics of drug addicts. *Ment Hygiene* 1925; 9:300–313.

Linton SJ. The socio-economic impact of chronic back pain: is anyone benefiting? *Pain* 1998; 75:163–168.

Maron J, Loeser JD. Spinal opioid infusions in the treatment of chronic pain of a non-malignant origin. *Clin J Pain* 1996; 12:174–179.

Maruta T, Swanson DW, Finlayson RE. Drug abuse and dependency in patients with chronic pain. *Mayo Clin Proc* 1979; 54:241–244.

McQuay HJ. Opioid use in chronic pain. *Acta Anaesthesiol Scand* 1997; 41:175–183.

Medina JL, Diamond S. Drug dependency in patients with chronic headache. *Headache* 1977; 17:12–14.

Moulin DE, Iezzi A, Rasheed A, et al. Randomised trial of oral morphine for chronic non-cancer pain. *Lancet* 1996; 347:143–147.

Nachemson A. A critical look at conservative treatment for low back pain. In: Jayson MIV (Ed). *The Lumbar Spine and Back Pain.* London: Pitman, 1979.

Pavelka K, Peliskova Z, Stehlikova H, Ratcliffe S, Repass C. Intraindividual differences in pain relief and functional improvement in osteoarthritis patients receiving diclofenac or tramadol. *Ceska Rheumatol* 1995; 3:171–176.

Perry S, Heidrich G. Management of pain during debridement: a survey of U.S. burns patients. *Pain* 1982; 13:12–14.

Portenoy RK. Opioid therapy for chronic non malignant pain: current status. In: Fields HL, Liebeskind JC (Eds). *Pharmacological Approaches to the Treatment of Chronic Pain.* Progress in Pain Research and Management, Vol. 1. Seattle: IASP Press, 1994.

Portenoy RK, Foley KM. Chronic use of opioid analgesics in non-malignant pain: report of 38 cases. *Pain* 1986; 25:171–186.

Portenoy RK, Foley KM, Inturrisi CE. The nature of opioid responsiveness and its implications for neuropathic pain: new hypotheses derived from studies on opiate infusions. *Pain* 1990; 43:273–286.

Porter J, Jick H. Addiction rate in patients treated with narcotics. *N Engl J Med* 1980; 302:123–131.

Rauck RL, Ruoff GE, McMillen JI. Comparison of tramadol and acetaminophen with codeine for long-term pain management in elderly patients. *Curr Ther Res Clin Exp* 1994; 55:1417–1431.

Rayport M. Experience in the management of patients medically addicted to narcotics. *JAMA* 1954; 156:684–691.

Savage SR. Addiction in the treatment of pain. Significance, recognition and management. *J Pain Symptom Manage* 1993; 8:265–278.

Schofferman J. Long-term use of opioid analgesics for the treatment of chronic pain of non-malignant origin. *J Pain Symptom Manage* 1993; 8:279–288.

Schug SA, Merry AF, Acland RH. Treatment principles for the use of opioids in pain of non-malignant origin. *Drugs* 1991; 42:228–239.

Sees KL, Clark HW. Opioid use in the treatment of chronic pain: assessment of addiction. *J Pain Symptom Manage* 1993; 8:257–264.

Shannon CN, Baranowski AP. Use of opioids in non-cancer pain. *Br J Hosp Med* 1997; 58:459–462.

Simpson RK, Edmondson EA, Constant CF, Collier C. Transdermal fentanyl as treatment for chronic low back pain. *J Pain Symptom Manage* 1997; 14:218–224.

Stjernsward J. WHO cancer pain relief programme and future challenges. In: Takeda F (Ed). *Cancer Pain Relief and Quality of Life.* Saitama: WHO Collaborative Centre for Cancer Pain Relief and Quality of Life, 1991, pp 5–9.

Sorenson HT, Rasmussen HH, Moller-Petersen JF, et al. Epidemiology of pain requiring strong analgesics outside hospital in a geographically defined population in Denmark. *Dan Med Bull* 1992; 39:464–467.

Taub A. Opioid analgesics in the treatment of chronic intractable pain of non-neoplastic origin. In: Kitahata LM, Collins D (Eds). *Narcotic Analgesics in Anaesthesiology.* Baltimore: Williams and Wilkins, 1982, pp 199–208.

Tennant FS, Uelman GF. Narcotic maintenance for chronic pain: medical and legal guidelines. *Postgrad Med* 1983; 73:81–94.

Turk DC, Okifuji EA. What factors affect physicians' decisions to prescribe opioids for chronic non-cancer pain patients. *Clin J Pain* 1997; 13:330–336.

Turk DC, Brody MC, Okifuji EA. Physicians' attitudes and practices regarding the long-term prescribing of opioids for non-cancer pain. *Pain* 1994; 59:201–208.

Turner JA, Calsyn DA, Fordyce WE, Ready LB. Drug utilisation pattern in chronic pain patients. *Pain* 1982; 12:357–363.

Urban BJ, France Rd, Steinberger DL, Scott DL, Maltbie AA. Long term use of narcotic-antidepressant medication in the management of phantom limb pain. *Pain* 1986; 24:191–197.

Volger A, Hayes M, Evans PJD. Tramadol hydrochloride—an open two week study of its use in chronic pain. *J Pain Soc Great Britain and Ireland* 1996; 12(1):27.

Yoshida GM, Nelson RW, Capen DA, et al. Evaluation of continuous intraspinal narcotic analgesia for chronic pain from benign causes. *Am J Orth* 1996; 25:693–694.

Zenz M, Strumpf M, Tryba M. Long-term opioid therapy in patients with chronic non-malignant pain. *J Pain Symptom Manage* 1992; 7:69–77.

Correspondence to: Peter J.D. Evans, FRCA, Consultant Anaesthetist, Pain Management Centre, Charing Cross Hospital, Fulham Road, London W6 8RF, United Kingdom. Tel: 44-(0)181-846-7016; Fax: 44-(0)181-846-7585; email: pj.evans@ic.ac.uk.

Opioid Sensitivity of Chronic Noncancer Pain,
Progress in Pain Research and Management,
Vol. 14, edited by Eija Kalso, Henry J. McQuay,
and Zsuzsanna Wiesenfeld-Hallin, IASP Press,
Seattle, © 1999.

23

Opioids in Headache

Flemming W. Bach

Department of Neurology, Aarhus University Hospital, Aarhus, Denmark

Despite the appearance of new and specific drugs for the treatment of headache, opioids are still frequently prescribed for this common condition. Critics argue that the danger of habituation and addiction is significant and that the analgesic effect of opioids is not well documented. Therefore, many headache experts strongly advocate that opioids should not be prescribed for headache patients. This chapter will address the controversial use of opioids in headache patients (discussed in detail by Ziegler 1994) and review clinical trials.

If headache differs from other types of pain with respect to opioid sensitivity, then perhaps one could argue that the pain mechanisms are different. This may well be the case for migraine, where the trigeminovascular interaction seems to be a specific phenomenon. Sicuteri (1982) proposed the "endorphin theory" of migraine. He emphasized that hypernociception, anhedonia, and autonomic disturbances occur in both primary headaches and morphine abstinence, and speculated that migraine is a "hypoendorphin syndrome." This idea initiated a series of studies that measured endogenous opioid peptides, first in plasma, then in cerebrospinal fluid, and later in immune cells (for review, see Bach 1997). Although several studies have found a decrease in some elements of opioid peptide systems during headache, it remains highly controversial whether decreased activity in endogenous opioid systems is an important factor in headache (Bach 1997). If, however, this should be the case, we would have a very rational argument for using exogenous opioids in treating severe headache.

EPIDEMIOLOGICAL DATA

How much are opioids prescribed for headache? No doubt this varies a lot in different countries and within various specialties, depending on regulations and traditions. A Danish population study (Sørensen et al. 1992) registered all prescriptions of strong opioids by general practitioners for 1 month in a region of Denmark inhabited by about 10% of the national population. Of the 480,000 inhabitants, 663 persons (not including registered drug addicts) were given prescriptions of strong opioids by their family physician. Twelve percent of these prescriptions were given for headache. Another Danish study counted 227 prescriptions of strong opioids by night-call doctors in a 2-week period (Christensen and Olesen 1997). Thirty-three percent of these prescriptions were for headache. Many patients received strong opioids from doctors other than their family physician, but in most cases the patients' own doctors agreed with the prescriptions (Christensen and Olesen 1997). In a Danish study of patients with prolonged severe headache, 12% of those admitted to a neurological department were taking prescription opioids (Langemark and Olesen 1984). Eighteen patients who had had been taking opioids for more than 11 weeks discontinued the drug during their hospital stay of 2 weeks or more, and of these 12 improved and 6 remained unchanged following discontinuation (Langemark and Olesen 1984).

These data show that headache is responsible for a significant part of the opioid consumption in Denmark, where prescriptions of opioids for headache are discouraged by experts, and that many opioid prescriptions are written by doctors other than the family physician.

TRIALS ON THE EFFECT OF OPIOIDS ON HEADACHE

Surprisingly few controlled studies on the effects of opioids on headache are available. The acute effect of opioid administration has been studied in both experimental and clinical settings. Nicolodi (1996) randomly assigned 13 patients suffering from severe migraine without aura to either intramuscular injections of morphine at 120 μg/kg or saline in a crossover design. Measured on a 5-point verbal analogue scale, the analgesic effect of morphine was zero. On the other hand, vomiting was worsened by morphine. Several studies have evaluated emergency room treatment of acute headache. Thirty patients visiting an emergency room with acute crises of different benign types of headache were randomly assigned to treatments with 50 mg meperidine plus 25 mg promethazine, 60 mg ketorolac, or saline (Harden et al. 1996). All three treatment groups showed the same degree of pain relief as evaluated by visual analogue scale (VAS) and the McGill Pain Questionnaire, short form (i.e., active treatments were no better than placebo). The authors argued that the placebo response in the emergency room setting is so predominant that it may be difficult to validate drugs in this setting, even those with high expected efficacy (Harden et al. 1996). These data are also relevant for interpretation of similar studies that included no placebo group.

In a double-blind study, twenty-eight patients were randomized to treatment in an emergency clinic with either 75 mg meperidine plus 75 mg hydroxyzine i.m. or 1 mg dihydroergotamine and 10 mg metoclopramide i.v. using a double-dummy technique. Headache improved in both groups, but improved least in the meperidine group (Klapper and Stanton 1993). An open study on 11 patients with cervicogenic headache (headache associated with neck pain, tenderness, and stiffness) showed that only 4 of 11 patients given 10 mg morphine s.c. had a VAS pain reduction of 50% (Bovim and Sjaastad 1993). Another migraine study evaluated the effect of a weaker opioid, dextropropoxyphene, as part of a combination compound called Dolerol, containing 65 mg dextropropoxyphene, 350 mg aspirin, 150 mg phenazone, 5 mg phentiazin, and 50 mg caffeine (Hakkarainen et al. 1978). Twenty-five patients were randomized to treatment) with either one tablet Dolerol, 1 mg ergotamine, or 500 mg aspirin. Patients could take one additional dose 30 minutes after the first dose. Patients crossed over after treating 21 consecutive migraine attacks with each substance. Both dolerol and ergotamine were superior to aspirin in alleviating migraine attacks, as evaluated by a point-score system.

Recurrent headache of an unspecified nature was treated in 31 patients in a crossover design with 16 mg codeine in combination with aspirin with or without doxylamine, or placebo. Both codeine combinations were better than placebo (Gawel et al. 1990).

Weaker opioids have also been studied in chronic headaches other than migraine. An older study used an unusual crossover design with self-randomization to 32 mg propoxyphene, 32 mg codeine, 600 mg aspirin, or placebo (Magee and DeJong 1959). Results, evaluated by pain ratings, were no better with propoxyphene or codeine compared with placebo. Twenty-four patients with nonmigrainous headache were randomized to treatment with 30 mg codeine, 1000 mg aspirin, or placebo in a crossover design with single dosing. Codeine was no better than placebo, although aspirin provided somewhat better relief (Graffenried et al. 1980).

CONCLUSIONS

It is clear that the popularity of opioids in the treatment of headache and particularly of acute exacerbations of headache is not founded on solid scientific documentation of the efficacy of either strong or weak opioids. Especially for strong opioids, it is hard to provide any evidence that may justify its use in migraine attacks or high-intensity crises in other types of headache. The efficacy of recently developed 5-HT (serotonin) agonists may make it impossible to perform large enough studies to gather sufficient data to enable evidence-based opioid treatment of headache. One could argue that it also makes that information unnecessary.

REFERENCES

Bach FW. Opioid peptides in primary headaches. In: Olesen J, Edvinsson L (Eds). *Headache Pathogenesis: Monoamines, Neuropeptides, Purines, and Nitric Oxide*. Frontiers in Headache Research, Vol. 7. Philadelphia: Lippincott-Raven, 1997, pp 193–200.

Bovim G, Sjaastad O. Cervicogenic headache: responses to nitroglycerin, oxygen, ergotamine and morphine. *Headache* 1993; 33:249–252.

Christensen MB, Olesen F. Ordination of opioid analgesics in the out-of-hours general practice service in the county of Aarhus, Denmark. *Ugeskr Laeger* 1997; 159:2381–2385.

Gawel MJ, Szalai JF, Stiglick A, Aimola BS, Weiner M. Evaluation of analgesic agents in recurring headache compared with other clinical pain models. *Clin Pharmacol Ther* 1990; 47:504–508.

Graffenried BV, Hill RC, Nüesh E. Headache as a model for assessing mild analgesic drugs. *J Clin Pharmacol* 1980; 20:131–144.

Hakkarainen H, Gustafsson B, Stockman O. A comparative trial of ergotamine tartrate, acetyl salicylic acid and a dextropropoxyphene compound in acute migraine attacks. *Headache* 1978; 18:35–39.

Harden RN, Gracely RH, Carter T, Warner G. The placebo effect in acute headache management: ketorolac, meperidine, and saline in the emergency department. *Headache* 1996; 36:352–356.

Klapper JA, Stanton J. Current emergency treatment of severe migraine headaches. *Headache* 1993; 33:560–562.

Langemark M, Olesen J. Drug abuse in migraine patients. *Pain* 1984; 19:81–86.

Magee KR, DeJong RN. An evaluation of dextropropoxyphene hydrochloride in the treatment of headache. *Univ Mich Med Bull* 1959; 25:74–78.

Nicolodi M. Differential sensitivity to morphine challenge in migraine sufferers and headache-exempt subjects. *Cephalalgia* 1996; 16:297–304.

Sicuteri F. Natural opioids in migraine. In: Critchley M, Friedman A, Gorini S, Sicuteri F (Eds). *Headache: Physiopathological and Clinical Concepts*. Advances in Neurology, Vol. 33. New York: Raven Press, 1982, pp 65–74.

Sørensen HT, Rasmussen HH, Møller-Petersen JF, et al. Epidemiology of pain requiring strong analgesics outside hospital in a geographically defined population in Denmark. *Dan Med Bull* 1992; 39:464–467.

Ziegler DK. Opiate and opioid use in patients with refractory headache. *Cephalalgia* 1994; 14:5–10.

Correspondence to: Flemming W. Bach, MD, PhD, Department of Neurology, Aarhus University Hospital, Norrebrogade, DK-8000 Aarhus C, Denmark. Fax: 45-8949-3300; email: akh.grp02s.fwb@aaa.dk.

Opioid Sensitivity of Chronic Noncancer Pain,
Progress in Pain Research and Management,
Vol. 14, edited by Eija Kalso, Henry J. McQuay,
and Zsuzsanna Wiesenfeld-Hallin, IASP Press,
Seattle, © 1999.

24

How Should We Measure the Outcome?

Henry J. McQuay

*Pain Relief Unit, Nuffield Department of Anaesthetics,
University of Oxford, Oxford, United Kingdom*

For a difference to be a difference it has to make a difference
— Attributed to Gertrude Stein, ca. 1920

WHAT IS THE QUESTION WE ARE TRYING TO ANSWER?

Among the complex strands that ran through the 1st IASP Research Symposium, one issue caused some confusion—establishing the distinction between the academic answers, for instance to the question "Do opioids work in neuropathic pain?" and the clinical answers, for instance to the question, "Will opioids work without too many adverse effects in this patient?" Approaches to academic questions and clinical conundrums may differ. To deal with the academic question, "Are opioids effective in this particular syndrome?" we need to consider the design and size of clinical trials.

THE PROBLEM OF SMALL SAMPLE SIZE
IN CLINICAL TRIALS

We have learned many lessons about clinical trial design recently, and some of these lessons have emerged from the systematic review of studies. Perhaps one of the most fundamental is that the size of trials is critically important (Moore et al. 1998). For many years if a small trial (group size <50) has produced a statistically significant result, for instance that women responded better than men to the particular intervention, then we have burrowed around trying to explain this unexpected difference. We must accept that such variations can occur randomly, and that the chance of obtaining an unexpected result is much greater with small trials.

For example, if we have a *very* large box of balls, half red and half blue, how many balls do we need to sample to be 99% sure that the true proportion of red balls is between 49% and 51%? The answer is 20,000. Of course, the number required would decrease if we were to relax our criteria, but the example shows how much bigger our samples need to be than is typical of current trials. If we wish to produce clinically credible results, not just statistical significance (which gives us the direction but not the magnitude of any difference), then in analgesic trials we may need group sizes as large as 500 patients (Moore et al. 1998).

OPIOIDS IN NONCANCER PAIN

Traditional reasons for not using opioids in noncancer pain include the political concern that medical availability would increase street drug problems, fear of creating an addict and of inculcating abuse behavior, and concerns about toxicity. Each of these problems can be dealt with separately. When oral opioids were introduced in Sweden for cancer pain there was no evidence of any resulting increase in opioid problems on the street. Toxicity with chronic pethidine use is indeed a danger, but with other opioids adverse effects (rather than toxic effects) can be managed for most patients. Historical anecdotal evidence of individuals who used opioids for long periods to control their pain, for instance Florence Nightingale, shows that it is possible to function over the long term on opioids without developing antisocial behavior. The parallels with alcohol use are obvious. In an ideal world one might argue that we should all be teetotalers. The reality is that many adults use alcohol as a recreational drug and do not develop addictive behavior that is a problem to them or to society. The tension then is between banning alcohol to protect the minority who do develop addiction, or protecting the rights of the majority while living with the knowledge that some cannot cope. In medicine the tension we face is between denying patients opioids to relieve their pain and thus protecting the few from addictive behavior, and allowing access to opioids in the knowledge that some patients will develop addiction.

The bottom line is that opioids should be considered for use in nonmalignant pain if they are the only effective remedy. This conclusion begs the question as to how we prove that the opioids are effective.

TESTING INDIVIDUAL PATIENTS
FOR OPIOID SENSITIVITY

A common clinical puzzle is to determine whether it is sensible to continue increasing the opioid dose for a patient whose pain has not yet responded to upward titration. Several different conditions require such a decision: (1) pain relief with adverse effects, (2) no pain relief and no adverse effects, and (3) no pain relief with adverse effects. In the presence of intolerable or unmanageable adverse effects, further increase in dose is unlikely to yield benefit, and the decision then is whether to change the type of opioid or route of delivery, or change the method of pain relief to something other than opioids. In the absence of either pain relief or adverse effects (condition 2), most clinicians would continue to titrate the dose upward.

Where then is the problem? The problem is that the situation is rarely as clear as these conditions infer. The patient may well be unsure in condition 1 that the drug is indeed making any difference. Ideally, a clinician might wish to administer an opioid "challenge," which would determine whether the pain was sensitive to opioids. Unfortunately, the logistics of such a challenge are not straightforward. If the patient has been taking large doses of an oral controlled-release formulation, how should the challenge be given? If by injection, how large a dose?

These problems have been considered at length in the parallel but different context of designing clinical trials to determine opioid sensitivity of particular pain syndromes (Jadad et al. 1992; McQuay et al. 1992). Multiple problems arise in designing such a test for an individual patient before we reach the interesting question about outcomes. First, we need to know: How long has the patient been on the present dose (and previous doses) of opioid? How much relief has the patient received? Which adverse effects (if any) have occurred, and what steps (if any) has the patient taken to control them?

JUDGING PAIN RELIEF

COMMON PAIN ASSESSMENT TOOLS

The most common assessment tools used are categorical and visual analogue scales (VAS). Categorical scales use words to describe the magnitude of the pain. In this earliest pain measure (Keele 1948), the patient picks the most appropriate word. Most research groups use four words (none, mild, moderate, and severe). Scales to measure pain relief were developed later. The most common is the five-category scale (none, slight, moderate, good or lots, and complete).

Numbers assigned to the verbal categories permit analysis: for pain intensity, none = 0, mild = 1, moderate = 2, and severe = 3; and for relief, none = 0, slight = 1, moderate = 2, good or lots = 3, and complete = 4. Data from different subjects are then combined to produce means (rarely medians) and measures of dispersion (usually standard errors of means). The validity of converting categories into numerical scores was checked by comparison with concurrent VAS measurements. Good correlation was found, especially between pain relief scales, by using cross-modality matching techniques (Scott and Huskisson 1976; Wallenstein et al. 1980; Littman et al. 1985). Results are usually reported as continuous data or as mean or median pain relief or intensity. Few studies present results as discrete data that give the number of participants who report a certain level of pain intensity or relief at any given assessment point. The main advantages of the categorical scales are that they are quick and simple to use. However, the small number of descriptors may force the scorer to choose a particular category when none describes the pain satisfactorily.

Visual analogue scales, which use lines with the left end labeled "no relief of pain" and the right end labeled "complete relief of pain," seem to overcome this limitation. Patients mark the line at the point that corresponds to their pain. The scores are obtained by measuring the distance between the "no relief" end and the patient's mark, usually in millimeters. The main advantages of VAS are that they are simple and quick to score, avoid imprecise descriptive terms, and provide many points from which to choose. They do require more concentration and coordination, which can be difficult postoperatively or for patients with neurological disorders.

Pain relief scales are perceived as more convenient than pain intensity scales, probably because patients have the same baseline relief (zero), whereas they could start with different baseline intensity (usually moderate or severe). Relief scale results are thus easier to compare. They may also be more sensitive than intensity scales (Sriwatanakul et al. 1982; Littman et al. 1985). A theoretical drawback of relief scales is that the patient must remember what the pain was like initially.

OTHER PAIN ASSESSMENT TOOLS

Verbal numerical scales and global subjective efficacy ratings are also used. Verbal numerical scales are regarded as an alternative or complementary to the categorical and VAS scales. Patients give a number to the pain intensity or relief (for pain intensity 0 usually represents no pain and 10 the maximum possible, and for pain relief 0 represents none and 10 complete relief). They are easy and quick to use, and correlate well with conventional VAS (Murphy et al. 1988).

Global subjective efficacy ratings, or simply global scales, are designed to measure overall treatment performance. Patients answer questions such as, "How effective do you think the treatment was?" by using a labeled numerical or categorical scale. Although these judgments probably include adverse effects, they can be the most sensitive discriminant among treatments. One of the oldest scales was the binary question, "Is your pain half gone?" Its advantage is that it has a clearer clinical meaning than a 10-mm shift on a VAS. The disadvantage, at least for advocates of intensive measures in small trials, is that all the potential intermediate information (1–49% or >50%) is discarded.

Judgment by the patient rather than by the caregiver is the ideal, because caregivers overestimate the pain relief compared with the patient's version.

RESTRICTING PAIN TRIALS TO PATIENTS WITH MODERATE AND SEVERE INITIAL PAIN INTENSITY

The trail blazers of analgesic trial methodology found that if patients had no pain initially, it was impossible to assess analgesic efficacy. To optimize test sensitivity, clinicians developed a rule to study only patients with moderate or severe pain intensity at baseline. Obviously, in testing for opioid sensitivity we should only test patients with pain of at least moderate intensity, but the rule is worth reiterating because it is broken so often. We know that a patient who records a baseline VAS score in excess of 30 mm would probably have recorded at least moderate pain on a four-point categorical scale (Collins et al. 1997).

TEST DESIGN AND VALIDITY

Pain measurement is one of the oldest and most studied of the subjective measures, and pain scales have been used for over 40 years. Even in the early days of pain measurement there was understanding that the design of studies contributed directly to the validity of the result obtained. Trial designs that lack validity produce information that is at best difficult to use, and at worst is useless.

PLACEBO

Patients in pain respond to placebo treatment and sometimes obtain 100% pain relief. The opioid sensitivity test must include some form of control for the placebo response. This could be a "positive" control, such as using two different doses of the challenge drug to assess dose response, or a "negative" control, a true placebo, with due provision for escape analgesia if needed.

RANDOMIZING AND BLINDING FOR THE INDIVIDUAL PATIENT TEST

One approach to an individual patient test is a classic single-patient or N-of-1 randomized design. Using five paired treatments, control(s) and test, it is possible to derive a statistical and perhaps even clinical indication of test drug efficacy. The reality, however, is that such tests are logistically complicated and time consuming.

LIKELIHOOD RATIOS

Most of us can become confused when trying to remember the sensitivity and specificity of a diagnostic test: will this challenge dose of opioid produce analgesia or won't it? The point of this digression into likelihood ratios is to emphasize the power of the clinical history in generating high pretest probability so as to exploit any additional power of a test. Sackett and colleagues (1991) state this well using the example of angina:

> Look at the relative size of the likelihood ratios for a brief, immediate, relatively cheap history and a much longer, delayed, and relatively expensive exercise electrocardiogram. There is no contest. Likelihood ratios for key points in the history and physical examination, both for this and for most other target disorders, are mammoth and dwarf those derived from most excursions through high technology.

My suspicion is that the clinical judgment of opioid sensitivity from the history is far more important in generating pretest probability than any test we could devise.

The example that follows uses likelihood ratios in diagnosing alcohol abuse (Moore and McQuay, Web site). The likelihood ratio (LR) can be calculated from the sensitivity and specificity of a test expressed as ratios rather than percentages. It expresses the odds that a given finding would occur in a patient with, as opposed to without, the target disorder or condition. The positive LR is derived as:

$$LR_{pos} = \text{sensitivity}/(1 - \text{specificity}).$$

With the LR greater than 1, the probability of the disease or condition being present increases; when it is less than 1 the probability of it being present declines, and when it is exactly 1 the probability is unchanged.

Negative LR can also be calculated. To determine the odds that a given finding would not occur in a patient without, as opposed to with, the target disorder or condition, LR is derived as:

$$LR_{neg} = (1 - sensitivity)/specificity.$$

EXAMPLE FROM ALCOHOL ABUSE

Patients can be screened systematically for drinking problems with a simple questionnaire. There are just four questions (known by the acronym CAGE), with one point given for each positive answer: Have you ever felt you should *cut down* on your drinking? Have people *annoyed* you by criticizing your drinking? Have you ever felt bad or *guilty* about your drinking? Have you ever had a drink first thing in the morning to steady your nerves or to get rid of a hangover (*eye-opener*)?

Researchers in Virginia applied these questions to patients older than 17 in the outpatient medical practice of an urban teaching hospital (Buchsbaum et al. 1991). Of 836 patients who met the inclusion criteria, 98% agreed to participate. Of these, 36% met criteria for a lifetime history of alcohol abuse or dependence as assessed by a highly reliable instrument. Likelihood ratios were calculated for patients who scored 0, 1, 2, 3, or 4 questions answered with yes (Table I). These ratios can be used on the nomogram (Fig. 1) to help determine the post-CAGE probability of alcohol problems.

The pretest probability could be calculated from prevalence figures without knowing the patient (or taking a history). U.S. data on alcohol abuse using the same instrument as the Buchsbaum study suggest a lifetime prevalence of 25% for men and 4.5% for women (Edwards 1996). For an individual patient we could determine the pretest probability from the history.

The analogy with opioid sensitivity testing is that, just as we asked at

Table I
Likelihood ratios with CAGE scores in 821 patients
attending general medical outpatient clinics

CAGE Score	Number of Patients		Likelihood Ratio
	Alcoholic	Nonalcoholic	
0	33	428	0.14
1	45	54	1.50
2	86	34	4.50
3	74	10	13.00
4	56	1	100.00

Note: Patients were defined as alcoholic or nonalcoholic according to *Diagnostic and Statistical Manual of Mental Disorders* criteria.

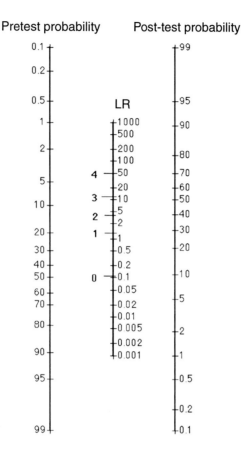

Fig. 1. Nomogram for pre- and post-test probability with likelihood ratio (LR) for alcohol abuse. To determine post-test probability, draw a line through pretest probability and LR to yield a CAGE score; e.g., if pretest probability is 70 and CAGE score is 2, then post-test probability is just under 90.

the start of the chapter, we have to know what we are looking for. My contention is that the history can indicate that a pain is unlikely to have "normal" opioid sensitivity. We know, for instance, that sensitivity may well be reduced in neuropathic pain. If the pain occurs in a numb area then our pretest probability of reduced opioid sensitivity should be high. Similarly, if the dose has been titrated up to the point of adverse effects with no glimmer of efficacy, again our pretest probability should be high.

   The obvious next stage would be to see whether we could devise a set of questions analogous to the CAGE questionnaire for alcohol abuse, but aimed at giving us similar points on the nomogram to fix our post-test probability. It would be marvelous if this could be achieved without the need for "invasive" challenge testing, with all its difficulties as described above.

JUDGING ADVERSE EFFECTS

Moulin and colleagues (1996) provided some intriguing data on adverse effects after 6 weeks of oral morphine dosing. Forty-six chronic noncancer pain patients were studied in a randomized crossover study, with 3 weeks titration and two 6-week treatment periods with a 2-week washout. The mean daily dose of controlled-release morphine was 84 mg/day, against benztropine "active" control. Adverse effects are summarized in Table II.

These incidences, derived in the context of a randomized trial, show that chronic opioid use has considerable potential for adverse effects. Our focus is often on the short term; indeed, in the context of an opioid challenge to determine sensitivity we are focused primarily on the short-term adverse effect burden. Patients on long-term opioids may have a different view, particularly if they take other medications to manage the adverse effects.

We thus confront at least two major issues. The first is our concern about whether a patient should be using opioids long term; it follows that our thoughts about adverse effects should focus on the long rather than the short term. The second is that it is the patient's thoughts about the adverse effects and not the doctor's that should be of greatest concern. The Moulin data are the best we have in this context, but the report does not mention the severity of the adverse effects. A common feature of adverse effect reporting is to report the incidence but not the severity (although that information is often collected). Superimposed on this important shortcoming is that we have little idea of which adverse effects are most important to the patient. This information can be collected by organizing focus groups of current opioid users.

Thus, two different challenges are adverse effect reporting as part of determining pretest probability in the context of the opioid challenge, and

Table II
Adverse effects of oral morphine

Adverse Effect	Patients Experiencing Adverse Effects (%)	
	Morphine	Placebo
Vomiting	39	2
Dizziness	37	2
Constipation	41	4
Poor appetite/nausea	39	7
Abdominal pain	22	4
Dose-limiting adverse effects	28	2

Source: Moulin et al. (1996).

the real-life assessment of adverse effects for long-term use of opioids. Both challenges face a further hurdle, which is that patients who are obtaining pain relief from the opioid may well tolerate adverse effects, whereas patients who receive no benefit would reject them. While it is clearly useful and important to know the absolute incidence and severity of adverse effects, the real-life assessment must consider the compromise between pain relief and adverse effects. This problem occurs in other therapeutic areas and has no easy solution. It is the adverse effect burden relative to the degree of relief that will determine the patient's decision whether to continue with the drug.

Fig. 2 attempts to balance these considerations in a two-dimensional form, with the most desirable outcome, less pain and less harm, in the upper left area, and the least desirable, more pain and more harm, in the lower right. This problem cries out for more thought. How do we best measure the benefit and risk, and how do we best combine them to allow us to contrast different therapies?

ALTERNATIVE OUTCOMES

There is a real and justifiable concern that by focusing on the purist outcome of pain relief or reduction in pain intensity we are excluding other dimensions. An example is the use of transcutaneous electrical nerve stimulation (TENS) machines. In acute postoperative pain and in childbirth the evidence of a true effect in reduction of pain intensity is quite thin (Carroll et al. 1996, 1997; Reeve et al. 1996). The lack of pain reduction does not

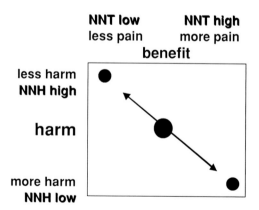

Fig. 2. Benefit/harm ratios. NNT is the number needed to treat, and NNH is the number needed to harm. Ideal interventions would reduce pain on the benefit axis without increasing harm.

exclude the possibility that these devices make people feel better. By focusing on the pain dimension to the exclusion of the important "make me feel better" dimension we are (arguably) not providing the full picture. Of course, reducing the pain should be our primary concern, but we need to be inclusive.

The satisfaction and quality of life scales are a fashionable way to bridge this gap, but another approach extends the efficacy dimension into real life. In one sense this approach can answer the tricky question of how much change on one of our measures of pain intensity or relief constitutes a worthwhile change for the patient. One method is to allow the patient to nominate several different areas in his or her life or activities that have been adversely affected by pain (Ruta et al. 1994). The Ruta Patient-Generated Index (PGI) specifies as its first stage that the patient should list the five most important areas or activities; a sixth item is all other areas or activities. In the second stage each area is scored from 0 to 100 in multiples of 10. A score of 0 means the worst a patient could imagine for him or herself, and a score of 100 represents the ideal in that area or activity. The third and final stage is that the patient has 60 points to improve the score in any of the areas or activities mentioned. The patient can award these points in any weighting up to the 60-point total. The PGI score is then calculated by multiplying each of the six ratings by the proportion of points allocated to that area and summing.

This scale was validated by comparing the results in 359 patients with back pain against the SF-36 (Ruta et al. 1994). The results of the study seemed sensible: patients referred to hospital had significantly lower (i.e., worse) PGI scores than those cared for by general practitioners, and the general practitioners' assessments of symptom severity tallied well with the patient's PGI scores. Used serially, the PGI might well prove a useful general audit tool in chronic pain, and specifically in this difficult area of opioid use in nonmalignant pain. It could widen the efficacy focus into the areas and activities of life that matter most to patients.

CONCLUSION

In the difficult area of opioid use in nonmalignant pain it is easy to confuse two separate themes—establishing the relative opioid sensitivity of different pain syndromes, and determining the treatment plan for an individual patient. The clinical trial approaches needed for the academic question of the first theme are different from those needed for the clinical question of the individual patient. The clinical trials should perhaps shift their focus from the intensive study of a small number of patients to simpler protocols studying much larger groups. The management of the individual patient presents the further problem of distinguishing the idea of a one-time opioid challenge from the longer-term question of the balance between risk and benefit. The chance of developing a worthwhile diagnostic one-time opioid challenge is slim. We are unlikely to produce a test that would improve on best clinical judgment. An area where we could make substantial improvement is the balance between risk and benefit for long-term opioids compared with other therapies.

REFERENCES

Buchsbaum DG, Buchanan RG, Centor RM, Schnoll SH, Lawton MJ. Screening for alcohol abuse using CAGE scores and likelihood ratios. *Ann Int Med* 1991; 115:774–777.

Carroll D, Tramer M, McQuay H, Nye B, Moore A. Randomization is important in studies with pain outcomes: systematic review of transcutaneous electrical nerve stimulation in acute postoperative pain. *Br J Anaesthes* 1996; 77:798–803.

Carroll D, Moore RA, Tramèr MR, McQuay HJ. Transcutaneous electrical nerve stimulation does not relieve labour pain: updated systematic review. *Contemp Rev Obstet Gynecol* 1997; Sept:195–205.

Collins SL, Moore RA, McQuay HJ. The visual analogue pain intensity scale: what is moderate pain in millimetres? *Pain* 1997; 72:95–97.

Edwards G. Drug problems as everyday doctor's business. *Oxford Textbook of Medicine,* 3rd ed. Oxford: Oxford University Press, 1996, pp 4623–4625.

Jadad AR, Carroll D, Glynn CJ, Moore RA, McQuay HJ. Morphine responsiveness of chronic pain: double-blind randomised crossover study with patient-controlled analgesia. *Lancet* 1992; 339:1367–1371.

Keele KD. The pain chart. *Lancet* 1948; 2:6–8.

Littman GS, Walker BR, Schneider BE. Reassessment of verbal and visual analogue ratings in analgesic studies. *Clin Pharmacol Ther* 1985; 38:16–23.

McQuay HJ, Jadad AR, Carroll D, et al. Opioid sensitivity of chronic pain: a patient-controlled analgesia method. *Anaesthesia* 1992; 47:757–767.

Moore RA, McQuay HJ. Bandolier Web site. Available at: http://www.jr2.ox.ac.uk/Bandolier. Accessed May 1999.

Moore RA, Gavaghan D, Tramer MR, Collins SL, McQuay HJ. Size is everything—large amounts of information are needed to overcome random effects in estimating direction and magnitude of treatment effects. *Pain* 1998; 78:209–216.

Moulin DE, Iezzi A, Amireh R, et al. Randomised trial of oral morphine for chronic non-cancer pain. *Lancet* 1996; 347:143–147.

Murphy DF, McDonald A, Power C, Unwin A, MacSullivan R. Measurement of pain: a comparison of the visual analogue with a nonvisual analogue scale. *Clin J Pain* 1988; 3:197–199.

Reeve J, Menon D, Corabian P. Transcutaneous electrical nerve stimulation (TENS): a technology assessment. *Int J Technol Assess Health Care* 1996; 12:299–324.

Ruta DA, Garratt AM, Leng M, Russell IT, MacDonald LM. A new approach to the measurement of quality of life. The Patient-Generated Index. *Med Care* 1994; 32:1109–1126.

Sackett DL, Haynes RB, Guyatt GH, Tugwell P. *Clinical Epidemiology: a Basic Science for Clinical Medicine.* Boston: Little, Brown, 1991.

Scott J, Huskisson EC. Graphic representation of pain. *Pain* 1976; 2:175–184.

Sriwatanakul K, Kelvie W, Lasagna L. The quantification of pain: an analysis of words used to describe pain and analgesia in clinical trials. *Clin Pharmacol Ther* 1982; 32:141–148.

Wallenstein SL, Heidrich IG, Kaiko R, Houde RW. Clinical evaluation of mild analgesics: the measurement of clinical pain. *Br J Clin Pharmacol* 1980; 10:319S–27S.

Correspondence to: Henry J. McQuay, MD, Pain Relief Unit, The Churchill, Oxford Radcliffe Hospital, Headington, Oxford OX3 7LJ, United Kingdom. Tel: 44-1865-226161; Fax: 44-1865-226160; email: henry.mcquay@pru.ox.ac.uk.

Index